How to Detect and Manage

Dyslexia

A Reference and
Resource Manual

Philomena Ott

NEWTON LE WILLOWS
LIBRARY

TEL 01744 677885,6,7

Heinemann

Heinemann Educational Publishers
Halley Court, Jordan Hill, Oxford OX2 8EJ
A division of Reed Educational and Professional Publishing Ltd

OXFORD   BLANTYRE
CHICAGO   PORTSMOUTH NH (USA)
MELBOURNE   AUCKLAND
IBADAN   GABORONE   JOHANNESBURG

© Philomena Ott. 1997

First published 1997

01 00 99 98
10 9 8 7 6

ISBN 0 435 104195

Text design by Jackie Hill
Typeset by Wyvern 21 Ltd, Bristol
Cover design by Miller, Craig and Cocking
Printed in Great Britain by Biddles Ltd, Guildford and King's Lynn

Acknowledgements

The Author and Publishers should like to thank the following for permission to
use copyright material.

'Toward a definition of dyslexia' by G. Reid Lyon, reprinted from *Annals of
Dyslexia, 1995, 45;* 3–27 with permission of The Orton Dyslexia Society, Inc.
September 1996; British Dyslexia Association (BDA) for the extract from *The
Dyslexia Handbook* edited by J. Crisfield; 'Adapting a college preparatory
curriculum for dyslexic adolescents; Rationale' by G. Morris, reprinted from
Annals of Dyslexia, 1983, with permission of the Orton Dyslexia Society, Inc.,
September 1996; Pauk, Walter, *How to Study in College,* Second Edition.
Copyright © 1974 by Houghton Mifflin Company. Adapted with permission; the
extract from *Study Skills: A Student's Guide for Survival* by R. A. Carman and
W. R. Adams Jr. © John Wiley & Sons, reprinted by permission of John Wiley &
Sons, Inc; the Associated Board of the Royal Schools of Music for the extract
from Guidelines for the Examining of Dyslexic Candidates; the Joint Forum for
the GCSE and GCE for the extract from Regulations and Guidance (1996); HMSO
for Circular No 4/96 (1996). Crown copyright is reproduced with the permission
of the Controller of HMSO. Anne Henderson for extracts from *Maths and
Dyslexics* (1989), St. David's College, Llandudno.

The Publishers have made every effort to trace the copyright holders, but if
they have inadvertently overlooked any, they will be pleased to make the
necessary arrangements at the first opportunity.

*Throughout this book, for simplicity, the pupil has been styled as 'he' and the
teacher as 'she'.*

Philomena Ott: Dyslexia Specialist and Educational Consultant

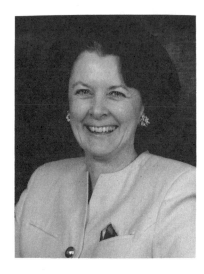

Philomena Ott was born in Dublin. She graduated from the National University of Ireland and went on to obtain a post-graduate teaching qualification there. Teaching experience was gained in both primary and secondary levels of education in the UK and abroad.

While working at a Child Guidance Clinic she embarked on what was to be a lifetime career as a specialist in teaching pupils with specific learning difficulties. Training involved courses at all the major centres in the dyslexia field in the UK including The Helen Arkell Centre, The Dyslexia Clinic at St Bartholomew's Hospital in London and The Dyslexia Institute at Staines, Middlesex.

In 1982 she was awarded a Churchill Travelling Fellowship in the category 'Everyone concerned with the integration of disabled children in normal educational establishments and employment'. She chose to study 'the latest techniques in the diagnosis and teaching of dyslexics' in the USA and went to the Scottish Rite Hospital in Dallas.

For many years she was an Executive Board Member of The British Dyslexia Association (BDA) and later became Chairman of its Local Associations' Committee. She has lectured throughout the UK to parents, teachers and students.

She is currently involved in running her own teaching centre, as well as counselling, assessing and acting as an educational consultant and adviser to a number of schools in the maintained and independent sectors.

Acknowledgements

I should like to thank my family, colleagues and pupils, whose encouragement was invaluable. The experience and opportunities provided by the Winston Churchill Memorial Trust, which financed my travelling fellowship, has been a lasting and pervasive influence. Special mention has to be made of Mr David Jefferson for reading the whole of the manuscript; to Mrs Felicity Nowell for word processing drafts of the book and amending it many times; to my publisher, Ms Janice Whitten; and to my editors, Ms Sarah Langman Scott, Ms Shirley Wakley and Ms Rachel Normington. Thanks are given to the following people for advice, support and their contributions and for helping to get the text into its present form:

Mr John Birkle, Mrs Violet Brand, Mrs Ann Brereton,
Mrs Liz Brooks, Dr Jill Carlisle, Dr Steve Chinn,
Dr Macdonald Critchley, Mr Steve Cuthbert, Mr Donald Davis,
Dr Angela Fawcett, Mrs Dorothy Gilroy, Mrs Gail Goedkoop,
Mr Jason Hazeley, Dr Bevé Hornsby, Mrs Jean Hutchins,
Dr Doris Kelly, The Honorable Sir Paul Kennedy,
Mr Graham Kitchen, Miss Alice Koontz, Mrs Jo Matty,
Mrs Elaine Miles, Professor Tim Miles, Mrs Carol Orton,
Mrs Jane Taylor, Professor Colin Terrell, Dr Michael Thomson,
Mr Guy Walters, Mr Bill Watkins, Mr Chris Woodwark.

*This book is dedicated to Michael, Jonathan,
Mélanie and Claire-Louise.*

Contents

With so many disasters in the world and so many highly-publicized horrors appearing in the world's media, many of the ills which are part of our everyday life can easily be overshadowed by the graphically illustrated visions we receive through television and print.

However much our hearts go out to the suffering that this modern world seems to produce continuously, we should not ignore what is happening often much closer to us, for example within our own families. Suffering does not necessarily come from violence, famine, or through natural disasters. The large majority of people will never know the anguish, the deep pain and the suffering which goes on in the mind of a young person in our own schools, where he or she may be mentally abused because they have a learning disability.

These youngsters can be healthy, energetic, many of them highly intelligent and desperately seeking to escape from the mental prison to which their minds seem to have so unfairly shackled them. Even in their own home, parents and family members 'do not understand' and may accuse them of not listening, not paying attention, not concentrating. They are made to feel second-class citizens because they may simply be unable to follow instructions which for others seem easy.

Broken bones mend, many horrifying wounds heal in hospitals around the world, but the damage inflicted on the minds of many young people who have dyslexia, or other forms of learning disabilities, leave scars which sometimes fester and spread.

It is therefore enormously important that more people, both professionally in the education system, and in the homes of young people who have dyslexia, more fully understand the condition. It is imperative that dyslexia is detected at the earliest possible age, then managed in a manner which will allow the young person to grow and develop in order to reach his or her true potential in life. There are so many examples of people, from past and present, who can 'give heart' to those youngsters and their parents. They know what it is to feel that they are being drowned in a sea of self-doubt, humiliation and frustration, with waves which tumble them into depths of despair, creating complexes and feelings of inferiority, which can result in many forms of human behaviour being manifested, some far from desirable.

Historically the large majority of our education systems have not recognized a specific learning disability as quickly as it might be identified these days. I was one who was never diagnosed as dyslexic until I was 42 years old! I left school at the age of fifteen having been mostly identified as stupid, dumb or 'thick' by my educators and also my peers.

Children can often be more cruel than adults. A young person put in front of a class of his or her own age and humiliated by not being able to read a simple passage from a book, then penalized by having to write a hundred lines of 'I will do my homework in future' neatly and precisely, can be subjected to unimaginable abuse and degradation in the playground; not to mention the giggles, the coughs and the spluttering that goes on in class whilst the painful ordeal is taking place.

Today I am not ashamed to declare that I cannot recite the alphabet nor spell, in some cases the simplest words; but in my childhood and adolescence I was ashamed and embarrassed. As I grew older and achieved success in competition clay pigeon shooting and later in motor racing, I glossed over it and compensated for my inabilities in a variety of ways. But it was a very thin, clear varnish in my own mind. To this day I still suffer from my lack of education and it may well be that even now, in my late fifties, I am striving for success and still have ambitions that drive me to reach the highest standards of which I am capable.

God blessed me with good hand/eye co-ordination. This allowed me to shoot competitively for Scotland and for Great Britain. The same gift let me drive racing cars successfully and by so doing gave me a springboard to other things. Not all young dyslexic people are blessed in this way. We must all, therefore, do what we can to help, to support, to give strength and to comfort them; but more than anything else, to try to understand their difficulties. We must allow them to build on the talents we all surely have by using, in some cases, unconventional routes, not only to survive, but to grow and to develop into people who can achieve in so many varied and talented ways.

I sincerely hope this book will encourage not only people of today, but also of tomorrow, to be more understanding of the problems that currently exist with dyslexia, and to use all possible endeavours and skills to build for the future.

Jackie Stewart OBE

Chapter 1

A century of delay and debate

- defining dyslexia
- historical perspective
- prevalence

Introduction

The word 'dyslexia' is in common use. Like many medical and scientific terms it is derived from the Greek. The prefix *'dys'* means 'difficulty' or 'malfunction', and the root-word *'lexis'* means 'language'. The literal translation is 'difficulty with words'. 'It implies that the problem is not simply with reading, but includes spelling, writing and other aspects of language' (Thomson, 1990). This broad, all-encompassing use of the word 'language' is fundamental to an understanding of the issues involved and implies that 'dyslexia' is more than just 'reading failure', which was at one time a frequent perception.

Dyslexia: The myths and the reality

When children first attend school their teachers and parents are keen to ensure that their reading and writing skills develop at the expected level. It soon becomes clear that children learn at different paces, but some children fall noticeably behind their peers. Although educationalists try to avoid labelling children it is extremely distressing for all concerned when a child, who may be bright in many other ways, is failing to learn to read.

There may be many reasons for the child's difficulty with reading, one of which is dyslexia. If a child is dyslexic, it is important that this is identified and addressed as soon as possible. In the past, parents' concerns may have been brushed aside with observations such as 'boys often develop later than girls' or that the child lacked concentration. The child may also have shown signs of behavioural problems which were sometimes given as explanations for his lack of progress.

It is important that outdated opinions such as 'dyslexia was the middle-class excuse for the stupid child' and the comment in a letter to *The Guardian* that 'if you live in Acacia Avenue you are dyslexic, if you live in Gasworks Terrace you are thick' (Crabtree, 1975) be replaced with a realistic and informed approach to the condition. People who are dyslexic require recognition and teaching to help them overcome their learning difficulties and it is inappropriate for critics to comment that the dyslexia lobby's 'new found vigour diverts funds and attention from children who have genuine disabilities' (Booth and Goodey, 1996).

The reality of the situation is that dyslexia occurs throughout the world, in all environments, and does not respect class boundaries. It can cause a great deal of anxiety and friction when an 'otherwise bright child' is still unable to read despite many attempts at teaching the skill using a variety of methods. The frustration this causes may then develop into antagonism between the parties involved. According to Pumfrey and Reason (1991), 'the situation is one in which friction between believers and sceptics, between parents and psychologists, between psychologist and psychologist can easily arise.'

Definitions of dyslexia

Dyslexia – What is it?

This is the question asked most frequently both by the lay person and the professional, and is usually followed by, 'Can you give me a simple definition?'. Many books and articles have been written and much academic and professional debate has been devoted to this topic. Scores of different definitions have ensued. Hammill (1990) was able to find 43. The accent and emphasis of the definition has often been influenced by the practitioner's professional background and what she saw as the underlying cause of dyslexia. There is still no universally accepted definition but dyslexia is officially recognized and accepted by governments and legislators in many countries worldwide.

World Federation of Neurology (1968)
This was one of the first working definitions and it is still regarded as a benchmark by many workers in the field. It defined dyslexia as:

> *a disorder in children who, despite conventional classroom experience, fail to attain the language skills of reading, writing and spelling commensurate with their intellectual abilities.*

Source: Waites L. (1968) Dyslexia International World Federation of Neurology. 'Report of Research Group on Developmental Dyslexia and World Illiteracy'. *Bulletin of the Orton Society*, 18: 21–2.

The Research Group on Developmental Dyslexia of the World Federation of Neurology was multi-disciplinary. 'On account of this, each word of the definition was chosen carefully to accommodate the requirements of the individual approaches to the subject.' (Critchley, 1996)

It also produced a definition of *'Specific Developmental Dyslexia'* as:

> *'a disorder manifested by difficulty in learning to read despite conventional instruction, adequate intelligence and socio-cultural opportunity. It depends on fundamental cognitive disabilities, which are frequently constitutional in origin.*

There have since been many criticisms of these definitions because of their use of exclusionary criteria. Snowling (1987) took issue with the 'check-list approach' and queried 'how many signs or symptoms must be present before a diagnosis is made?'. But she approved of the medical diagnostic approach of looking at a 'particular constellation of difficulties [which are] atypical'.

These definitions influenced the legislation in the USA. The Education for All Handicapped Children Act (Public Law 94-142) in 1968 stated:

> *The term 'specific learning disability' means a disorder in one or more basic psychological processes involved in understanding or in using language, spoken or written, which may manifest itself in an imperfect ability to listen, speak, write, spell or do mathematical calculations. The term includes such conditions as perceptual handicap, brain injury, minimal brain dysfunction, DYSLEXIA [emphasis added], and developmental aphasia. Such terms do not include children who have learning disabilities which are primarily the result of visual, hearing, or motor handicaps, of mental retardation, of emotional disturbance, or of environmental, cultural, or economic disadvantage.*

Source: US Office of Education (1977): 65083 *The Education for All Handicapped Children Act (Public Law 94–142).*

The Orton Dyslexia Society's definition (1994)

The quest for a valid definition of dyslexia continues one hundred years after its first 'discovery'. Reid Lyon (1995) described how the *Orton Dyslexia Society Research Committee* collaborated with various National Research Organizations, as well as scientists and clinicians in the USA, and in 1994 came up with a working definition:

> *Dyslexia is one of several distinct learning disabilities. It is a specific language-based disorder of constitutional origin characterized by difficulties in single word decoding, usually reflecting insufficient phonological processing. These difficulties in single word decoding are often unexpected in relation to age and other cognitive and academic abilities; they are not the result of generalized developmental disability or sensory impairment. Dyslexia is manifest by variable difficulty with different forms of language, often including, in addition to problems with reading, a conspicuous problem with acquiring proficiency in writing and spelling (The Orton Dyslexia Society Research Committee April, 1994).*

Source: Reid Lyon G. (1995) 'Toward a definition of dyslexia'. *Annals of Dyslexia*, 45:9

BDA definition of dyslexia (1996)

> *Dyslexia is a complex neurological condition which is constitutional in origin. The symptoms may affect many areas of learning and function, and may be described as a specific difficulty in reading, spelling and written language. One or more of these areas may be affected. Numeracy, notational skills (music), motor function and organizational skills may also be involved. However, it is particularly related to mastering written language, although oral language may be affected to some degree.*

Source: Crisfield J. (ed) (1996) *The Dyslexia Handbook*. BDA, Reading

What is the problem?

A wide range of symptoms

Dyslexia is perhaps best characterized as a syndrome with a wide range of symptoms. It is a much broader issue than simply a 'specific reading retardation'. Often pupils do not have the same cluster of symptoms and this can make diagnosis difficult. Naidoo's (1979) findings showed that 'we did not find a single, common pattern which typifies all these children'. There is unevenness and variability in their performance. They do not constantly make the same mistakes when reading or writing or spelling. They have good and bad days. Their errors are often compounded by tiredness, stress, or illness. Miles (1974) commented that 'it is important, therefore, to look out for inconsistencies of dyslexia'.

Masland (1989) said that 'differences appear to relate to the location and extent of the primary neurological dysfunction at the root of dyslexia'. The medical fraternity has learned much about dyslexia, particularly with the developments in neuro-imaging and genetic studies and much is now known about the function of different parts of the brain.

Characteristics of dyslexia

Some educationalists take issue with the use of medical terminology to describe the symptoms of dyslexia, but the following terms are useful characteristics of dyslexia:

- congenital – people are born with it

- genetic – inherited and runs in families, more males than females

- constitutional – there is a neurological basis

- problems with phonological awareness – difficulties with letter sounds when reading and spelling and writing

- problems with language – such as verbal naming or word retrieval or pronunciation

- problems with short term memory – which particularly affect auditory sequential memory (such as for the repetition of digits) or visual sequential memory (such as used in coding skills).

It would be unusual for an individual to have all these difficulties. Usually he will have a cluster of symptoms. The prognosis depends on individual strengths and weaknesses, on the individual learning strategies, on the degree of the dyslexia, on when the diagnosis was made and on appropriate tuition.

The road to discovery

Critchley (1996) commented that 'the first description of dyslexia I have come across was by Thomas Willis in his *De Anima Brutorum* in 1672', where Willis said that there were certain young men who were late in learning to read. The man usually credited with first using the word *'dyslexia'* to describe the dyslexic condition in patients was Professor Rudolf Berlin, an ophthalmologist working in Stuttgart in 1887.

Adolf Kussmaul

In 1877 the German physician, Adolf Kussmaul, noticed that following a stroke the brain could function well in many areas but that, 'a complete text-blindness may exist, although the power of the sight, the intellect, and the powers of speech are intact'. He coined the phrase *'word-blind'* to describe those stroke patients who, although they had normal eyesight, had lost the ability to recognize written words.

James Hinshelwood

Dr James Hinshelwood, an opthalmologist and assistant surgeon at the Glasgow Eye Infirmary, described in an article entitled 'Word-blindness and visual memory' (Hinshelwood, 1895) the case of a patient, a teacher of French and German, who one morning discovered that he could not read an exercise book given to him by a pupil to be marked. He could still read 'any number of figures quite fluently and without any mistakes whatever'. Hinshelwood concluded that 'his inability to read was thus manifestly not due to any failure of visual power but to the loss of visual memory for letters'. Today his condition would be described as 'acquired dyslexia'. Hinshelwood continued to study and write on the subject. He wrote numerous articles for medical and ophthalmic journals over a period of almost twenty years. In 1912 he concluded that 'the study of the cases of acquired word-blindness is necessary to the proper understanding of congenital word-blindness' (Hinshelwood, 1912). In his final book, *Congenital Word-Blindness*, published in 1917, he stressed that the condition should be described as such. He noted 'that it tended to affect more males than females, that there was often a family history of literacy problems and that it required different teaching methods'.

William Pringle Morgan

On 7 November 1896 the British Medical Journal published an article entitled 'A case of congenital word-blindness' by a Sussex GP called Dr Pringle Morgan. Pringle Morgan described fourteen-year-old Percy as 'a bright intelligent boy, quick at games and in no way inferior to others of his age' but who spelt his own name 'Precy'. 'Words written or printed seem to convey no impression to his mind' and he 'was quite unable to spell the name of his father's house, though he must have seen it and spelt it scores of times'. According to Critchley (1970) this is the first description of what we today speak of as 'developmental dyslexia'.

James Kerr

Coincidentally, as with many medical discoveries, in 1896 James Kerr, the Medical Officer of Health for Bradford, reported on cases of children who could not learn to read. He described them as having 'congenital word-blindness' Kerr (1897).

Samuel Torrey Orton

Samuel T Orton's work with children who had learning difficulties dates back to January 1925 when he directed a 'mental hygiene' clinic in Iowa. He examined 125 school children and found that 'fifteen appeared to be retarded in reading' and 'to show certain similarities in the errors which they made'. 'He was impressed with a specific characteristic of reading impairment in the children he studied – the instability in recognition and recall of the orientation of letters and the order of letters in words, which he termed "strephosymbolia" meaning "twisted symbols".' (J. L. Orton, 1966)

In his paper 'Specific reading disability – Strephosymbolia' (1928) he wrote 'one of these cases would fit the measure for the congenital word-blindness of Hinshelwood'. He had studied the papers of British and German workers as well as those of workers based in the USA and, in the words of June Orton (1963), 'was unusually well-prepared for such investigations ... for he had studied more human brains post mortem by laboratory methods than anyone else in the country'. He was a neurologist and a psychiatrist 'whose results convinced him that investigation of brain physiology would lead to a scientific understanding of the severe reading disability then known as "congenital word-blindness"' (J. L. Orton, 1963). Orton became Professor of Neurology at Columbia University in New York and in 1937 his landmark text *Reading, Writing and Speech Problems in Children* was published.

Orton realized that what he had discovered in his own patients was not some rare condition but a 'common cause of failure in the course of early education' (Geschwind, 1982). He was one of the first medical practitioners to appreciate the importance of education in Paediatric Neurology. According to Tomkins (1963), 'Orton's theory provoked widespread opposition among reading authorities in the education field'. Yet today he is hailed as a brilliant diagnostician and pragmatist who championed the rights and needs of his patients. Orton died in 1948. To ensure that his work continued, a group of his associates formed the Orton Society in 1949. It later changed its name to the Orton Dyslexia Society. It is the American national organization for dyslexia and has branches in every state. The society organizes annual conferences and produces a professional journal called *Annals of Dyslexia*, with conference proceedings including papers by the leading researchers in the USA and the rest of the world.

Anna Gillingham and Bessie Stillman

In the 1930's Orton's masterstroke for the dyslexic pupil was to ask his research assistant, an educational psychologist called Anna Gillingham, to devise a method for the teaching and remedying of the problems he had identified in the children he had examined. Later Gillingham collaborated with an experienced teacher named Bessie Stillman, who was dyslexic herself, to devise a programme to overcome the word-blind child's problems. They began work in 1946 and published their programme privately, called *Remedial Training for Children with Specific Language Disability in Reading, Spelling and Penmanship,* in 1956. The book became the classic teaching text worldwide and was revised many times. The multi-sensory teaching techniques outlined in their programme were linked to the underlying weaknesses and difficulties experienced by the pupils and which Orton had identified. This programme, known colloquially as the *Gillingham–Stillman Manual*, became a bible for those working in the field and many later teaching programmes have been influenced by or have their origins in this text.

Anna Gillingham was an outstanding teacher and understood the frustration often experienced by teachers 'over their failures to teach certain pupils to read, particularly when these children appeared to be bright and could do well orally' (J. L. Orton, 1966). 'She found both the "why" and "how" answered to her satisfaction' when working with Orton and, according to June Orton (1966), 'devoted the rest of her life' to training other teachers in her ways.

Multi-sensory teaching

The simultaneous use of the eyes, ears, hands and lips to utilize all the pathways to the brain when learning.

Gillingham and Stillman (1956) said that multi-sensory teaching 'is based upon the constant use of all of the following: how a letter or word looks, how it sounds, how the speech organs or the hand in writing feels when producing it'. The pupil uses the visual channel (eyes), the auditory channel (ears) and kinesthetic (motor memory) and tactile (hands) to learn.

A historical perspective of the growth of the dyslexia movement in the UK

1940s and 1950s

A small number of doctors such as Critchley, White Franklin and Strauss were seeing children with reading difficulties. These children were referred to Maisie Holt, a psychologist at St Bartholomew's Hospital in London. She taught the children and incorporated much of the Gillingham-Stillman and Edith Norrie methods into her work at what was to become known as the Dyslexic Clinic at Barts. Bevé Hornsby joined Maisie Holt as a student in 1969.

1962

The Invalid Children's Aid Association (ICAA) held an international conference in London. 350 delegates attended. The ICAA conference established 'that there were people who had undue difficulty in learning to read'. This meeting was 'crucial to the development of the dyslexia movement in Britain' (McNair-Scott, 1991).

1964

In 1964 the Word Blind Centre for Dyslexic Children was established as a research project by the ICAA in London. 'One of its many functions was to carry out research into the nature and causes of specific developmental dyslexia – an elusive learning disorder.' (BDA, 1979) It did outstanding work both in the field of research and teaching, organizing conferences and kindling an interest in the study of the teaching and assessment of dyslexic children that lead to a cross-fertilization of ideas between the medical and educational world. It was closed in 1972 because of a lack of funding.

1966

The Bath Association for the Study of Dyslexia was founded by Marion Welchman. Sally Child, Anna Gillingham's heir, was invited from Dallas to run two-week teacher training courses. Kathleen Hickey, Bevé Hornsby and Kathy Moorhouse went to Dallas for further training at the Scottish Rite Hospital.

1970

The British Council for the Rehabilitation of the Disabled (REHAB) set up a centre to teach adults.

The Chronically Sick and Disabled Persons Act was passed and the word 'acute dyslexia' was first mentioned in the House of Commons.

1971

The Helen Arkell Dyslexia Centre opened in London to teach children and train teachers.

1972

The British Dyslexia Association (BDA) was founded by members of eight Local Dyslexia Associations. It was run by Jennifer Smith from her home from 1982, helped by an enthusiastic and dedicated band of unpaid volunteers and assisted by various professionals – medical practitioners, psychologists, teachers and businessmen and women.

In 1986 the then Chairman of the Association, Tony Davies, found permanent office accommodation at 98 London Road, Reading. He was instrumental in raising the funds to pay professional staff, rather than having to rely solely on the goodwill of voluntary workers, which made it more efficient and enabled it to offer a full-time service to the increasing demand for help. Public awareness was increased. Corporate donors became involved and their help was often given on the condition that it was used to train teachers.

Guinness PLC opened the door to wide-scale teacher training courses with a generous contribution in 1985 and were responsible for the formation of the Dyslexia Educational Trust.

Kathleen Hickey began to teach children for the North Surrey Dyslexia Association. This lead to the opening of the Dyslexia Institute in North Surrey with Kathleen Hickey as its first Director of Studies and Jean Augur as its first teacher. It moved to Staines in 1974 and accepted pupils on a fee paying basis for assessment and tuition. It also began to train teachers. Later Dr Harry Chasty became its psychologist and he was to become prime mover in putting dyslexia to the forefront through the country.

From the 1970s Bangor Dyslexia Unit, which was part of the University of North Wales, was doing innovative work under Professor Tim Miles and his wife Elaine Miles. They worked in partnership with their Local Education Authority (LEA). This was virtually unheard of in this period when many specialist teaching centres were not recognized or accepted by LEAs.

1973
The BDA had its first official meeting with the Department of Education and Science (DES).

1974
Alpha-to-Omega by Bevé Hornsby and Frula Sheer was published privately.

The Cambridge Conference was chaired by Professor Oliver Zangwill and he and Beryl Wattles founded the Cambridge Specific Learning Disabilities Group.

1975
Lord Radnor and Lord Renwick spoke about dyslexia in their maiden speeches in the House of Lords.

1976
The Aston Index by Margaret Newton and Michael Thomson was published.

1977
Kathleen Hickey's programme *A Language Training Course for Teachers and Learners* was published.

1981
Violet Brand founded the Watford Dyslexia Unit. It ran teacher training courses and taught dyslexic children and adults.

The Education Act 1981 was passed.

Dyslexia was on the agenda not just in the Houses of Parliament but also in schools and homes. Throughout the 1980s the whole movement grew.

1983

The Education Act 1983 was passed. It recognized that some children have Special Educational Needs (SEN).

1984

The Hornsby Centre opened in Wandsworth, London.

1985

The Dyslexia Education Trust helped fund teacher training courses, such as the RSA and BDA diploma courses.

1987

The BDA was asked to submit a memorandum to the House of Commons Select Committee on Education concerning the implementation of the 1981 Education Act. Government Minister Robert Dunn said in the House of Commons on 13 July that 'the Government recognizes dyslexia ... the important thing is to be sure that something is being done about the problem'.

1989

The Scottish Dyslexia Association was one of the group of eight local associations that was involved in the setting up of the BDA in 1972. Because the legal and educational systems in Scotland differ from those in England and Wales, the Scottish Dyslexia Association decided to form its own national organization in 1982. Affiliated branches are located throughout Scotland and offer support, help and information. The Headquarters of the Association was established in Stirling in 1995 and now boasts a resource centre which is open to the public.

The Dyslexia Computer Resource Centre was initiated at the Department of Psychology at the University of Hull.

The BDA held its first international conference in Bath and attracted participants and lecturers from around the world.

1990

An awareness campaign was launched by the BDA which resulted in 20 000 telephone calls to the helplines set up throughout the UK.

1992

Marion Welchman, the matriarch of the self-help organizations, was awarded an MBE in the New Year's Honours List, in recognition of her tireless crusade for dyslexics. She is known in the USA as the 'Bath Bombshell'. She has been a splendid ambassador for the BDA, both at home and abroad and has steered the organization admirably by her ability to listen and to avoid confrontation.

1994

1994 was designated the Year of the Young Dyslexic Adult. It aimed to increase the awareness of their needs and the support that they require after they leave school.

The prevalence of dyslexia

Lack of precise agreement on definition makes it impossible to know the extent of the prevalence of dyslexia in the population. Miles and Miles (1990) stated that 'the absence of consistent selection criteria makes the matter very much one of guesswork' and 'moreover, it is for these reasons that no satisfactory figures are available for the incidence of dyslexia'. If you can't measure it, you can't manage it. 'Based on government-sponsored studies, the British Dyslexia Association estimated that 10 per cent of children have some degree of dyslexia. Appropriate teaching and the use of coping strategies may moderate its effects significantly.' (Crisfield, 1996) The UK government stated that 'nationally, only two per cent of children have special educational needs' (Code of Practice, 1994).

Varying degrees of dyslexia

Knowledge about the extent and severity of the problem is important for educationalists and government officials who are charged with budgetary and fiscal decisions, including provision for people with special educational needs.

Many experienced teachers and researchers comment on the wide variations in the skills and weaknesses found in the dyslexic person. Dyslexia can manifest itself in severe, moderate or mild forms.

It is these categories that are at the core of the arguments about the prevalence of dyslexia. Pumfrey (1994) illustrated this with an example:

Pupil of 10.0 years IQ 120		
The scores would be as follows		
Degree of Dyslexia	**Reading Age**	**Spelling Age**
Severe dyslexia	6.3 years	6.4 years
Moderate dyslexia	8.3 years	7.4 years
Mild dyslexia	10.6 years	8.6 years

These scores would not be considered in isolation but would be linked to other known dyslexia sensitive factors that would have indicated the dyslexia profile, including varying degrees of weakness in some or all of the following tests:

Digit Span
Coding
Auditory Sequential Memory
Rapid Naming
Phonological Awareness
Laterality
Arithmetic
Creative Writing

Vail (1990) divided dyslexics into two groups: the middle group and the low group. The 'middle group' might not even be diagnosed dyslexic as their intelligence covers the dyslexia and their dyslexia conceals the intelligence, but undiagnosed dyslexia can be a constant source of internal worry and strain. The 'low group' experiences severe difficulties with even the mechanics of reading, writing, spelling, and pencil arithmetic. Critchley (1981) drew attention to yet another category, the borderline dyslexic, when he said 'there exist incomplete cases of dyslexia – dyslexia variants. In other words, the triad of late reading, poor spelling, and inability to communicate easily on paper, does not of necessity always occur in combination. "Formes frustes" (variants) of dyslexia are quite often encountered among the relations of a person who is known to be a fully fledged dyslexic'.

It is essential to be aware of this wide spectrum and herein lies the crux of the vexing question – the prevalence. The figures quoted on the prevalence of dyslexia are no more than 'guesstimates' because there is not a consensus on how to count heads and who to include, resulting in statistics that are unreliable and fundamentally flawed. The way forward is for a properly funded national enquiry to be taken of a large sample of the population to establish the prevalence of dyslexia in the population. These results could then help the planners allocate funding for special educational needs and teacher training.

Management – Medical or educational?

There has been much debate over whether dyslexia should be considered a medical or an educational concern and over whether doctors or educationalists should make the assessment. In 1961 Critchley lectured on 'Disorders of reading of central origin' at the invitation of London County Council and 'it was on that occasion I discovered I had unwittingly stirred up controversy, mostly from school teachers in the audience' (Critchley, 1996). His assessments were criticized by medical colleagues and educationalists until finally the British Medical Association (BMA) became so incensed by his work that it issued a statement which said 'as a learning disability, its certification was the province of the educational psychologist' (BMA, 1980) and that dyslexia and its diagnosis and treatment was essentially an educational matter. Despite this censure Critchley continued his battle: 'I have always insisted that the diagnosis of specific developmental dyslexia is a medical responsibility. This view is not popular among certain educational psychologists, but its truth can scarcely be denied' (Critchley, 1981). Miles and Miles (1990) felt 'that one of the original reasons for this hostility seems to have been that the dyslexia concept came from medical specialists, who thus seemed to be encroaching on education's "patch"'. The work of medical researchers such as Galaburda and Geschwind in the USA confirmed this view and 'strengthens the case for neurological involvement' (Pumfrey and Reason, 1991). The advances being made by modern technology, including the work of doctors studying genes and the brain, are providing fresh evidence about the causes of the condition.

There is still debate over whether dyslexia should be considered a medical or an education concern. During the debate on the Education Bill in 1981 the Under-Secretary of State drew attention to the fact that 'the baffling condition popularly known as dyslexia is difficult to pin down' and 'certain educationalists presume that it does not exist'. At the time this came as no surprise to dyslexic people, their parents or their teachers who had long battled with the education system and were fully aware that 'the situation is one in which friction between believers and sceptics exists' (Pumfrey and Reason, 1991). The European Dyslexia Association (1994) stated that 'dyslexia is a medical term: specific learning disability (or difficulty) is an educational one'. Miles and Miles (1990) agreed with this when they said 'there is, in our view, a good case for saying that it is a medical matter in origin and an educational matter in its treatment'. Rawson's view (1986) coincided with this and when considering the strategies for management she suggested that we look at the Orton Dyslexia Society's four part analysis:

1   The differences are personal.

2   The diagnosis is clinical.

3   The treatment is educational.

4   The understanding is scientific.

The psychologists' role in identification and assessment

Psychologists have had the main responsibility for the assessment of pupils who fail to progress in school.

During the late 1940s and 1950s, the trend among psychologists was to explain learning problems in terms of 'family dynamics'. These attitudes prevailed and affected the work in Child Guidance Clinics. Critchley (1966) observed that educational psychologists 'regarded the problem of learning difficulty as something which ranged from intellectual inadequacy at one end of the scale to neurosis at the other'. Miles and Miles (1990) said 'there was a tendency, whenever this seemed plausible, to attribute children's reading and spelling difficulties to tensions within the home'. Miles (1993) quoted from a letter he received from the mother of a child who had all the symptoms of dyslexia. The mother wrote that 'he has just been seen by the educational psychologist, who says he is not dyslexic, it is due to the jealousy of his younger sister'.

Burt and Schonell were the two most influential educational psychologists. Naidoo (1972), an educational psychologist herself, gave a succinct overview of her colleagues' underlying philosophies when she wrote, 'Following Burt's investigation (1921) into back-wardness with their emphasis on environment and psychological factors, interest in congenital word-blindness waned' and congenital word-blindness was not included in the training of educational psychologists or in teacher training colleges and universities.

A survey of 882 psychologists conducted by Pumfrey and Reason (1991) found that 87 per cent of them preferred to use 'specific learning difficulties' when writing reports and only 30 per cent found the use of the word 'dyslexia' appropriate. It is a war of words. Another reason sometimes put forth by the combatants is their dislike of labelling children. The BDA (Crisfield, 1996) said that dyslexic people often think it [specific learning difficulty] derogatory.

Changes in education policy – The way forward

There have been many changes in education throughout the 1980s, including the Education Reform Act 1988, which resulted in The National Curriculum. The *Education Act 1993* required the Department of Education to issue a *Code of Practice* on the *'Identification and Assessment of Special Educational Needs'* for Local Education Authorities, schools and all those who help in them and work with children with special educational needs, including the health and social services. The Code is advisory rather than mandatory. It states that 'a child has special educational needs if he has a learning difficulty which calls for special educational provision to be made for him'. A child has a learning difficulty if he has 'significantly greater difficulty in learning than the majority of children of his age' and it states 'that the needs of most pupils will be met in the mainstream and without a statutory assessment or statement of special educational needs'.

Summary and conclusions

1   There is a welter of definitions used to describe the dyslexic condition which has many variances. According to Pumfrey and Reason (1991) 'the terminological confusions were (and remain) attributable to the complexities of the issues, the involvement of different professions' and 'some have the clarity of oxtail soup'.

Dyslexia implies vastly more than a delay in learning to read, which is but the tip of the iceberg. The etymology of the term 'dyslexia' expresses admirably a difficulty – not in reading – but in the use of words, how they are identified, what they signify, how they are handled in combination, how they are pronounced, and how they are spelt. The term 'specific reading retardation' is therefore not appropriate as it indicates an isolated symptom, whereas developmental dyslexia is a complex syndrome.

Source: Critchley M. (1981) 'Dyslexia – an overview'. In Pavlidis G. Th. and Miles T. R. (eds) *Dyslexia Research and its Applications to Education.* John Wiley and Sons Ltd, Chichester.

Yet Pennington (1989) said that 'dyslexia may be simply defined as unexpected difficulty in the acquisition of reading and spelling skills'.

2   Lack of precise agreement on definition makes it impossible to know the extent and prevalence of dyslexia in the population. In 1991 Miles stated his opinion that 'we still do not know with any degree of precision how many people in the general population are dyslexic'. *The figures most frequently quoted by the BDA and others is that 4 per cent of the population is severely dyslexic and up to 10 per cent have some degree of the difficulties.*

3   The BDA and many professionals working in the field often use 'specific learning difficulties' synonymously with dyslexia. Snowling (1987) said 'the "unexpected" failure of a child to acquire written language skills can be referred to as specific developmental dyslexia but it is usually called "dyslexia" for short'. The reason given is that some professionals will not use the word 'dyslexia' but are happy with the concept of specific learning difficulties. (Newton, 1996), when speaking of assessment of pupils for LEAs, said 'they still won't let us write the word dyslexia in our reports'.

4   There is still debate over whether dyslexia should be considered a medical or an educational concern. Miles and Miles (1990) said 'there is, in our view, a good case for saying that it is a medical matter in origin and an educational matter in its treatment'.

5   Gargantuan steps have been taken in the recognition of the problems of dyslexia. Parents have become more enlightened and their expectations of the educational system have been raised, as a result of the implementation of the *Education Act 1993* and the *Code of Practice 1994*.

Chapter 2

Early identification

- screening tests
- who is responsible for the assessment of special educational needs?
- early warning signs

Introduction

The knowledge and understanding of dyslexia has broadened as people become better informed. There is a growing number of people who were diagnosed as dyslexic as children. As a result, we are now seeing a second generation of children whose parents were diagnosed as dyslexic. The pressure for recognition and help has often been parent driven, with the help of the voluntary and the specialist organizations. The media, too, has helped to raise public awareness and acceptance of dyslexia. The professionals are trying to find reliable ways of diagnosing dyslexia and they are striving to ensure that the dyslexic child is identified as early as possible.

The earlier the better

In the last ten to fifteen years more teachers have been trained to recognize the evidence of dyslexia, and awareness courses have been organized by dyslexia organizations and by LEAs. The findings of the experimental psychologists have focused on early childhood. Increasing awareness and evidence of difficulty at an early age has been documented and reported by parents, teachers and researchers. A number of signs (see pp.25–32) have been identified which can point to problems in a child. The BDA ran a very successful Early Recognition Campaign which helped to give many parents confidence in their own intuition that 'something was not quite right' about their child's development.

A number of researchers now claim that it is possible to identify areas of weakness and difficulty from around the age of three to four years, which may indicate children who will experience problems when they begin to learn to read. The work of the researchers Bradley and Bryant (1983) resulted in evidence to substantiate these claims: 'The performance of the pre-schoolers on this phonological [sounding out] awareness task was found to be a good predictor of their reading and spelling ability over three years later.' Bryant (1985) advanced the debate when he stated that 'there is no point in anyone trying to prevent children ever becoming dyslexic without having a precise way of detecting which child among a group of three or four year olds is likely to do much worse at learning to read [...] the problem is however that no such measure exists'.

Diagnostic tests for early identification

There are now two diagnostic tests for early screening: the *Dyslexia Early Screening Test* (DEST) and the *Cognitive Profiling System* (CoPS 1).

Dyslexia Early Screening Test (DEST)

Nicolson and Fawcett, researchers at Sheffield University, became aware that early screening could prevent the cycle of 'cumulative and corrosive' damage and 'emotional scars' that dyslexia imposes on many sufferers. They argued that 'the cost of administering screening tests has been high, involving lengthy procedures for each child by educational psychologists' (Nicolson and Fawcett, 1995). They set about devising a test which could be administered by the pupil's own teacher or a school health professional who could test all pupils on entry to school, in the same way that children have routine sight and hearing tests. Their early research has been piloted on pupils nationally and is currently being evaluated by Southampton and Newcastle universities. The features of the DEST are:

- It is suitable for children aged from 4.6 to 6.5 years.
- It consists of ten simple sub-tests which allow the tester to check for strengths and weaknesses.
- It is a pencil and paper test which means all schools can use it.
- It takes about 30 minutes per pupil to administer.
- Is it modestly priced.
- It can be administered by teachers and health care professionals with no previous experience of psychological testing.
- It will be useful to the Special Educational Needs Co-ordinator (SENCO) because the *Code of Practice 1994* requires that schools must show that 'there is clear, recorded evidence of clumsiness, significant difficulties of sequencing or visual perception, deficiencies in working memory, or significant delays in language function'. This must be done before a child is formally assessed or Statemented.

The Cognitive Profiling System (CoPS 1)

CoPS 1 (The Cognitive Profiling System for Assessment of Dyslexia and Special Educational Needs) was a project funded by Humberside County Council and was developed by Singleton and colleagues at the Psychology Department of the University of Hull. It consists of a number of computer-based tests. Its chief features are:

- It is suitable for children aged between four and eight years.
- It can be carried out using the school's existing computer hardware.
- It takes about 45 minutes to administer.
- It is designed to be used by qualified teachers and educational professionals.
- The interpretation of the results requires professional expertise.

The process of screening

The process of screening needs to be carefully thought through before there is a headlong rush to mass screening. What is going to be done to help these children who may show features of the 'dyslexia' syndrome? The words of the paediatrician White Franklin (1979) are as rational and relevant today as they were twenty years ago: 'A screening programme will make matters worse unless associated with it is a course of action that will avoid what the screening predicts.'

Who are the key players in the detection of dyslexia?

Many people are involved in the care of a child. Miles and Miles (1990) said 'at least in the straightforward cases [however] it is now clear that the presence of dyslexia will be obvious to anyone with the appropriate experience, whatever their "paper" qualifications'.

The parents

'Those who have round the clock experience of living with dyslexic children often form a very different view of their skills than do researchers' (Nicolson and Fawcett, 1994). This strongly supports the view that parents are usually the best placed to be on the alert for early warning signs.

Parents often realize that there is something 'different' about their child. He may appear very bright but has great difficulties with some basic skills, such as learning to dress, or he may be clumsy, or his speech development may be poor. Parents may be alerted by a delay in acquiring skills that his siblings master easily and often spontaneously. Family life may have become fraught because the child has become aggressive, or subject to sibling rivalry because a younger sibling is able to master skills of which the dyslexic elder is incapable. The family doctor may not be able to find anything wrong with the child.

Health care professionals

Family doctor

Dr Jill Carlisle, previously Principal Clinical Medical Officer for North Warwickshire, set up a model Developmental Screening Programme for the North Warwickshire Health Authority. For many years she spearheaded an almost personal crusade to increase awareness and understanding among her medical colleagues in recognizing dyslexia at an early age. As chairman of the BDA's Medical sub-committee she emphasized the important role of the health visitors and doctors who are performing developmental and health screening checks on pre-school children.

Health professionals can refer a child to the appropriate specialist who may be able to prevent or strengthen, or at least to minimize, the areas of weakness and the learning difficulties which may develop on entry into school.

Health visitor

The health visitor in the UK plays a vital role in identifying children who may have dyslexia as they, in theory, see all children and are therefore uniquely placed to monitor all children's progress. Other countries tend only to monitor the development of sick children.

It is important that health visitors should be aware of those specific weaknesses or unexpected failures in a child's developmental profile which suggest that the child may be 'at risk' of subsequent specific learning difficulties at school. These signs are particularly significant if coupled with a family history of dyslexia.

Speech therapist

The speech therapist has a central role in the identification of children at risk, and their early intervention can minimize or prevent later problems for many children. In the first half of this century speech therapists were mostly concerned with spoken language disorders, such as delays in the acquisition and use of language and particularly with the treatment of aphasia. Nowadays speech therapists are often involved with pre-school children when the language difficulties become obvious, and they are trained to diagnose and treat disorders of communication (see Chapter 3). Hamilton-Fairley (1976) pointed out that 'faulty speech patterns in the young may accentuate reading and spelling difficulties as the child matures'. The speech therapists use many tests which can identify known areas of weakness in dyslexic children, for example, delays in speech and language, word-naming difficulties. Some of the best practice in the field of identification and remediation of learning disorders has been developed by and from the work of the speech therapists. The demands for their services are set to increase dramatically if the early screening programmes, now available, are widely used.

According to the *Code of Practice* the help of a speech therapist should be provided by district health authorities and GP fundholders, but their services are in demand. If the NHS cannot provide help, then, according to a court ruling known as the Lancashire Ruling, the child's LEA must provide and pay for the speech therapy – if the language impairment has resulted in educational difficulties. Some LEAs have a policy not to provide help for children over the age of seven or eight.

Education professionals

The nursery teacher and the play-group leader/supervisor

The nursery teacher and play-group leader/supervisor, if they are trained and know what to look for, are well placed to recognize the early signs of an irregular pattern of development in a child. They can then begin to develop and use some form of remedial programme for the child who is not reaching his developmental milestones at the 'normal' time or who is showing some delays in specific areas of his development ('milestones' is something of a misnomer because it implies that a child suddenly acquires a skill on one day, or even that each child should do so at exactly the same age – 'stepping-stones' would be more appropriate).

In 1993 Baroness Warnock became the President of the BDA. As a mother, former Headmistress and a distinguished educationalist she was very much aware of the problems that surround the whole issue of dyslexia. She said that 'by far the best way to tackle educational failure is to have mandatory nursery schools; for a structured nursery is the best place both for identification and successful intervention' (Warnock, 1993). She was also concerned about the 20 per cent of young adults who are illiterate and suggested that 'one needs a whole body of teachers who can identify children who need early and intense help, in this way we can reduce this 20 per cent'.

In 1996 a pilot voucher scheme was introduced to three London boroughs and Norfolk in which parents were supplied with vouchers that could be used to buy nursery education for their children. The objective of the scheme was to provide universal availability of high quality nursery education for three- and four-year-old children. According to Schools Minister Robin Squire (1996), 'for some children the scheme could actually mean the early identification of their learning difficulties' with providers having 'to have regard to the principles of the Special Educational Needs Code of Practice'.

The teacher

Children who have been identified as possibly 'at risk' and who may have special educational needs before they come to school are best served if their teachers are made aware of their problems as soon as possible. It prevents hours of wasted time and energy spent on tasks that are not within the ability of the child. It also enables the teacher to use the most appropriate method of teaching the child, preventing the terrible self-perpetuating chain of failure, frustration and refusal that can occur for the dyslexic pupil.

The *Code of Practice 1994* clearly states that teachers have duties as do LEAs, health services and social services [who] must have regard to the Code from 1 September 1994 (see Chapter 13). 'The importance of early identification, assessment and provision for any child who may have special educational needs cannot be over emphasized.' (Code of Practice, 1994)

The politician

Politicians are clearly well placed for campaigning to ensure that enough funding is available to provide for the services required.

The BDA reported to the House of Commons Select Committee on Education in 1996 and 'in a nutshell, we said that several issues need to be addressed if the commendable Code is to become a reality: issues such as the prompt identification of dyslexia by properly trained teachers, investment in Individual Education Plans, consistent and fair treatment at Tribunal hearings' (Cann, 1996).

Benefits of early diagnosis for remediation

There is plenty of research evidence which shows that the earlier the problem is detected the better the prognosis. Bradley (1989) demonstrated that 'the younger the child, the more effective the remedial intervention'. Gardner (1994) reinforced this and said 'good nursery education can help the child with certain underlying weaknesses'. Much work is needed to improve 'the spoken language skills and the child's awareness of it' (Snowling, 1987) because of its importance to the child's later acquisition of literacy. According to Brady et al (1994), there are 'numerous prediction studies [which] demonstrate that the greater a child's awareness of the phonological structure of words prior to reading instruction, the greater will be that child's success in learning to read.'

Multi-disciplinary approach

'The nature of the deficit changes with development' (Snowling, 1987). This implies that changes can be brought about by the appropriate intervention of all those associated with bringing up the child (parents, play-group leader, teachers, speech therapists). Problems that may serve to identify dyslexia are often observed before the appearance of reading difficulties. Appropriate reaction to such pointers could save such children having to endure the 'experience of academic failure and the negative consequences of failure' (Catts, 1989). Yet some authorities still believe that it is not appropriate or sensible to diagnose dyslexia formally by assessment much before the child is six or seven years old (Gardner, 1994). Hornsby (1993) said 'one is not attempting to diagnose dyslexia in pre-school years, merely to indicate those that could be "at risk" and to take suitable intervention measures'. This seems to encapsulate the views of many practitioners in the field.

Advantages of early intervention

Miles and Miles (1984) were commissioned by the Department of Education and Science (DES) to examine the effect of early intervention. They found that 'it is particularly advantageous if special teaching can start no later than age seven'. They concluded that 'if dyslexic children are caught early, less time is needed for catching up, while in many cases they can be helped before frustration sets in'. The research of Badian (1988) replicated these findings. She reported that 'when diagnosis of dyslexia was made in the first two grades of school, over 80 per cent of the students could be brought up to their normal classroom work'. Chasty (1996) stated that 'at the age of seven, a child with mild to moderate dyslexia/specific learning difficulties (i.e. 80 per cent of all children with such difficulties) can be helped within the classroom situation by the class teacher or class assistant allocating one hour – in short and frequent sessions throughout the week. However, if the child's difficulties are not recognized and the necessary support not given, then within a few years these difficulties will have accumulated to a level requiring eight hours a week, in teaching and support – both within the classroom and outside'.

Dyslexia cannot be prevented or cured. Early identification can lessen the long term effect of the symptoms when it is accompanied by appropriate remediation, sympathetic understanding and an awareness that there may be weaknesses and lateness in acquiring fundamental life skills. Secondary emotional and behavioural problems can be prevented or avoided if appropriate intervention is made in early childhood.

Identification often brings relief

Miles (1993) pointed out that dyslexia need not be a calamity, but 'in the first place, if dyslexic children are not told the nature of their difficulties they readily come to believe that they are "thick" or "stupid" and it is clearly very frustrating to find that other children can easily cope with tasks which they themselves find difficult'. Although many authorities hold the view that children should not be given labels, those who have experience of working with dyslexics say that the benefits of being told they have a recognized condition far outweigh the disadvantages of being labelled 'dyslexic'. Parents often say that 'not knowing is far worse than knowing'.

Early diagnosis should help to take away the burden of blame from the child, his parents and his teachers. Those people connected with the child (parents, baby-sitter, child-minder, grandparents, Brownie or Cub Leader, play-group supervisors) should be made aware of the child's difficulties. Carlisle (1995) stated that 'any adults spending much time with the child can be encouraged to follow advice on helpful activities but alarm or anxiety must not be caused'. It is important that parents and others associated with the child are counselled and that they are given encouragement and constructive practical advice on matters such as play activities, games and management. All involved must be mindful of the old adage that 'diagnosis without remediation is unethical'.

Early warning signs that may predict learning difficulties

In a child aged between two and six there are a number of early warning signs that indicate that the child may experience learning difficulties later. Before considering this subject it is important to be mindful that 'dyslexics [do not] fall neatly and tidily into a small number of different sub-types, [...] and any attempts to force them into mutually exclusive categories distorts the nature of the dyslexic reality' (Ellis, 1993). Richardson (1989) reminded us that the diagnostician or specialist 'each reflects the particular school of thought in which he or she was trained' and 'the remedial strategies each chooses will depend in kind on the theoretical base subscribed to by the therapist'. This highlights the importance of a multi-disciplinary approach to diagnosis, assessment and remedial intervention.

It is difficult to be age specific about some of the early warning signs. It is also important to be aware that an individual child will not have all of the symptoms as cited below. 'One of the advantages of the word "syndrome" is that it can be used when one is aware that certain signs "belong together"' (Miles and Miles, 1990). The diagnostician must be on the lookout for the 'unexpected failure' in the otherwise normal child. She should also note that 'dyslexia is a disorder with a number of different manifestations' (Snowling, 1987).

Family history and genetic evidence

There is much anecdotal evidence to support the view that dyslexia may run in families. There is also much well-documented research from as long ago as Thomas (1905) to substantiate this. Hinshelwood (1917) stated that 'Dr Thomas called special attention to the fact that congenital word-blindness may assume a family type and that a heriditary tendency is probable. The present example [in the article] of four members of the same family with congenital word-blindness is a brilliant confirmation of the correctness of Dr Thomas's observation'. 88 per cent of the 112 families studied by Hallgren (1950) contained at least one dyslexic member. This figure was almost replicated in the study by Finucci et al (1976) which found that 81 per cent had 'at least one affected parent'.

A most striking vignette underlines the fact that it is not just parents and their children who are affected. Grandparents, uncles, aunts, first and second cousins may also be. The mothers of two boys who were at a boarding school in the south-east of England were talking on the touchline of the playing field one day. They began to compare notes on the progress of their offspring. It emerged that both boys were very bright, with IQs in the 130s. Both were doing very well in mathematics – one boy being top of his class in this subject – but neither boy could read, despite having specialist teaching for a considerable period of time. Each of the mothers mentioned that other cousins in their families had problems with literacy. One of the boys had a sister who also had learning difficulties. Finally it emerged that the mother of one boy was a long lost first cousin of the second boy's father. The parents of the first boy had emigrated to South America and lost contact with their eleven brothers and sisters in Yorkshire. The common link was their dyslexia. But a much more striking, and even more interesting, feature was the similarity of the symptoms displayed by the two boys. Smith (1992) confirmed that 'large extended families provide valuable information about the inheritance pattern of complex traits'.

- Research shows that children whose parents are dyslexic 'are significantly more likely to have reading problems themselves' (Vogler, De Fries and Decker, 1985). They also 'found the risk to a son of having an affected father is 40 per cent and of having an affected mother is 35 per cent. For daughters, the risk for dyslexia of having an affected parent of either sex was 17–18 per cent.'

- Anecdotal evidence underlines the fact that if both parents are dyslexic, there is a high chance that some or all their offspring will be dyslexic. If one parent is dyslexic and the non-dyslexic parent has relatives who are, the odds are higher that they will have a dyslexic child. The research of Finucci and Childs (1976) confirmed that 'the number of affected children increased when both parents were clearly affected'.

- The Colorado Family Reading Study was initiated in 1973 and is one of the most influential research projects. It found in the 250 families tested that the gender ratio of dyslexics was 3.3:1 males to females (De Fries, 1991). Other studies suggest that dyslexia affects 3.5–4.0:1 males to females. The Colorado Research on twins, both identical and non-identical, strengthens the case for accepting dyslexia as being heritable. 'Taken together, however, these previous studies do support the hypothesis that dyslexia is a symptom of a genetically determined neurological disorder with immunological components.' (Galaburda, Sherman and Rosen, 1989)

- Smith et al (1983) found 'significant evidence for linkage between dyslexia and chromosome 15' in 20 per cent of the dyslexic families. Lubs et al (1993) have been studying three generations of families with dyslexia to 'evaluate the effects of the presumed gene or genes leading to the diagnosis of dyslexia'. Their findings to date show that from the eleven families in the study, 74 family members have 'a gene leading to dyslexia' and 'the severity of the defect in reading and spelling may be greater in males'. They have identified chromosome 6 as the one carrying a specific abnormality.

- Some specific developmental dyslexics have no family history of dyslexia. This group includes those with the 'secondary' or 'acquired' dyslexia, but who have the same symptoms as the child with the specific developmental dyslexia. It is important that these people know, or are told, that their children are not likely to be dyslexic (unlike those with a positive family history). According to Carlisle (1994) the following factors can be significant when making a diagnosis of acquired dyslexia:

a)   A history of placental dysfunction 'small-for-dates- baby'.

b)   Difficult birth with anoxia (lack of oxygen).

c)   Head injuries as a result of an accident.

d)   Brain tumour.

Speech and language

Most researchers agree that language development is the most significant feature that has to be examined in the identification of dyslexia. Snowling (1987) said that 'the predominant view to date is that dyslexia is associated with phonological difficulties originating within spoken language processes'. A child with language problems may experience some or all of the following difficulties:

- Word-naming problems.
- Word mispronunciation.
- Jumbling words.
- Poor use of syntax.
- Difficulties with rhyme and alliteration.
- Tendency to use circumlocutions.
- Hesitant speech.
- Needs frequent presentation of a word before being able to use it accurately and consistently.

Sequencing

Many children have initial difficulties with some of the tasks described below, but the dyslexic child's problems will be greater and more persistent. A dyslexic child will make mistakes frequently that other children make only occasionally.

Visual difficulties

- The child may be poor at drawing – some are excellent and have a good use of colour.
- The child may find it difficult to track through a maze.
- The child may find it difficult to sort beads by shapes.
- The child may have difficulty learning to dress himself – what goes on first? Shirt or vest? He may also be very slow at dressing and changing his clothes, or put his clothes on inside out.
- The child may put shoes on the wrong foot.
- Some find it difficult to turn on and off taps because they cannot remember which way the thread goes.

- Buttons can cause problems because of being unable to remember where to start. Some lack the manual dexterity to cope with finding the buttonhole and then putting the button through it.
- The child may have difficulty turning door handles, particularly door knobs.
- The child may find doing jigsaw puzzles or making models difficult.

Auditory sequential memory difficulties

- The child may not be able to learn or repeat nursery rhymes or childish ditties.

- The child may not be able to repeat messages – when he takes a telephone call he may forget the name of the speaker, or when given the message 'Dad will be home late, he has missed the train and will be on the next one' he will perhaps only remember that 'Dad will be late'.

- The child may have difficulty in following a series of instructions – he goes up stairs to look for something and forgets what he has been sent to find. He may have difficulty remembering a series of instructions, for example, from the teacher on the playing field. This will often be exacerbated by directionality confusions. Catts (1989) confirmed that 'dyslexics have been shown to perform less well than normal individuals in the short term recall of lists of letters, words, digits and sentences'.

- The child may often find it hard to string a few sentences together to describe a recent event – 'What did you have for lunch today?' He may begin at the end of the story and seem to lose his way. He may also struggle to find the words to convey his meaning.

- The child may find clapping or beating time to music difficult. Wolff, Michel and Ovrut (1990) showed that dyslexic children have persistent problems in tapping rhythm, specifically when asked to tap the hands asynchronously.

- The child may have difficulty with remembering common sequences – the alphabet, days of the week, months of the year. He finds it difficult to tell whether it is morning or evening. Phrases like 'next week' 'in a month's time' may confuse him. He may neither be able to remember his own address nor often the date of his birthday nor his telephone number. Badian's (1995) research confirmed the importance of letter naming as a predictor and of the role of phonemic awareness in early reading acquisition.

- The child may find counting difficult – particularly counting backwards (see Chapter 7).

- The child may show signs of poor auditory discrimination. He may hear the sound but be unable to identify what he hears, just as the colour-blind person can see the colour but is unable to recognize the colours. Such a child will often be accused of not listening or being inattentive.

Motor skills

Motor skills are so called because the muscles that perform these skills work like a motor controlled by the brain.

Fine motor skills

Fine motor skills are those associated primarily with the fingers and hands.

Lenneberg (1967) pointed out that 'the appearance of increasingly complex speech and language behaviour paralleled milestones in motor development. A sense of rhythm is important to help improve motor co-ordination'. Some children have no difficulty acquiring these skills while others do so late, or with difficulty. By the age of six the child should normally have acquired most of these skills. Rudel (1985) found that 'there is evidence of early difficulties in newly acquired [motor] skills, but these difficulties are largely outgrown by nine to ten years'.

- The child may have difficulty learning to use cutlery. Some are messy eaters who frequently spill and knock things over at table.

- The child may find it difficult to use a pair of scissors – especially if he is left handed.

- The child may find it difficult to trace.

- The child may not be able to use a rubber effectively.

- The child may hold his pencil awkwardly.

- The child may find it difficult to tie shoe laces.

- The child may find learning to do a tie extremely difficult.

Gross motor skills

Gross motor skills are those associated with the arms and the legs.

- The child may find hopping difficult.

- Skipping is even more difficult for some because it involves balancing while moving.

- The child may have difficulties catching, throwing or kicking a ball because he finds it difficult to put his hands in the right place. Others find it difficult to anticipate the velocity of the ball.

- The child may be constantly bumping into people and objects. In games he often collides with others. He may bump into other children on the stairs at school because the child who is going up the stairs does not realize that another child is coming down the stairs on the left, at the same time.

- The child may have a tendency to knock things over or to drop things.

- Going up steps may prove difficult – some children have a tendency to do so one at a time. When coming down the stairs they tend to continue to jump off the final step.

- Learning to ride a bicycle can be a tortuous process.

- Setting the table may be difficult – knives and forks may be put on the wrong side.

- Learning to swim can be difficult for some children, especially the breaststroke because the arms and leg movements must be synchronized. Others find bilateral breathing required for the overarm can be difficult: when the right arm comes out of the water the head has to be moved to the left and vice versa.

- Playground games may be difficult, especially if they involve words such as left/right, up/down, backwards/forwards, in front/behind.

- Learning to dance may be difficult for some children, particularly if there is a sequence of steps to be remembered, as in country dancing.

- There is anecdotal evidence of a child slipping down inside his sleeping bag and being unable to find his way out because of directionality confusion.

- The child may experience difficulties with co-ordination in the gym when climbing the ropes, crawling through apparatus, standing on one leg or walking along a bench. The child who has very pronounced difficulties in this area can be assessed by an occupational therapist who will use tests and make a clinical observation. This may result in a diagnosis of dyspraxia, which implies poor co-ordination and difficulty in the planning and carrying out of fine and gross motor skills.

Laterality

Laterality describes the side of the body used for certain tasks. Many children have a lack of cerebral dominance (a preference for the left or right side of the body for carrying out certain functions involving the eyes, ears, hands or feet). For example, someone who is right-side dominant will use his right hand, right eye, right ear and right foot to perform most tasks. Someone who is cross-lateral will use different parts of the body for different tasks, for example, his left foot to kick and his right eye to look through a camera lense. Inconsistencies are often evident in the young child. Researchers have 'observed higher rates of weak right handedness among a spectrum of developmental disorders' (Duane, 1991), thus a child may throw a ball with his right hand but may use a knife with his left hand when eating. It is well-established that certain people who are predominantly right handed can be left handed for specific tasks, for example, when playing cricket. This is not regarded as dysfunctional as long as the person is consistent in their handedness. It is essential to realize that cross-laterality is not in itself a diagnosis of a learning difficulty.

- Lack of consistent handedness or ambidexterity can lead to greater difficulties when the child begins to use crayons, felt pens or a pencil.

- One of Orton's early observations was that there was a high frequency of left handedness in dyslexics and in their families. Geschwind (1982) cited that he and Dr Peter Behan 'completed a study on a large group of strongly left-handed people and confirmed that this population has a much higher rate of dyslexia and other learning disabilities than a control population of strongly right-handed individuals'.

Practical suggestions

to help the child who has motor difficulties

- Colour code shoes on the sole or inside with a bright symbol to help distinguish between left and right.

- Buy or make a tie that is permanently knotted on a piece of elastic. The child can learn how to tie the tie without undoing the knot later.

- Mark the toes of socks with bright cotton to prevent the child from fumbling while attempting to put his toe into the heel of the sock.

- Make use of commercially available aids, such as a card to help the child learn to tie shoe laces.

- When teaching a child to button a coat or a cardigan, teach him to always begin at the bottom where he can easily see what he is doing.

- Stand behind the child to teach him to do a tie or bow. (If the child is left handed and the teacher right handed, face the child.) Get him to begin with the wide end, which should be twice as long as the narrow end.

- Buy velcro fastening shoes and trainers whenever possible.

Summary and conclusions

1   The clamour for early recognition is becoming louder and has been marshalled by the dyslexia organizations. Parents are better informed, many have had to struggle with dyslexia themselves and are therefore quickly alerted to similarities between their own and their child's development.

2   There is a body of opinion, and research evidence, which shows that children who are 'at risk' can be identified before they go to school or shortly after they start school.

3   Screening tests, such as the DEST or the CoPS 1, have been developed which can alert those who deal with children whose progress is uneven or who are slow at acquiring certain skills. These may turn out to be the children who later struggle when learning to read.

4   Caution needs to be exercised in the use of such screening tests. Counselling and practical advice will need to accompany any screening programme to reduce any alarm or anxiety that may be raised. White Franklin (1979) gave cautionary advice when he said 'screening is all very well if it is linked with prevention. A screening programme will make matters worse unless associated with it is a course of action that will avoid what the screening predicts'.

5   Early identification of a learning difficulty must be accompanied by the appropriate measures to help remediate the problems. Chasty (1996) said that 'schools represent the most critical period for diagnosis. The earlier the diagnosis, the more immediate the help – and the less serious the damage to the child'.

6   The Education Act 1993 and the *Code of Practice 1994* clearly state that the teacher and the school have statutory duties and responsibilities to identify and assess the child with special educational needs as soon as possible. Parents have to be consulted and informed about all decisions relating to their child.

7   There is much evidence to support the idea that the earlier the identification of a problem, and the sooner appropriate intervention is begun, the better, quicker and more cost effective it will be for child, parent, school and society. It may prevent years of humiliation, frustration and despair.

8   There is evidence that there is a genetic link in dyslexia and that it reappears in succeeding generations of families. Pennington (1989) argued that 'family history could be used to help screen for children at high risk for this disorder'. This has important implications for fiscal management and for those in control of the budgets for the provision of funds for children with special educational needs. Early recognition and intervention can be cost effective.

9   There is a wide spectrum of difficulties. The symptoms of dyslexia vary. Inconsistency, unpredictability and unexpectedness are its most consistent features.

10 The euphoria surrounding early screening and intervention must not lull educators into a false sense of security. The dyslexic pupil's problems are not solved once he has learnt to read at school as a result of early screening and help. Fawcett (1994), the co-author of DEST, maintained that 'with early help dyslexics can learn to read as well as anyone else, although perhaps not as quickly. They will probably always have trouble with spelling however' and many will also have life long handicaps in many other aspects of their lives because of their dyslexia.

11 Miles (1974) stated that 'in my experience cross-laterality is of no special use, even as a diagnostic sign, since there are plenty of people who are cross-lateral without being dyslexic and plenty of people who are dyslexic without being cross-lateral'. Yet in a survey of learning support teachers Reid (1990) found that 'the issue of cerebral dominance appears to be the most frequently cited cause [of specific learning difficulties] raised by the sample'. 'But despite extensive research the relevance of laterality to dyslexia [...] remains a matter of dispute.' (Hiscock and Kinsbourne, 1995).

Chapter 3

Spoken language

- identifying the problem
- how parents and teachers can help

Introduction

Language is universally acquired by humans. Most children learn to speak and require very little help to do so, but 'some children have to work harder and for a longer time than others at learning language' (Bloom, 1980). Masland (1990) stated that 'dyslexia is a disorder of language'. The US government's definition of learning disabilities Public Law 94–142 states that 'children with specific learning disabilities exhibit a disorder in one or more of the basic psychological processes involved in understanding or in using spoken or written language. These may be manifest in disorders of listening, thinking, talking, reading, writing, spelling or arithmetic' (US Office of Education, 1977).

Geschwind (1982), when surveying the contributions of Orton, reminded us that 'in his [Orton's] original observations he pointed out the frequency of slowness in the acquisition of spoken speech in dyslexic children thus laying the groundwork for the important concept that dyslexia appears on a foundation of delay in the development of the entire system devoted to language'.

Duane (1991) made an optimistic contribution when he reminded us that, 'despite the very strong correlation with oral language, there are children with reading difficulties who seem to have little or no problem in speech perception or speech production'. But for those who do, the earlier the problem is identified the better the prognosis and 'the prognosis depends primarily upon the extent of the child's phonological disorder, that is, its severity' (Snowling, 1987). The predominant view of the researchers as to the underlying cause of specific learning difficulties has been described as 'the phonological deficit hypothesis', which in plain English means an inability to analyse speech into the sounds that it is made from.

Spoken language in the pre-school child

Parents, or the child's primary carer, are often aware that their child is late or slow in talking. Other children are identified by the health visitor, general practitioner (GP) or speech therapist. Early screening tests (see Chapter 2) will help to identify the child needing help. Pre-school language impairment, or the late acquisition of speech, are important and useful early indicators of dyslexia.

When are speech therapists needed?

A pre-school child may need help from a speech therapist if he is experiencing difficulties in the acquisition and use of speech. Speech therapists have long been involved with children with language problems, particularly disorders of articulation and communication, voice disorders, delay in speaking and use of language and dysfluency (stuttering).

If the answer is 'yes' to the following questions the child should be referred to a speech therapist for an assessment:

- Does the child say very few words by the age of two years?
- Are the phrases or speech of a three-year-old child unintelligible to his primary carer?
- Is the child's speech unintelligible by the age of four years?
- Does the child mispronounce words or substitute sounds by the age of seven years?

The repercussions of a spoken language problem

If the child cannot speak or understand language, learning to read and write will present a great problem. 'A child who has a problem in learning language in pre-school years will be a child with a learning disability in the school years.' (Bloom, 1980) The Bullock Report (Bullock, 1975) stressed that children learn by talking and writing just as much as they do by listening and reading. Some children have expressive language difficulties and they will have poor vocabularies, difficulty in naming people, places and objects, incorrect grammar and poor syntax. This results in problems, particularly when the child enters school where 75 per cent of the day is spent in listening and speaking. Hamilton-Fairley (1976) commented that 'faulty speech patterns in the young child may accentuate reading and spelling difficulties as the child matures'. Quite a large number of children do have problems. A report in *The Guardian* stated that 'nearly 250,000 children of school age have some degree of speech and language impairment or disorder ... and 10 per cent of those of school age have difficulties which could interfere with their educational development' (Croall, 1995). The Royal College of Speech and Language Therapists (1996) reported that 'one in five children are entering school with a communication problem'. It is important to identify and address the difficulties in order to prevent more problems for the child later in life, which may affect many other areas of his development.

Proficiency in spoken language, or what some professionals refer to as 'oral' language, is the foundation to further success in acquiring and using all other language skills. Most researchers agree that language development is the most significant underlying feature in the identification of dyslexia and has to be examined carefully.

What are the main speech and language difficulties that children experience?

Dyslexic children often display a variety of symptoms. Snowling (1987) said 'dyslexia is a disorder with a number of different manifestations'. This applies as much to their language skills as to any other functions. Calfee (1983) argued that 'a number of scholars have proposed that dyslexia results from a form of minimal language disability or "dysphasia"' and 'so it seems quite reasonable to suggest that the child with subtle language problems might encounter more than unusual difficulty in learning to read'. But 'it would be wrong to suggest that all children with reading and spelling problems have a speech and language disorder' (Bishop and Adams, 1990). Many do not and often they are identified as 'bright' because of their good verbal skills.

Pre-school attainments for language development

A child should be able to:

- say first words – at 12 months
- speak 5–20 words – at 18 months
- use 50 words and understand more as well as use simple sentences – at 24 months
- use full sentences, answer and ask questions, give his full name, use plurals and pronouns, listen to stories, know several nursery rhymes (if taught them) – at 36 months.

Failure to reach the goals which identifiy satisfactory language development can help to identify a child who may have problems later. By the time a child is four he should be able to make himself understood when he speaks to people outside his own family. If he cannot, then, according to Danwitz (1975), he has a language problem. Danwitz (1975) pointed out that for a normal five year old 'the typical verbal output is 10,000–15,000 words per day from a vocabulary of 5,000 words'.

Auditory problems of the Primary School child

Rhyme and alliteration

Alliteration describes words which begin with the same sound or letter, for example 'Sing a song of sixpence', or a group of words that begin with the same sounds, for example, ship/shop/shed.

Some dyslexics may have a difficulty with rhyme and alliteration. Out of a set of rhyming words, such as mat/fat/pat/bed, the child may find it difficult to hear and identify the odd one out. Similarly, when given a task involving alliteration, such as chat/chum/chip/shop, he may have difficulty picking the odd one out.

Bradley and Bryant (1983) carried out a study of 400 children aged between four and five years and found that some had difficulty with alliteration and rhyme in words such as 'bat', 'bun', 'bed', 'gap', 'rig', 'big', 'wig', 'dot'. These children were tested four years later and '28.5 per cent of our weak categorizers went on to become weak readers'. They found that ability to perceive and discriminate incoming sound was the most powerful predicator of later reading achievement. Lundberg, Frost and Petersen (1988) 'showed that pre-readers who were trained to segment speech into phonemes before they received any reading instruction, learned to read and spell better than control subjects who did not receive this training'.

Long-term repercussion of weak auditory skills

Weak auditory language skills have many long-term repercussions. Rome and Osman (1985) used the analogy of a tape recorder in the ear. 'A person with a very good ear memory can listen and play back to himself what he or she has just heard' (Sheffield, (1991). Chasty (1985) said that 'in the classroom, reading, writing, studying, comprehension exercises, note taking, essay writing, using tables, number facts, drawing maps, handling chemical formulae, learning foreign languages may all be affected'.

Oral problems of the Primary School child

Difficulty with syllables

The child may have difficulty with breaking words into syllables when reading, spelling and in speech, saying perhaps 'amlance' for 'ambulance' or 'butrfy' for 'butterfly'. Being able to break words into syllables is very important, particularly for spelling. Some children have difficulty in repeating multi-syllabic words (Miles, 1974). They may find the repetition of some words, for example 'preliminary', almost impossible. This is evident when they are tested on the repetition of polysyllabic words, as in the *Bangor Dyslexia Test* (Miles, 1983).

Pronunciation

The child may mispronounce words, saying, for example 'Farmer Christmas' for 'Father Christmas'. Longer words of more than two syllables, such as 'specific', create even greater problems (Miles, 1983). Blacock (1982) pointed out that 'specifically, dyslexics have often been observed to show misarticulations in their speech'.

Jumbling words

The child may sometimes jumble words, for example 'iced chops' for 'choc-ices', 'padmington' for 'badminton', or produce spoonerisms. A **Spoonerism** takes its name from the scholar, the Reverend W. A. Spooner (1844–1930), who had a tendency to accidental or deliberate transposition of initial letters in two or more words, and in 1879 in the chapel of New College, Oxford announced the hymn 'Kinquering Congs Their Titles Take'.

Sequencing

Many parents report that dyslexic children have difficulty saying nursery rhymes. They seem to lose the sequence. As a result they may find it difficult to join in playground or party games because they forget words in the ditty which tells them what to do next. 'Rhyming experience should be a main focus in pre-school years onwards.' (Stackhouse, 1985)

Auditory sequential memory

Dyslexics often have auditory sequential memory difficulties which are often interpreted by parents and teachers as owing to a lack of attention or carelessness. A frequently-heard comment of a teacher, faced with the pupil who has forgotten his PE kit for the third week running, might be, 'Oh! I know he is dyslexic and can't spell but this boy is just plain careless and doesn't care.' The child 'has an organizational problem caused by a retrieval problem, that is dyslexia' (Sheffield, 1991).

The child may need to be presented frequently with a word before he can use it accurately and consistently. According to Catts (1989), 'upon hearing a new word, dyslexics often need multiple presentations of the word before they can accurately and consistently produce it'. Anecdotal evidence comes from the child who is unable to remember his new baby brother's name.

Expressive language problems

Dyslexics often express themselves clumsily in oral language. According to Heisler (1983), 'the child with language delay may experience stress and frustration in communicating with others, either in understanding or in trying to express himself or both.' As a result, these children can become shy or withdrawn. How frustrating for child and parent when the simple question, 'What did you do in school today?' or 'Tell me about the school trip in London' elicits a one- or two-word answer. Gauntlett (1978) called it 'mental fright'. It can be difficult to get dyslexics to talk about a subject, even one they know well. Sheffield's (1991) experiences confirmed this: 'Almost every dyslexic I've ever worked with has found it difficult to express in words all the fine ideas that he has in his mind'. Dyslexics also have difficulty following a sequence of verbal instructions. On the playing field, one talented rugby player was sent off because he could not follow or remember what the team coach was telling him to do. He was dismissed as being inattentive.

'Some on the other hand are extremely articulate.' (Hornsby, 1988) Evidence of this can be seen in the performances of the many successful, dyslexic actors and actresses. Michael Heseltine's rhetoric performance at the annual Conservative Party Conference does not appear to have been affected by his dyslexia.

Syntax and spelling

The rules concerning the grammatical ordering of words in speech or written language to make sentences are known as **syntax**.

The child's use of syntax may be poor, for example, he may confuse the tenses (especially the irregular past tense) coming out with 'The dog satted on the chair' or 'She teached me how to do it.'

Children are asked to do 'free' writing at a very early stage in their school career. They are often required to write about their weekend activities. Some dyslexic children may be able to describe events orally but have enormous difficulties putting what they have just said onto paper. They may find it difficult to remember the names of the places they visited. They often confuse the tense of the verb, for example 'We went to London and we are going yesterday.' They confuse personal pronouns. They may start the story in the third person and intersperse it with the first person, for example 'He went to Thorpe Park with his Mum and Dad and I went on the roller coaster.'

Some dyslexic children use a very restricted vocabulary because of a subliminal tendency to use only words they know how to spell. The Bullock Report (Bullock, 1975) said that 'some find it virtually impossible to communicate their ideas in writing because their spelling vocabulary is so limited, but a substantial number are unable to read their own writing back because their spelling is so unlike the spelling of the words they have learned to recognize in books'. Others write an approximation of what they hear, for example in a

Geography examination one child wrote 'the 10's' for 'the Thames' [flows through London], which is what the word sounded like to him.

Word-naming problems

Many researchers have found that dyslexic children have great difficulties in 'naming' things. When he starts school he can't remember his grandparents' names, class teacher's name or a place he has been on holiday for two weeks. He may know the colours and he can point out a red car if asked, but if the question is put the other way and he is asked, 'What colour is that car?' he may not be able to answer it (Denckla and Rudel, 1976).

The child may have a tendency to use circumlocutions, for example, 'This is a thingummyjig' or 'The thing you look in to see yourself' for a 'mirror'.

'Naming latencies [slowness or lateness] for a variety of materials illustrate that access to a verbal code is slower in dyslexic children' (Snowling, Stackhouse and Rack, 1986). They are also slower than non-dyslexic children at performing these tasks. An understanding of their difficulties is important, particularly in the light of the demands of the National Curriculum, which says 'children should participate as speakers and listeners in a given task. They should be able to describe real or imaginary events. They should listen to stories and poems and talk about them. They should be able to listen to, ask and answer questions. They should respond appropriately to more complex instructions and be able to give simple instructions themselves'.

Dyslexics may not be able to remember frequently-used words and they may say 'amimals' for animals, 'pagetti' for spaghetti or 'contiments' for consonants. Henry, when asked 'Have you done a test like this before?' replied, 'Yes, at the diluke's institute' [Dyslexia Institute]. According to Sheffield (1991), 'this retrieval problem is crippling for many dyslexic youngsters'. How frustrating in an examination when the child is asked to underline the verb, and has to ask, 'What's a verb?' When he has an opportunity to revise the word, he can often complete the exercise correctly. Sawyer and Butler (1991) reminded us that much information, such as address and date of birth, is recalled automatically yet 'young children, and children with limited language skills, may have considerable difficulty in retrieving from long term memory the acceptable definitions or descriptions of words or objects'. The pioneer researcher in this area of verbal deficit hypothesis was Vellutino (1979) who hypothesized that 'written language problems are caused by difficulties with language processing in general'.

Figures of speech

Figures of speech and literary devices cause the child with a specific learning difficulty great problems. They are literal thinkers. When asked, 'What are battery hens?' Paul responded that 'they are hens who have been battered'. Aylett Cox (1982) gave a charming example: The teacher asked the pupil, 'How many p's in "apple"?' The pupil's answer was, 'None! p's are in a pod.' Their literal mindedness makes it difficult for the dyslexic to comprehend or see the irony in proverbs or idioms. Edward, when asked to explain what 'roaring trade' meant, answered 'loud shoppers'. They have to be taught the meaning of these, as well as puns. Analogies, for example mutton is to sheep as pork is to pig, also cause them great difficulties.

The language of mathematics

Chasty (1985) said that '70 per cent of dyslexics experience difficulties with number language words' such as sum, total, odd, take away, power. This was confirmed by Miles and Miles (1992) and Chinn and Ashcroft (1993). Dyslexics have difficulty both with the technical terms and the deceptively familiar words that have totally different associations when used in a mathematical context. They have difficulty with direction and the words 'up/down', 'backwards/forwards' confuse them. (See Chapter 7.)

Comprehension

Comprehension is obviously at risk both because of receptive and expressive language difficulties. Children with language delay, limited vocabulary or low verbal intelligence will struggle with reading comprehension. The child, because he is a poor reader, may have limited experience and consequently a small vocabulary. He may never have experienced the word: therefore, he does not know what it means. Often the understanding of a whole passage may depend on the meanings of one or two keywords or phrases. Another problem for the dyslexic child is that weak reading skills result in all his effort being expended on the mechanical aspects of reading. He then often forgets the content of what he is reading. Freud (1891) said 'understanding becomes impossible once reading itself has become difficult'. See Chapter 4.

How can parents and teachers help pupils with language problems?

'Try to relax and not be too worried or anxious... Anxiety very soon rubs off on to the child, and may set up undesirable reactions' (Hornsby, 1989). Many children say they love the 'talking part' of their lesson because they find it enjoyable and fun. This is perhaps because the stress and pressure of having to make written responses has been removed. Games come into their own and play can form an important role. As long ago as the first century Quintilian said, 'Much can very profitably be done by play long before a child enters school.' (Haarhoff, 1920)

The following guidelines and suggestions may be useful. An imaginative parent/teacher will devise many of her own methods and ideas.

Recommended books
Before Alpha: Learning Games for the Under Fives (Hornsby, 1989)

Language Remediation and Expansion. 100 Skill-building Reference Lists (Bush, 1979)

Developing Spoken Language Skills (Borwick and Townend, 1993)

Phonological (sound) awareness

There are a number of ways to help improve an awareness of sounds (phonological awareness).

- Play 'I spy'. Ask for words beginning with a particular letter sound. Then later go on to the sound of the letter that the word ends with. Then do the sound in the middle of the word.
- Play 'Odd-man-out' when the child is asked to say what word does not belong: shop/chip/shot/ship.
- Work on alliteration. Ask the child to say which word is the odd man out: sap/sun/pig/sad. Do this using different initial letters. Then go on and do it with consonant digraph words: hat/chat/chop/chip; and also the blends: blot/stop/stun/stem.
- Make finger puppets or individual stickers for each of the five short vowels (the child needs to be taught that they say their sound). This is a very useful way of helping to establish the vital concept of discrimination between the short vowels. Small thimbles with the five short vowel sounds written on them are also useful. Children love to show the puppet for /e/ when asked what sound can they hear at the beginning of the word 'egg' or in the middle of the word 'bed'. Duane (1991) said,

'the motor theory of speech perception suggests that the production of speech sounds is an essential concomitant to the comprehension of speech sounds that are heard', and underlined the importance of work on oral skill, with the help of both parents and of teachers.

The above approaches improve and help auditory perception and auditory discrimination. Research by Goswami (1991) shows that children 'find it much simpler to break words up into 'onsets' and 'rimes' than into single phonetic units': d/ash rather than d-a-s-h. This is something that many teachers have guessed instinctively for a long time. They tie in with what the child hears and the aural cues he receives.

Understanding syllables

An understanding of syllables is very important when learning to read and spell (see Chapter 6). We know, from the work of Liberman and Shankweiler (1985) and Treiman (1985), that children are able to break words into syllables, for example bat/man, before they can break them into phonemes, for example b-a-t-m-a-n. Rehearsal and practice takes away the fear of long words and breaks up the task into small manageable steps. There is often a look of delight on the child's face when he makes the discovery that he can write '/re/mem/ber/' or read 'car/pet', or 'den/tist'.

- Clap and count syllables. The young child needs to learn to count the number of syllables in a word. Begin with one syllable words and gradually, as the child's confidence increases, go on to two, three and four syllable words. Train him to say the word first and then to clap each syllable out with his hands. He needs plenty of practice doing this. The teacher can clap out words in syllables, asking the child to repeat the words and/or to clap them with the palm of his hand on his thigh. This also helps short term auditory memory.

- Another helpful method is to teach the child to put his hand directly under his chin. Ask him to repeat the word, for example 'batman'. Then ask him how many times his chin touched his hand – twice – this tells him how many syllables there are in the word.

Rhyme

Bradley and Bryant (1983) found that 'teaching children to categorize words by sounds definitely improves their reading' and 'it is something all pre-school children enjoy. They revel in nursery rhymes'.

Nursery rhymes

The last statement may not have universal application but it is certainly worth teaching nursery rhymes, such as the old favourites 'Three Blind Mice', 'Baa Baa Black Sheep', 'Ring-a-Ring of Roses'.

Rhyming sentences

Sentences with integral rhyme are also fun and help the awareness of similar sounding words. Ask the child to fill in the missing rhyme:

The nurse had a ? (purse)
We will go in a train to ? (Spain)
The pink ink is in the ? (sink)
Never run with a ? (bun)
The fish is on the ? (dish)

Rhyming synonyms

Older children may be asked to give rhyming synonyms:
enjoyable sprint (fun run)
broken down lorry (stuck truck)

Expressive language

Expressive language is very important. In 1982 Phelps wrote that 'It is a repeated observation during treatment that, if oral discussion precedes writing, instead of the other way round, the written form is more mature, fluent and stable.' These skills have to be structured.

The National Curriculum places strong emphasis on spoken language skills. Snowling (1987) concurred when emphasizing 'the important point is that the spoken language system, and the child's awareness of it, influence the acquisition of literacy'. For the dyslexic this is another skill that must be taught, as many do not acquire spoken language spontaneously.

- Ask the child to complete a sentence:
  Jack and Jill went up the? (hill)

- Play the Memory Game:
  'I went to the supermarket and I bought … , … '
  'Tom had a birthday and he got a computer, felt tips, … , … '.
  These games help to develop auditory sequential memory.

- Play 'Simple Simon Says . . . take two steps forward, then sit down' This helps with direction and orientation.

- Do the 'Hokey-Cokey'. ('Put your right arm out and shake it all about.')

- Play 'Old Macdonald had a farm'. This helps with the awareness of sound ('On his farm he had some ducks, with a quack quack here and a quack quack there.')

- Play 'Silly Sentences'. The child has to repeat the sentence, then say what is wrong and give a suitable word in its place:
The shop sailed out to sea.
I like baked beams.
The telephone is singing.

- Cut out a picture and ask the child to tell you about it. Help him to tell you what happened before and after the picture was taken or drawn.

- Give the child three or four words and ask him to make a sentence about them:
witch – cat – broomstick
haunted – ghost – fright
accident – bicycle – traffic

  This also makes the child aware that a sentence must make complete sense and that it must have a subject and a verb.

- Work on categories and classification:
labradors – corgies – terrier
tulips – daffodils – roses

  Ask the child to give the names of four different drinks, sports or vegetables.

Instructions

Teach the child to give instructions. Choose a favourite possession, for example the video recorder, and ask, 'How do you use it?' (It often helps if you tell the child to pretend the questioner is an alien, someone who has just arrived from Mars and has never seen a television or a video recorder before.)
Bike – 'How do you mend a puncture?'
Favourite food – 'How do you make scrambled egg or beans on toast?'

Descriptions

Role play scenarios and drama provide good opportunities to help people overcome speech and language difficulties. To unlock the tongue of the shy or withdrawn child, suggest to him that he is a reporter for BBC Six O'clock News:
This is ... reporting from the scene of the aeroplane crash/ burglary/ fire.

Teach him how to describe an object. Here are a few key questions that can be asked to help describe a chair, a sock, a bicycle:

'What is it made from?', 'What shape is it?', 'What size is it?', 'What weight is it?', 'What is its main purpose?'

Teach him to describe a person. Pretend he has to make a 'Photofit' picture of a bank robber because he was a witness at the scene of a crime. Here are a few useful words to describe a person: figure, face/head, nose/forehead, hair, eyes, skin, mouth/lips/teeth, character, clothes, habits, mannerisms, voice, age.

It is useful to put these words on a card index. Then the parent/teacher and the pupil can provide the appropriate answer. Later, ask the pupil to describe someone to you – almost charades. It can be great fun, guessing the identity of a favourite sportsman, pop star, television personality, politician.

Figures of speech

It is often the figures of speech (idioms, proverbs, similes, antonyms) that cause most problems for dyslexic children. They are often literal thinkers and interpret words verbatim.

Idioms

It is useful to treat these in categories and build them up in a systematic way on a card index so that the parent and teacher can review them frequently. The child can illustrate the meaning with drawings.

- Food
  'A finger in every pie'
  'In a real stew'
  'Salt of the earth'
- Animals
  'Dark horse'
  'Pig-headed'
  'Fish out of water'
- Body
  'Level-headed'
  'Pick your brain'
  'Lost my head'
- Colours
  'Red tape'
  'Green with envy'
- General
  'Chip off the old block'

'The grass is always greener on the other side of the fence'
'Burn the midnight oil'

Proverbs

Will sociologists tell us that with the decline of the nuclear family
went children's knowledge of proverbs? This great store of
knowledge that has enriched our language does not now appear to
be in such common use. Linguistic interaction is an important part
of childhood development which is developed by play. Changing
social habits mean that many of the traditional games which were
part of our heritage have been lost, as a result of which many
children do not know the meaning of:
'Don't count your chickens before they are hatched'
'Too many cooks spoil the broth'
'People who live in glass houses shouldn't throw stones'

Similes

Similes have to be taught:
'As poor as a church mouse' (why was he poor?)
'As blind as a bat'
'As old as Methuselah' (who was he?)

Antonyms

Antonyms help to enrich the expressive language skills. Play 'Snap'
by putting on cards words:
'last', 'first'
'easy', 'hard'
'arrive', 'depart'

Riddles

Riddles make children aware of the hidden meaning in words and
help with comprehension skills:
'I have numbers on my face, I have two hands, I sometimes chime.
What am I?' (a clock)
'I am hot, I sometimes spray or give off steam, I move over clothes.
What am I?' (an iron)

Poetry

Poetry is helpful for some children. Some dyslexics enjoy it and love
to make up their own poems. Others find it very difficult. Some
children can be totally flummoxed by the meaning of the words
which the poet may have used.

Summary and conclusions

1   It is now well established that many dyslexics have difficulties or delays in acquiring spoken language, but not all do. For those who do the earlier the problem is identified the better the prognosis. The prevailing view of the researchers suggests that 'a deficit in phonological coding is at the core of dyslexia' (Pennington, 1990). Pre-school language impairment or the late acquisition of speech are useful early indicators of dyslexia.

2   The speech therapist has an important role to play in the diagnosis and remediation of dyslexia. If a child can communicate easily and effectively, then his cognitive growth, personal development and academic achievement will benefit.

3   Reading and spelling are dependent 'on proficiencies already available in the primary (spoken) language system' (Sawyer and Butler, 1991).

4   Some dyslexic people are articulate and good communicators – others are not.

5   Most children acquire language skills osmotically, the dyslexic often needs formal instruction to reach the same level of competence.

6   Language deficiencies can be remedied and can be developed. A solid foundation of oral skills on which to build the higher language skills of reading and spelling and writing is necessary for all learners. It is essential to develop a bedrock of spoken language skills. This can be done at home and in school with the help of games, drama and imaginative play.

7   The National Curriculum (1995) has focused attention on the importance of teaching spoken as well as written language.

Chapter 4

Reading

- tests and assessment by teachers and SENCOs
- the multi-sensory teaching of reading
- how to overcome the dyslexic reader's problems

Introduction

Literacy is necessary for survival in daily life – whether it is to read road signs, to shop in a supermarket, to know how to work the video or to read directions on the medicine bottle. In all advanced cultures the ability to read, write and spell is vital for communication and employment. Proficient reading is an essential tool for learning a large part of the subject matter taught at school.

Over the past decades there has been widespread concern over reading standards. Some university tutors are so concerned at the standard of literacy of some of their students that they have instigated remedial reading classes. Employers have been aware for some time that there is a reading problem amongst the workforce. In 1993 a report in *The Independent* said that 'one in four recruits are functionally illiterate and unable to read and interpret basic instructions'. This widespread concern about standards of literacy has fuelled much debate over how reading is taught.

The key issues in the debate can be found in the 'polarized and controversial positions of the advocates of the "real book" versus those favouring the use of phonics and graded series' (Pumfrey and Reason, 1991). 'Real books' may generate enthusiasm but those who work with dyslexic children know to their cost the futility of putting a book in the hands of a child who simply cannot decipher most of the words on the page. The National Curriculum (1995) now encourages teachers to use a variety of methods within 'a balanced and coherent programme' to ensure children gain 'phonic knowledge'.

This chapter outlines various methods used to teach reading and then goes on to outline specific methods used to help people with dyslexia.

Teaching methods

There are four main methods that may be used to teach reading. The proficient and successful teacher will be familiar with all these methods and will incorporate elements of each in her teaching. Teaching reading successfully demands a mixture of strategies.

Each of the methods used to teach reading has a role to play in the teaching of the dyslexic pupil. The vast majority of pupils learn to read whatever the method used but about 20 per cent of pupils fail to learn effective reading. It is difficult to be age specific because dyslexic pupils' reading abilities differ widely. Whatever the chronological age of the pupil the same basic teaching methods apply, although there may be differences in the chosen reading books because of the differences in the individual interests and maturity. The nature of the dyslexic pupil's strengths or weaknesses, and whether they are auditory or visual, should be taken into account when a teaching programme is devised for him.

The 'Whole Word' or 'Look and Say' method

This involves the pupil being taught by being shown whole words or even whole phrases. The idea is that repeated visual inspection helps the child to memorize and read the word.

In the past the pupil was shown whole words, or even whole phrases, on flashcards. Pictures giving contextual cues accompanied the flashcards. The emphasis was on continuous exposure to words that were usually meaningful, to help build a sight vocabulary. The pupil learned over a period of time to recognize the word without the help of the pictures.

The Look and Say method encourages the pupil to recognize words immediately as visual units. It does work very effectively for many pupils but for some it is disastrous. The method ignores the fact that different individuals can learn to read in different ways and it assumes that a pupil can recognize words for automatic recall.

Hinshelwood sowed the seeds of a century of debate concerning the most effective methods to use for teaching failing readers when he said that many pupils could not be taught to read using the Look and Say method. He preferred to diagnose the reading difficulties of his patients then prescribe very exact methods to teach them to read dependent upon the results. 'I advised that the boy should be taught to read on the old method, beginning with the letters of the alphabet ... then he should be taught to spell, and then to read the simple words in a child's first primer, spelling them out letter by letter' (Hinshelwood,

1912). The 'old method' is what is now called the phonic method and involves the pupil learning letter names and sounds.

Rutter, Tizard and Whitmore (1970), in a survey of the Isle of Wight school population, found that for '20 per cent of the population, the Look and Say method is futile'. Hickey (1977) described it as the 'Look and Guess' method. She said that the dyslexic looks at a word but cannot say it until he knows the meaning (the pictures are useful here). He cannot progress to recognizing the word without the picture cue.

'It is commonly proposed that in the very earliest stages of reading development, written words are identified purely on their visual appearance' (Ellis, 1993), hence words with distinct features are often more easily recognized – television, McDonalds. But for many dyslexics the printed word makes no impression on their visual perceptual system, therefore they do not remember the word when it is seen in isolation or out of context. Nor is English a language made up of pictograms, it consists of letters with names and sounds. Sheffield (1991) observed: 'when taught by whole words, natural readers abstract rules and categories. Our [dyslexic] children learn hopelessness, passiveness and avoidance'. Thomson and Watkins (1990) reinforced this when they claimed that an 'approach such as look-say, does not work with the dyslexic because it calls for areas of skill in which the dyslexic is essentially deficient'.

The 'Phonic' method

With this method the pupil is taught the relationship between the letter names and the sounds of the letters. The pupil learns to sound out each letter in the word. This is useful for deciphering unfamiliar words.

This method is successful when the pupil uses his knowledge of the individual letter sounds to help sound out a word. The US Department of Education's researchers (Anderson et al, 1985) found that 'an explicit phonic approach [produced] larger than average gains on first and second grade reading tests'. According to Ellis (1993), 'a child possessed of some phonic reading skill is a much more independent reader'.

Muter's (1994) research showed that 'a possible reason for the failure of the letter-name training programs to improve reading acquisition is that a minimal level of phonological awareness [of the sounds] must be achieved by children before they can derive much benefit from knowledge of letter names'. Smith (1973) argued that phonics teaching can lead to too deliberate decoding and as a result the meaning of the text will be lost. Some pupils find it difficult to blend and synthesize sounds, that is, they find it hard to run together the sounds to make a word. Some may be able to say /m/ /a/ /t/ but then be unable to say 'mat'. They may read 'blot' for 'bot'. How do they deal with words such as 'cough' and 'eight'? Pupils with severe phonological difficulties often find this method hard.

The 'Whole Sentence' method or the 'Language Experience' model

With this method the pupil learns to read sentences and it is the content of what is read that is of primary importance. He is encouraged to use the meaning of the sentence to help him to make sense of (or guess) the individual words. An extension of this method is the *Cloze procedure* which involves using a text where letters, words or phrases are omitted and a gap is left. The pupil has to read the text and insert a suitable word so that the sentence makes sense. The pupil is given a multiple choice. For example:

The boys run/jump/hop over the hurdles.

The disadvantage of this method is that when a pupil meets an unfamiliar word, he is stumped.

The 'Alphabetic Multi-sensory' method

This method teaches the pupil to 'see, hear and feel' letters and sounds simultaneously. The pupil, and especially the dyslexic pupil, is better able to make the arbitrary connection between the sound and its symbol which is the crux of learning to read.

What is reading?

Reading is the decoding of symbols on the page. What we read should make sense. Letters have names, sounds, shapes and a feel (written representation). Most people do not remember how they learned to read. Many people look at a word, they recognize it and they can identify it the next time they see it. The dyslexic pupil does not and this explains why some dyslexic people were called 'word-blind'. They did not recognize a word however many times they saw it.

The three phases in early literacy development

Influential researchers such as Frith (1985) break down early literacy development into three distinct phases: the logographic, the alphabetic and the orthographic. It is important that those who teach reading are aware of these progressions as the pupil learns to read.

The logographic phase

The pupil recognizes written words that he has encountered in spoken language, he makes use of visual recognition of overall word patterns, just as he recognizes words with significance for him, such as Toys 'R' Us. This explains why sometimes a child will be able to read very long words, such as 'television', while still stumbling over easy words, such as 'was'. 'Dyslexics do not possess any skills with which to decipher unfamiliar words.' (Snowling, 1987) The pupil will be building a sight vocabulary during the logographic phase.

The alphabetic phase

The pupil begins to recognize letter–name–sound correspondence. He begins to understand the relationship between the sound of words and the letters used to represent those sounds. Phonic knowledge becomes important.

The orthographic phase

This stage is reached when the pupil automatically recognizes the word and he uses cues and context to help him.

Assessment of reading difficulties

For children with reading difficulties it is important to assess whether the reading problem is specific or related to poor general intellectual abilities.

According to Thomson (1990), 'the appropriate assessment of intelligence is one of the most crucial factors in the diagnosis of dyslexia'. 'Intelligence is a very significant influence on reading because it can contribute a great deal to a child being able to read better than most others of his age, as well as having the opposite effect' (Doyle, 1996). It is therefore essential to know something of the child's cognitive skills and underlying ability. However, Chasty (1981) said 'be careful about making assumptions or predictions on the basis of IQ scores. They may vary over a period of time in response to changes in the child's background, schooling, emotional adjustment or learning difficulty'.

IQ tests

Intelligence and intelligence testing is a thorny issue and has been the subject of much discussion and argument. Is intelligence heritable? Are some races more intelligent than others? Can it be influenced by nurture?

Much of our knowledge about intelligence comes from the work of psychologists. Some of the earliest work in the development of intelligence tests was conducted by Alfred Binet and his co-workers in the early 1900s. They devised methods for the identification of 'slow learning' children through the comparison of mental age with chronological age. Based on Binet's work, Lewis Terman produced the Stanford–Binet test in which the intelligence quotient (IQ) – mental age divided by chronological age times 100 – was first used.

$$\frac{\text{Mental Age (MA)}}{\text{Chronological Age (CA)}} \times 100 = \text{Intelligence Quotient (IQ)}$$

Educationalists frequently refer to mental age rather than IQ. This is based on the assumption that if a child is of average intelligence he will have a mental age (MA) equivalent to his chronological age (CA).

In 1949 Dr David Wechsler produced the tests bearing his name which are now used worldwide to test people's IQs. These tests measure the many subsidiary skills that go to make up the amalgamation of abilities that psychologists regard as the components of intelligence.

The most popular tests are the following:

- The Wechsler Pre-school and Primary Scale of Intelligence (WPPSI–R). For children aged between three and seven.
- The Wechsler Intelligence Scale for Children (WISC–R). For children aged between seven and sixteen.
- The Wechsler Adult Intelligence Scale (WAIS–R). For adults between the ages of seventeen and seventy.

These tests are used internationally and predict educational attainment. They may only be administered by suitably qualified psychologists.

The value of IQ tests for the dyslexic pupil

The educational world is increasingly aware of the value of knowing something about a pupil's intelligence. Many schools use verbal reasoning (VR) tests, such as the NFER's Nelson Verbal Reasoning Test Series (1996). These are very useful but verbal reasoning tests may not provide an accurate reflection of the overall intellectual abilities of a child with dyslexia. The WISC–R, which provides a much wider and more comprehensive measurement of ability, is likely to provide a better reflection of the child's intellectual ability. Thomson (1990) cautioned, 'I have sometimes found a discrepancy between my assessment of the child's IQ [on the WISC–R] and the school assessment' and 'it emerged that the intelligence test used in the school was one which required the child to read the questions and write the answers'. These are precisely the skills that the dyslexic child is weak at; consequently the results obtained on such tests can be misleading and unreliable for the pupil with a learning difficulty. The VR tests have a huge verbal/language basis. Stanovich (1991) pointed out that 'an extremely large body of research has demonstrated that reading skill is linked to an incredibly wide range of verbal abilities ... Verbally loaded measures are allegedly unfair to dyslexic children'. Parents and teachers must have a clear understanding of what tests are being used and what they are measuring so that confusions and misunderstandings do not arise.

The WISC–R

The WISC–R measures oral abilities (Verbal Scale) and practical abilities (Performance Scale).

- The Verbal Scale consists of the following sub-tests:

  Information

  Similarities

  Arithmetic

  Vocabulary

  Comprehension

  Digit span

  The results obtained from these tests give the Verbal IQ score. The verbal IQ is regarded as one of the best measures of academic potential because much in education relies on good verbal skills.

- The Performance Scale consists of the following sub-tests:

  Picture completion

  Picture arrangement

  Block design

  Object assembly

  Coding

  The results obtained from these tests give a Performance IQ score.

- The results of both tests are used to work out a Full Scale IQ.

The table below shows the classification of the Full Scale IQ scores that are obtained from the WISC–R.

Full Scale IQ score	% of population in category	Description
130 and above	2.2	very superior
120–129	6.7	superior
110–119	16.1	high average
90–109	50	average
80–89	16.1	low average
70–79	6.7	borderline
69–below	2.2	mentally retarded

For most people there is little variation in the score across sub-tests with perhaps a small difference between the Verbal and the Performance IQ scores. A wide scatter of sub-test scores or a significant discrepancy between the Verbal and Performance Scale scores often indicates an underlying learning difficulty, which may then need further investigation to determine what that difficulty is.

The pendulum has now swung against blind faith in the result of IQ tests. Singleton (1995) warned 'it is a mistake to imagine that conventional IQ measures are necessarily reliable indicators of the intellectual potential of dyslexics' because 'dyslexic people typically have a very uneven intellectual profile'.

Other intelligence tests

Many psychologists now use WISC–III[UK] (Wechsler, 1992) which was validated for the UK population in 1992 to give information about a pupil's intelligence. It also includes the Weschler Objective Reading Dimension (WORD) reading tests which can show how a child's reading compares with others of similar age or ability. Others prefer to use the British Ability Scales (BAS II) (Elliot, 1996) which has an age range of 2 years 6 months to 17 years 11 months.

IQ tests which SENCOs and teachers may use

Teachers and SENCOs may use *Raven's Progressive Matrices and Vocabulary Scales* (Raven, 1988). Thomson (1990) regarded them as 'particularly useful as they provide a measure of non-verbal intelligence and are not loaded against children who have language difficulties.' They are suitable for individual and group administration, and the results may be used in the Individual Education Plan (IEP).

Standardized reading tests

Standardized reading tests can help to identify the problems that a pupil with reading difficulties is having. They can also be used to monitor progress, report on attainment and establish his reading ability compared with others of a similar age. For these reasons it is important that standardized tests, rather than informal tests, are used. A standardized test is one that has been tested on a large sample of pupils and therefore a scale of averages can be worked out. For example it might show that the average eight-year-old pupil can read 40 words on the test. A pupil's reading age should correspond to his mental age level, though in practice it is usually regarded as acceptable if it matches the pupil's chronological age, either because the mental age is not known or because it is LEA policy to use the chronological age as a benchmark. The base age of many reading tests is five years because it is assumed that it is at the age of five (when the pupil begins school) that a pupil starts to learn to read. The results of the tests may show that the pupil has a reading problem. Reading tests alone are not enough to identify dyslexia in a pupil (see Chapter 2). They may alert the teacher to a problem but to make an accurate diagnosis of a pupil's reading problems it is essential also to analyse the errors a pupil has made while reading.

There are many different standardized reading tests available. The selection given below is for illustrative purposes.

Four basic tests

If possible, at least four different basic tests should be used, to provide information about a pupil's word attack skills, his knowledge of phonics, how he has been taught, and what strategies he uses when reading sentences and prose. Kline and Kline (1975) say that 'it is our opinion that no one reading test is sufficient for accurate identification and diagnosis of a reading disability'.

A word recognition test

The pupil is presented with lines consisting of words of increasing difficulty and asked to read them. The test is continued until the pupil is unable to read further words. The test is exacting as it involves reading words which are more demanding in isolation. There are no cues. According to Turner (1993), 'the identification of single words out of context forms a vital stage – perhaps the most vital – in the acquisition of reading'.

Word recognition tests
Graded Word Reading Test. The Macmillan Test Unit (NFER–Nelson, 1985)

Wide Range Achievement Test 3 (WRAT 3) (Wilkinson, 1993)

A reading accuracy test
The pupil reads a story which has a picture beside it to give cues. This test provides information about the pupil's reading strategies. A record of the errors made by the child should be kept for later analysis and to help plan the remedial programme.

Reading accuracy tests
Neale Analysis of Reading Ability. Revised British Edition (Neale, 1988)

New Macmillan Reading Analysis (Vincent and de la Mare, 1990)

A reading comprehension test
This test establishes how much the pupil can remember of what he has just read by asking him questions about the contents of what he has read. It reveals how much the pupil assimilates and how good his retention of information is (particularly important in the classroom).

Reading comprehension tests
Neale Analysis of Reading Ability. Revised British Edition (Neale, 1988)

NFER–Nelson Group Reading Test. The Macmillan Test Unit (NFER–Nelson, 1990)

A sentence completion test
The pupil reads a sentence silently and chooses the correct word from a selection and underlines or circles his choice. These tests can be given to a group of pupils in a classroom, whereas most of the other tests have to be administered individually. They reveal how quickly and well the pupil can cope when reading to himself.

Cloze Reading Tests (Young, 1992) *Suffolk Reading Scale* (Hagley, 1987)

When should a pupil be tested?

If there is a positive response to the following questions it may help in establishing whether there is evidence of a learning difficulty, in which case further tests will be useful. The analysis of errors should take into consideration the pupil's age, ability and reading methods. Many pupils may initially make some of the following errors but the dyslexic continues to do so, sometimes erratically, long after his peers and it is this which is diagnostically significant.

Does the pupil:

- read in a staccato-like way (word for word), with little expression and with little understanding of what he is reading?
- lose his place when reading?
- need to use his finger to keep his place?
- misread the simple, familiar words – 'a' for 'and'?
- omit endings from words – 'play' for 'playing'?
- confuse words of similar appearance – 'house' for 'horse', 'of' for 'off'?
- omit syllables from words – 'rember' for 'remember'?
- truncate the letters in a word – 'dont' for 'downstairs', 'active' for 'attractive'?
- add letters to words – 'breast' for 'beast'?
- tend to look at the initial letters of the word and guess the rest – 'interrupted' for 'intercede'?
- make bizarre guesses at words – 'downest' for 'downstairs'?
- read the word correctly on one line and then misread the same word on the next line?
- reverse whole words – 'on' for 'no', 'was' for 'saw'?
- invert letters – 'pig' for 'dig'?
- reverse letters – 'bud' for 'dub', 'brown' for 'drown'?
- omit letters from words – 'very' for 'every'?

Stanovich (1985) pointed out that 'systematic studies of the distribution of error types across reading ability have indicated that poor readers make more errors of all types, but that their number of reversal errors as a proportion of the total number of errors is no higher than that displayed by good readers'.

What can affect test results?

The individual scores on the test results are good indicators of the pupil's attainments but should not be accepted as infallible. The following factors can affect the test results:

- The personal interaction with tester and pupil – for example the pupil may become anxious in the test situation.
- The pupil may have an uneven pattern of performance – on good days he will do better and on bad days he will make more errors.
- The pupil's state of health – if he is suffering from a bad cold or hay fever, it can affect his performance.
- The pupil's underlying cognitive ability – his level of intelligence.

- Test results can vary if different tests are used or even if different forms of the same test are administered.

- Familiarization with a specific test can negate the object of the test – six-monthly intervals is the usual minimum time that should elapse before a test is repeated. It is better if parallel forms of a test are used, if they exist.

- Emotional difficulties, such as parental problems, poor housing, bereavement, abuse or neglect, may affect the pupil's performance.

- If English is the pupil's second language he may perform less well.

The interpretation of the test results is the chief concern of the diagnostician because this will affect the provisions in the Individual Education Plan (IEP) that will need to be devised for the pupil.

Guidelines and criteria
when choosing reading tests to assess for dyslexia

1 Will it provide the information required about the pupil (for example his strengths and weaknesses, his knowledge of phonics, his word recognition skills or the strategies he uses to read)?

2 Is the age range appropriate?

3 How long does it take to administer?

4 What is the purpose of test – to identify a problem or monitor progress?

5 Is it a group or individual test? SENCOs will need to use individual tests to identify SEN.

6 Are parallel forms available to monitor progress?

7 Are the norms reliable and up to date?

Tests and the Code of Practice

The implementation of the *Code of Practice 1994* has meant that the results of IQ tests and other tests, such as reading age scores, have become even more important for parents and teachers. A Statement of Special Educational Needs (SEN), for the purpose of funding and allocation of resources to schools, is based on the criterion that there has to be a discrepancy between the pupil's reading age and chronological age and not his mental age. In practice this means that a pupil might have to wait until it can be shown that he is two or three years behind his peers before he can receive help. Crombie (1994) asserted that 'a child cannot be discovered to have a reading age which is two years behind his chronological age unless that child is at least seven years of age as reading tests will not score below five years. By the time a child is seven, the child is aware of failure and motivation and self-esteem are probably suffering'.

Often very intelligent yet needy pupils are excluded from the help they need (and should have as a right). The BDA (1996) deplores this and says 'unnecessary underachievement should not be tolerated'.

Are dyslexic readers' problems different from other poor readers?

There is a whole body of poor readers, whom Gough and Tunmer (1986) described as the 'garden variety', whose below average reading is predictable from their general low levels of intelligence, whereas the dyslexic child has an unexpected difficulty because there is a mismatch between his reading skill and general intellectual ability. An additional component in the controversy over dyslexia is whether 'developmental dyslexia is qualitatively different from other forms of reading disability'. According to Aaron, Kuchta and Grapenthin (1988), 'dyslexic and non-dyslexic poor readers may resemble each other symptomatically and in overall reading achievement, but the immediate cause of developmental dyslexia is poor grapheme–phoneme [letter names and sounds] conversion skill (decoding) whereas the primary cause of general reading backwardness is poor comprehension ability'. The longer the child is left struggling to learn, the harder the problem is to overcome. Stanovich (1988) called this the 'Matthew Effect', based on the biblical text from St Matthew's gospel Chapter 25 which says, 'unto him that hath, more shall be given, unto him that hath not, even that which he hath shall be taken away' – that is, good readers get better whilst bad readers get worse. This may explain why some pupils fall more and more behind their peers. They cannot keep pace with the curriculum as they are unable to read the instructions or information for much of their work, so the whole of their education suffers. According to Fielding, Wilson and Anderson (1986), 'the knowledge acquired from today's text enables the comprehension of tomorrow's'. The dyslexic's confidence is sapped and behavioural or emotional problems may arise as a consequence of failure to learn to read.

Practitioners and researchers, particularly in the US and the UK, have produced a cornucopia of clinical and experimental evidence on the most effective way to teach children who are retarded readers. There is no 'best method' of teaching reading. The Bullock Report (1975) stated that 'there is no one method, medium, approach, device or philosophy that holds the key to the process of learning to read'. Some of the most forceful of the personalities who have written programmes for teaching dyslexics have often been gifted teachers themselves and insisted that their methods must be followed infallibly and to the exclusion of other methods. This is in some ways not so surprising because 'it is a human tendency to teach as we ourselves have been taught' (Sheffield, 1991). This applies to teacher trainers and to classroom teachers. It is important to be open to innovation and cross-fertilization of ideas.

Orton–Gillingham method

Anna Gillingham and Bessie Stillman devised the original multi-sensory teaching programme to teach dyslexic pupils based on the pioneering work of the founding father of the dyslexic movement, Samuel Orton. The techniques became known as the Orton–Gillingham method. The method has been gaining popularity. During a debate in the US Senate on the National Literacy Act in 1989, it was suggested that teachers should be trained using multi-sensory methods. 'The issue is no longer as it was several decades ago, whether children should be taught phonics.' (Anderson et al, 1985).

Programmes based on the Orton–Gillingham method
There is a large selection of books and programmes which are based on the philosophy of the Orton–Gillingham method.

In the UK the programmes used most frequently and regarded as suitable for teaching children with specific learning difficulties are as follows:

- *Alpha-to-Omega* (Hornsby and Shear, 1994)
- *The Bangor Dyslexia Teaching System* (Miles, 1993)
- *The Hickey Multi-sensory Language Course* (Augur and Briggs (eds), 1992)
- *Dyslexia: A Teaching Handbook* (Thomson and Watkins, 1990)
- *Units of Sound* (Bramley, 1996)

Teaching reading to dyslexic pupils

Every teacher who has tried to teach reading to a pupil with a learning difficulty has a favourite theory about how to do so. There is an abundance of information and research evidence about reading principles and methodology. But there is no doubt, according to Thomson and Watkins (1990), that 'in reading, the reader simultaneously synthesizes information from a number of sources. Briefly, these will include previous experiences, knowledge of syntax, semantics, orthography, sound-to-symbol mapping and phonetic information'. The reader needs a multiplicity of skills which integrate to help him to read. Reid (1993) concurred with this and said 'both the phonic method and the "whole-language" movement have many commendable aspects – both should be utilized in relation to the needs of the individual reader'.

The underlying principle of teaching dyslexic children, and one of the main differences between it and remedial teaching, is that a multi-sensory method of teaching is used. The justification for this comes as a result of many studies of remedial reading and Pumfrey and Reason (1991) said that 'by the 1970s doubts had been cast on the efficacy of the long-term effects of the short-term remedial teaching of reading'. The traditional methods have been shown not to be successful.

What is multi-sensory learning?

'It is learning by the simultaneous use of the eyes, ears, speech organs, fingers and muscles. The aim is for the learner to learn the names, sounds and shapes of all phonograms so he has permanent and automatic response.' (Augur, 1985)

Multi-sensory learning has been paraphrased in a vivid and lucid form by Sheffield (1991) who described it as 'an aid to a flagging memory for words, the student learns to articulate sounds and words as he writes them. When he is learning a new bit of language, he hears the teacher's voice first saying a sound, a word, a sentence. Then he hears his own voice repeat it. He concentrates on what his mouth is doing. He moves his own hand and then sees what he has written [then he reads it]'.

Hickey (1977) said that 'the value of multi-sensory learning is that it enables the individuals to use their own approach to the tasks through utilizing their strong areas and at the same time, exercising their faulty ones. They use their visual, auditory, tactile, kinaesthetic and oral-kinaesthetic perceptual systems to make learning secure'. In layman's language this means using the eyes, ears, the hands and muscles to write and read and say the word simultaneously. Chasty, cited in Townend (1994), reminded us that 'if they can't learn the way we teach, we must teach the way they learn'. Hornsby (1994) said that we must draw attention to the fact that 'currently teachers who teach "phonics" only teach sounds and no names, which is as much of a disaster for the dyslexic as the whole word method is'.

Evidence suggests that the teacher needs more than a single theory and the techniques derived from it to be able to teach reading. The teacher needs to know, and have at her disposal, all the different methods. 'The manuals are gold mines of materials, concepts and lists of words.' (Sheffield, 1991)

Guidelines

for the multi-sensory teaching of reading

1   The pupil learns the alphabet and simultaneously learns that letters have:

a) names (26)

b) sounds (44)

c) shapes (A a *a*)

d) feel – what the letter looks like when he writes it.

These are put on index cards. The pupil is given a specific word which is depicted on the card to help trigger the letter name and sound. In practice a picture of a bus is drawn and the pupil will be taught, when shown the picture of the bus, to give the letter its name ('b') and to say its sound (/b/). The words used on the cards are known as 'keywords' because they help to 'unlock' the name and sound of the visual representation of the letter. The pupil practises these sounds on a daily basis.

2   The pupil learns the consonants and must know how to make the sounds correctly. Some pupils have difficulty in remembering sounds that are sometimes confused, such as /d/ and /t/ or /m/ and /n/, particularly at the ends of words. Consonants such as these sound the same because 'they are produced by a similar motor touch of the tongue to the gum ridge behind the teeth' (Sheffield, 1991). They can be helped by using the *Edith Norrie Magnetic Letter Case* (1994). Looking in a mirror often helps to heighten awareness and may help to overcome the difficulty. Use workbooks and worksheets to reinforce this such as *Alpha-to-Omega Activity Packs Stages 1, 2 and 3* (Hornsby and Pool, 1990/1991/1992).

- Don't ask a pupil to read books at a level beyond his current skills. Some reading experts, such as Cox, Child and Gillingham, said that the pupil should be given no books until a certain level of proficiency is attained. Then teach him:

    a) the short vowels

    b) consonant digraphs

    c) consonant blends

    d) magic 'e'

    e) the long vowels.

    (See Chapter 6 for further explanations.)

- It is advisable to follow a chosen programme, preferably one that is easy to use or one that has involved training in the specific techniques used. This should be done in a 'structured, sequential, cumulative and thorough' manner (Rawson, 1968). The pupil should use carefully graded reading books which reinforce what he has been taught.

- The pupil is learning to read, write and spell at the same time. Sheffield (1991) affirmed that 'our youngsters often learn to read best by writing first'.

- When the short vowels have been mastered, introduce the concept of syllables. Syllables can be a revelation for the poor reader because, if properly taught, they help to eliminate the fear of long words and can almost overnight increase the reading skills of the pupil. Syllables and syllable division techniques are complicated and need to be taught step-by-step. They can take a long time to teach. The pupil needs to learn the following:

a) what a syllable is

b) counting syllables in words

c) the diacritical marks – these are the code marks used on the vowels. Short vowels are coded with a breve:

For example, hăt, pĕt, rĭg.

Long vowels are coded with a macron:

For example, trāin, wēed.

d) closed syllables

e) open syllables

f) vowel consonant 'e'

g) prefixes and suffixes which the pupil can instantly recognize and use to take the fear out of long words

h) syllable division techniques.

Syllable division techniques are very useful with the adolescent and adult reader and, once mastered, lead to a great improvement in their reading attainments. 'The concept of syllable division is so very important, because it theoretically allows children to attack new and unfamiliar words knowing that they have a fair chance of success' (Thomson and Watkins, 1990). (See Chapter 6.)

• The pupil needs daily reinforcement through reading, spelling and writing to lead to mastery. 'He needs to feel the muscles of his throat and mouth producing a sequence of sounds. He needs to write letters and words as he sounds them. He needs opportunity to overlearn until all three channels fire off simultaneously so that retrieval can become instantaneous' (Sheffield, 1991). He should never move on until the concept has been mastered. He should never be asked to do anything unless he has learned it in the programme he is following. Chall (1987) said that 'syntheses of the research evidence over the past 70 years have concluded that early systematic teaching and learning of word recognition and decoding produces better results than emphasis on meaning at the beginning'.

- Having mastered a particular sound, the pupil is then introduced to reading only words whose sounds and letter names he has learned and can recognize. This ensures that he is building sound–word recognition, using his newly acquired phonic skills and eliminating the need for guesses. He can begin using materials such as *Phonetic Word Cards (Jewel Case)* (Gillingham, 1956) and phonic readers, for example *Let's Read* (Bloomfield, Barnhart and Barnhart, 1964) and *Primary Phonics* (Makar, 1976).

- It is vital that the pupil is also taught a sight vocabulary (using carefully graded books). The pupil needs to learn to recognize at sight an ever-increasing number of words because it is on these that his fluency as a reader depends. Stanovich (1988) confirmed this with his view that 'lack of exposure and practice on the part of the less-skilled reader delays the development of automaticity and speed at word recognition level'.

- There are two pitfalls to beware of:
  a) too much emphasis on building a sight vocabulary may mean that the pupil fails to establish the necessary word recognition techniques
  b) stressing word recognition and neglecting the building of a sight vocabulary encourages the child to become a slow, laborious and over-analytical reader.

Helping the dyslexic pupil to read at home and in school

Daily reading

The pupil must read on a daily basis to a parent, teacher or classroom assistant, but remember that 'reading is a stressful experience for many dyslexics' ... 'and the approach taken to reading with them is very important.' (Thomson and Watkins, 1990) Until the 1960s parents were not encouraged to help their child read in case the child became confused and it interfered with what the teacher was doing. Douglas, Ross and Simpson's (1968) report changed this assumption. Parents now help in many classrooms by listening to pupils read. 'Since 1967 there has been much official endorsement of the parental role in education' (Carless and Hearn, 1990). The movement has gained momentum and the old attitude that 'teachers teach and parents rear' has finally been laid to rest. The *Code of Practice 1994* puts parental involvement in their children's education centre stage. LEAs, parents and school must now work more closely together.

Parental help

Hewison and Tizard (1980) showed that seven year olds whose parents regularly listened to them read at home were 'definitely better at reading than children who did not have help at home'. The Haringey Project (Tizard et al, 1982), conducted in a deprived, London inner city area, confirmed that listening to children reading improved their reading skills and furthermore 'outstripped the effects of extra help in school'.

Paired reading

Paired reading has been introduced in many schools. Teacher, parent (or classroom assistant) and pupil sit side by side and read aloud together. Morgan (1983) described its special features:

a) there is emphasis on the fact that the pupil chooses the book he wants to read, not what the parent feels he should be reading

b) the value of time spent with the adult's full attention

c) there is praise and feedback

d) the child decides what and when he reads

e) the book should be well below the pupil's reading age.

Source: Morgan R. (1986) *Helping Children Read. The Paired Reading Handbook.* Methuen Children's Books, London.

This is also known as the Pause, Prompt and Praise method.

Reading should be fun – if the pupil has to labour over every word, he will forget the meaning of what he is reading. 'It does not matter how interesting or exciting the book is if the child cannot read it' (Thomson and Watkins, 1990). We read for meaning and understanding, so that the pupil must not get bogged down in the mechanics of reading, and texts used should be within the pupil's capabilities.

There are a large number of texts on the market suitable for use in paired reading, for example the Ladybird Series of Puddle Lane readers by Sheila McCullagh.

Physical appearance of the book

A number of factors can contribute to making a book more easily readable: it should have large print, good line spacing and a suitable typeface (for example, Times Roman). According to Pumfrey and Reason (1991) 'it follows that considerable care is needed in the selection of books in relation to their typefaces and other presentational attributes'. Research evidence of Simpson, Lorsback and Whitehouse (1983) showed that 'poor readers were affected more by degradation [difficult-to-read texts] than good readers'.

Interest level

The pupil should be interested in the subject of the book. It is a joy to see children romping through a book because it is related to their hobby. Children have become keen and enthusiastic readers when allowed to read comics or magazines connected to a special interest, for example the pupil who brought in *Nature Times* each week learned all sorts of interesting things at the same time as developing a sight vocabulary.

- The synopsis of the story, if read to the pupil before he starts to read it, will help to whet his appetite. He will also know what to expect.
- He should also read the chapter headings.
- If the pupil is finding a particular book difficult or his interest is waning it often helps to read alternate pages to sustain his interest and the story content – in other words do paired reading.

Carefully controlled vocabulary

To begin with, the books should have a carefully controlled vocabulary. Finding these is one of the greatest challenges in teaching people with reading difficulties. According to Cooke (1993a) 'if sentences are long and complex and vocabulary difficult, the immediate task of reading the words requires a disproportionate amount of concentration'. The long term damage caused by attempting to read books that are too difficult haunts many people.

The more the merrier

Pupils should aim to read one book per week. The evidence of the researchers underline the fact that the more the reader reads the better he becomes. Janet and Allan Ahlberg, Enid Blyton and Roald Dahl are all popular. Anecdotal evidence suggests that poor readers begin many books and rarely finish any of them. 'I have a book case of books at home, but I never read any of them' is a common remark. According to Cooke (1993a), 'getting right to the end of a book can set a momentum of reading, with the child feeling he wants to start another one [book]'. The pupil should be encouraged to finish one book before beginning another. He should avoid getting into the habit of not finishing a book.

Graded texts

All books should be carefully graded according to reading ages. Beware of the reading ages that publishers give, many are inaccurate and unreliable. The National Association for Special Educational Needs (NASEN) publishes a useful guide *The NASEN A–Z Graded List of Reading Books* (Hinson and Gains, 1993) which gives the reading ages of various reading series. Peer (1996) described the Fogg Index which can be used to calculate the level of reading materials:

Step 1   Take a sample piece of writing of approximately 150 words.

Step 2   Calculate the average number of words per sentence.

Step 3   Count the number of words that contain three syllables or more. Express them as a percentage of the total number of words.

Step 4   Add the two figures together and divide by 2.5.

i.e. Average number of words per sentence: 12

Percentage of words with 3 syllables: 18

Fogg Index would be:

$(12+18) \div 2.5 = 12$

Research shows that:

50% of readers will get lost if a sentence exceeds 14 words

80% of readers get lost if it exceeds 20 words. A Fogg Index of over 12 is too high for most reading/writing passages.

Source: Peer L. (1996) 'Reading difficulty' (Fogg Index). *The Bulletin, BDA Newsletter*, May.

Pupils should also read from a phonic reader to help them develop word recognition skills and to make them into accurate readers. Misreading a word can have dire consequences – especially in the examination room if 'do' is read for 'don't'.

A combination of reading methods

Richardson (1990) confirmed that 'probably the most successful approaches, to beginning reading as well as in remediation, have been in the combination approaches'. Using the approaches outlined in this chapter the pupil is learning to read: by simultaneous learning and reading books that help build a sight vocabulary (Look and Say methods); by using a phonic reader

(Phonic method) and by library books (Whole Word or Sentence method to build on the other skills). His reading skills should be reinforced simultaneously by his multi-sensory training when he writes spellings or sentences of dictation from whichever programme his teacher is following to teach him.

Variety of authors

Pupils should read the work of different authors. Some schools ban certain books such as the horror literature found in the *Goosebumps* series because they disapprove of the contents and the style of writing. Many 'favourite' authors, such as Roald Dahl, include nastiness and the macabre.

Reading aloud

The pupil should read aloud until fluent to a teacher or parent otherwise he can skip and misread the words and then he won't improve. Greenwood (1983) urged that we 'keep required silent reading to a minimum. Only the visual channel is stimulated'.

Difficult words

The pupil should be told difficult words if he does not know them. Carless and Hearn (1990) make an important comment: 'unless there is frequent praise, emphasis may be given to the child's errors and it can become a negative activity'.

Punctuation

Teach the pupil to use and recognize punctuation. A useful way to increase awareness of this is for the teacher to read a paragraph using no punctuation or inflection. Then read the passage again correctly to illustrate the point.

Suggestions on how to overcome specific difficulties with reading

Earlier writers believed that faulty eye movements caused reading disability. They are, however, only symptoms of a reading disability, not causes. Stanovich (1985) said that 'general plausibility and a few case reports are not enough' and 'the idea that deficient eye movements cause reading problems has continually reappeared in the literature, but the data put forth in support of the hypothesis has either not proved adequate or has not been replicable' (see Chapter 14).

Difficulty keeping place on the page

- Use a finger as a guide across the page.
- Use a book mark two lines under the line being read.

- The older reader can feel less embarrassed if he uses a ruler to help him keep his place.

These are crutches. Try to wean the pupil off these because he can develop the habit of using his finger and thus reading word for word with little comprehension.

Expert opinion is divided on the efficacy of using **tracking** to improve the ability to scan, to help orientation skills to develop and to improve letter recognition. Tracking, which is following lines of print in a left-to-right direction, can involve matching and following the lower case letters of the alphabet which are embedded in perhaps ten lines of print. There are many commercially produced variations of tracking exercises available in varying print sizes and with different objectives, for example tracking 'high frequency words'.

Rapid word recognition

Some pupils find it difficult rapidly to recognize known words that are already in their sight vocabulary. Games and exercises can be used to overcome this.

- The pupil is asked to look at a line of words. Then he is asked to 'see how fast you can draw a line around the things that can run'. Words might include, for example:
  horse, house, girl, pig.

- The pupil is given a selection of known words on index cards that can be sorted into categories, for example clothes, animals, trees, food. The person who completes the set fastest is the winner.

- Ask the pupil to read a short paragraph where he has to say the missing word, for example:
  Billy caught the ball, then he th... to his dad. Dad ca... the ball.

  This also helps to develop the guessing strategies that are vital tactics for the dyslexic reader.

- Riddles encourage the pupil to guess and reinforce the idea that what we read should make sense, for example:
  I am strong, I wear a helmet, I have a hose pipe. What am I?
  (fireman)

  Researchers such as Pring and Snowling (1986) have shown that 'unskilled readers in particular, make use of context to compensate for their decoding difficulty'.

Difficulties with word endings or similar sounding words

Some pupils may have difficulty reading the first, middle or final letters in a word. Many tend to look at the initial letters of the word and guess the rest.

- Use multi-sensory exercises in workbooks, for example:
Ask pupils to fill in 'f', 'v', 'th' in the words 'an', 'in', 'un'. Have a picture of the correct word beside the unfinished word.

  Sheffield (1991) sounded a word of caution about workbooks. 'They [the teachers] give youngsters workbooks and expect the workbooks to teach. Sometimes even the teaching of phonics is left to workbooks. A student is expected to pull from a picture a sound he does not hear.' Ensure that the pupil rehearses the sound orally before he begins to write or read the word. Dyslexic children learn little from filling in worksheets if only their visual channels are being used to learn the sound or the name of the letter or word.

- Multiple-choice exercises are useful for increasing awareness of, for example:

Initial errors
The man put on his ...

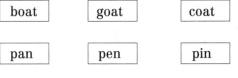

| boat | goat | coat |

Medial errors
The pig was in the ...

| pan | pen | pin |

Final errors
What rhymes with 'call'? The boy was playing with the ...

| band | back | ball |

To increase reading speed

There are a variety of ways in which the very slow reader can be helped to increase his speed:

- Use a tape recorder. The pupil can read a short passage on to the tape. Then he can replay the tape, listen carefully to his own voice and follow what he has read with a pencil. If he makes an error, he underlines the word. Then he repeats the process. He keeps a record of how long each reading has taken and tries to beat his own record.

- Cooke (1993a) suggested that the very slow reader, who has a tendency to read 'one-for-one', can be asked 'Tell me the words you have just read.' If the child responds in a normal speaking voice, he should then be told, 'It can be read that way too.'

- Hickey's suggestion to help improve reading the small words accurately is to make two columns, one for the pupil 'P' and one for the teacher 'T'. Give a point to the pupil for each line read correctly. Every time the pupil makes a mistake, the teacher gets a point.

- The Pause, Prompt and Praise method described by Glynn and McNaughton (1985) is based on the work of Clay. It encourages the child to develop independent strategies for reading unknown words. This method is described by some as paired reading and has become enormously popular in schools in the 1990s as more and more parents are being actively encouraged to help their child read either in the home or school setting. The idea is that when the pupil hesitates or stops, the parent allows him five seconds for self-correction. If the pupil still cannot read the word the parent gives one of three different prompts:

a)   semantic – meaning – related to the story

b)   visual – the way the words look – look at the first two letters again – chip/ship

c)   context – ask the pupil to finish the sentence – then guess the missing word.

This method also advocates that praise is given at all times, not only for correct responses but also for good guesses that may not be quite right. The pupil is encouraged to choose his own reading material and the adult gives the pupil as much help as he needs to read the book of his choice. The parent can read some of the text to the pupil. This helps with understanding and gives the pupil examples of how to pronounce difficult words.

• The Cloze procedure (see page 53) is also most useful to help the pupil use contextual cues to make sense of what he reads.

Suggestions

for choosing suitable books for children

Appearance

The book must look attractive. It is not only young children who like good illustrations. Initially it may be the cover of the book which attracts the child. The modern child expects well-illustrated books, with good, clear, colour pictures. A well-bound book with print that is large enough to read is a more inviting proposition.

Selection

Allow the child to help select the book, remember the child's personality and preference (whet his appetite by reading the synopsis on the cover). The parent should choose a selection of books that the child will be able to read, but the child should make the final decision. Do not be tempted to choose the books you have always wanted to read during your childhood and never did. Remember that parent and child may have different tastes. Try to guide the child to different authors. Some children get 'hooked' on a particular author or series, so try to vary the diet. Some dyslexic children enjoy the modern 'Choose Your Own' adventure/mystery type of books. Others find them disconcerting and are unable to remember the sequence of events because of the different options they are given. Some schools ban pupils from reading these. Allow the dyslexic child to read whatever he shows an interest in.

Length

Younger children have shorter spans of concentration. Some of them like to read the story all at once. Beware of reading a story with a very complicated plot or many different characters. If it is going to take too long to read the story, both parent and child may lose interest and forget the plot by the end of the week.

Contents

This is a very personal decision. The parent has the great advantage of knowing exactly what the child's special interests are. They should be guided by these. Some children love poetry, others adore science fiction and some like non-fiction. The gateway to personal reading for many reluctant readers has been opened by a parent reading an article to the child from his favourite hobbies magazine. The very bright child may enjoy the mental stimulation of an author who uses a broad vocabulary (but remember that some dyslexics are literal thinkers). The language in the unabridged versions of the classics may be totally confusing to some children. Books with colloquial speech or dialect, such as *The Secret Garden*, can also be a source of confusion.

Summary and conclusions

1   There has been increasing concern about literacy standards in recent years.

2   Many dyslexic pupils learn to read successfully but some, even as adults, 'remain inherently slow readers, taking longer to learn and comprehend a passage than their non-dyslexic peers' (Thomson and Watkins, 1990).

3   There have been many different theories about the causes of reading failure and methods used to teach people who have reading difficulties have varied widely. Stanovich (1985) pointed out that 'researchers should be concerned with communicating not only the latest facts about reading disabilities, but with providing critical information about the process'.

4   Failure to learn to read can cause social, emotional and financial problems. There is a known connection between problems with basic literacy and some delinquent behaviour.

5   There are many tests available to help the diagnostician identify the reading problem. The test results should not be taken at face value. It is important to record and analyse the reading errors and then to compare these with other test measures. Stanovich (1991) pointed out that 'the diagnosis of reading disability should be multi-dimensional'.

6   IQ tests are helpful in establishing the child's potential. A measure of the child's intelligence is crucial when establishing his level of retardation in reading. In the ideal world all children should have their IQ established by psychometric testing. This is not always possible because of the national shortage of chartered psychologists as well as the financial consideration. Teachers can assess and identify pupils who have special educational needs, including dyslexia, if they are trained to do so. More and more will need to because of the requirements of the *Code of Practice 1994*.

7   There are many different programmes available to help the dyslexic pupil to learn and there is no 'best method' of teaching reading.

8   The teacher needs to have a theoretical knowledge of all the main reading methods. Ideally the teacher should use a combination of all the methods simultaneously. An inquiry by school inspectors in 26 LEA schools concluded that reading 'problems are likely to arise when teachers rely on one technique alone'. The teacher must take account of the different learning styles of individual learners.

9   The researchers have shown that multi-sensory teaching methods are the most successful with dyslexic learners.

10 Reading improves with practice. Parents have a significant part to play in helping their child's reading both by reading to the child and by listening to their child read. They can help develop phonological awareness with games which make it easier for the child to learn when he begins to read, despite his core deficits in the relationship of speech sounds to words.

Chapter 5

Handwriting

- why and how to teach cursive handwriting
- practical suggestions to help the dyslexic
- how to manage the specific needs of the left hander

Introduction

Handwriting used to be regarded as a very important skill. It was considered to be a sign of education and culture. In certain societies, it bestowed respectability and status. In the Middle Ages very few lay people could read or write. These skills were nurtured by the Church, and as a result many priests rose to positions of temporal power. The Victorians spent a great deal of time and effort in perfecting a 'good hand' because the expansion and prosperity of the era led to an enormous need for clerks.

The advent of the telephone, typewriters, word processors and fax machines has meant that handwriting as a skill has become less important but it still has its uses. Some employers stipulate that job applications should be handwritten, and, according to Johnson (1984), 'employers reject potential personnel because their job applications are illegible'. Graphologists claim to be able to describe an individual's personality by studying his handwriting. The police occasionally use a handwriting expert to help them find or identify a criminal, for example in cases of forgery, poison pen letters or ransom notes. With the diminishing importance of handwritten correspondence, there has been a coincidental decline in the teaching of handwriting in the classroom. This decline began during the 1960s when some educationalists dismissed the teaching of many traditional skills. The trend was summed up by the headmistress of a leading girls' school (which was always top in league tables). When asked whether she had a policy for teaching handwriting in her school, her response was that she certainly did not. She replied that she did not want 'all her girls to write in a uniform style' and that 'writing should express each child's own individuality and personality'. Others, such as Brown (1992), would argue that 'a well-thought-out and consistently applied policy for handwriting from the start is the sure way to avoid piling up such damaging problems (poor writing) later in a child's school career'.

National Curriculum

The Bullock Report noted that '12 per cent of six year olds and 20 per cent of nine year olds spent no time on handwriting practice *per se*' (Bullock, 1975). Furthermore, it observed that 'if a child is left to develop his handwriting without instruction, he is unlikely to develop a running hand which is simultaneously legible, fast flowing and individual and becomes effortless to produce'. We have now seen a whole generation of pupils, and many of their teachers, who were never formally taught handwriting skills. In 1993 'A' Level examiners complained that the handwriting of the most able eighteen year old pupils had fallen to a new low.

The National Curriculum (1995) is seeking to address this. Key Stage 1 (for five to seven year olds) gives the targets:

> *Pupils should be taught to hold a pencil comfortably, in order to develop a legible style that follows the conventions of written English including:*
>
> • *writing from left to right and from top to bottom of the page*
> • *starting and finishing letters correctly*
> • *regularity of size and slope of letters*
> • *regularity of spacing of letters and words*
>
> *They should build on their knowledge of letter formation to join letters in words.*
>
> Source: The National Curriculum (1995). Department for Education and Employment. HMSO, London.

The National Curriculum has reinstated the teaching of cursive writing (which it calls 'joined up' handwriting) as a core skill but it fails to give specific guidelines on how to teach it. As a result, there is still disagreement among educationalists about what is, and is not, 'joined up' writing.

Different styles of handwriting

There are a number of different styles of handwriting. The lack of formal teaching of handwriting has meant that a number of teachers in schools use 'no specific style' of handwriting and that often individual teachers use different styles within the same school. This can lead to a great deal of confusion for any pupil; for the dyslexic pupil it can be catastrophic.

One of the reasons this happens is that there are many styles of handwriting. Adults can choose and develop their own style but children need guidance and consistency so that the foundation of the techniques of handwriting can be laid.

Cursive

The quick brown fox jumps over the lazy dog.

Example of cursive handwriting style.

The word cursive comes from the Latin '*currere*' meaning 'to run'. A dictionary definition says:

> *... it is writing written with a running hand so that the characters [letters] are rapidly formed without raising the pen, and in consequence have their angles rounded, and separate strokes joined and at length become slanted.*
>
> Source: Murray J. A. H., Bradley H., Craigie W. A. and Onions C. T. (eds) (1970) *The Oxford English Dictionary*. Oxford University Press, Oxford.

Cursive writing was the term traditionally used for what is now known in the vernacular as 'joined up' writing. This expression evolved from the classroom and was used by the teacher to explain to the pupil the process he was using to write. It has entered common parlance and the National Curriculum uses the words '"joined up" writing' consistently.

Italic

The quick brown fox jumps over the lazy dog.

Example of italic handwriting style.

The italic style was devised by Italian printers in the sixteenth century. It is angular and accentuates sharp directional changes and has different line thicknesses. In the early twentieth century

Edward Johnston was responsible for reviving an interest in it and for bringing back the use of the square-cut pen developed by the poet and craftsman of the Arts and Crafts period, William Morris (1834–96). It enjoyed great popularity for some time and is still being taught in schools. Some people feel it should belong to the art of calligraphy rather than be used daily at school.

Stick and ball

The stick and ball style, sometimes referred to as the 'manuscript style', was introduced by Margaret Wise (1924).

The quick brown fox jumps over the lazy dog.

Aa Bb Cc Dd Ee Ff Gg Hh Ii

Jj Kk Ll Mm Nn Oo Pp Qq

Rr Ss Tt Uu Vv Ww Xx Yy Zz

Example of stick and ball handwriting style.

Rosemary Sassoon calls it 'print script'. It is a printed script which consists of straight lines, circles and parts of circles and was favoured by those who said that it equated with the print in books. It is still widely used. Hickey (1977) argued that 'this broken rhythm intensifies the tendency to reverse or confuse letter shapes'. Its main disadvantage is that the child does not learn where or how to join the letters.

Marion Richardson

The quick brown fox jumps over the lazy dog.

Aa Bb Cc Dd Ee Ff Gg Hh Ii

Jj Kk Ll Mm Nn Oo Pp Qq Rr

Ss Tt Uu Vv Ww Xx Yy Zz

Example of Marion Richardson handwriting style.

Marion Richardson (1935), who was aware of the shortcomings of the stick and ball style, published *Writing and Writing Patterns* in which she put forth her ideas and demonstrated a style of writing which was better than the stick and ball but still did not address the problem of where the letter begins or how to join some of the letters when a 'joined up' style is introduced.

Despite the acknowledgement of its underlying faults by its creator, this crossbreed has remained universally popular in many British schools.

Difficulties that may be associated with handwriting

The teaching of handwriting is important for all pupils, for two reasons, but it has even greater significance for the pupil with specific learning difficulties. Firstly, he may have great difficulty learning to write and his work may remain very poor; secondly, cursive handwriting is an integral part of all the well-known and successful multi-sensory teaching programmes devised to help these pupils.

Gross and fine motor co-ordination problems and dyspraxia

'Children with gross and fine motor co-ordination problems are given a variety of labels: for example, they may be referred to as perceptually or minimally handicapped, clumsy, experiencing learning difficulties or dyspraxic.' (Alston and Taylor, 1987) Dyspraxia is a term used to describe a small number of poorly co-ordinated people who have difficulty performing familiar and unfamiliar motor skills. They know how to do something, for example rub their nose, but when *asked* to do it may be unable, and yet a few minutes later may do so spontaneously. It is the ability by which we figure out how to use our hands and body in skilled tasks. There are three stages involved in carrying out an action, for example:
'Take the lid off your lunchbox.'
1) the thinking about and knowing what to do
2) the actual movements or actions that will be needed
3) physically taking the lid off the box.

The child may have difficulty with all of these stages, both in their planning and execution.

Can solving these problems help?

Many of the programmes designed to help these children have been developed from and influenced by the work of Strauss and Lehtinen, as described in *The Psychopathology and Education of the Brain-injured Child* (1947), and of Kephart described in *The Slow Learner in the Classroom* (1960). Many dyslexic pupils, however, are described as of average or above average intelligence.

Dyspraxic pupils display some or all of the following symptoms:

- They are clumsy or accident prone and may fall over or bump into objects.
- Handwriting is poor, slow and illegible.
- They have problems with tracing or copying, particularly diagonal lines.
- Their fine motor skills are poor, for example threading beads, doing up shoe laces.
- Gross motor skills may also be poor, for example hopping, skipping, learning to ride a bike or to play a musical instrument.
- PE and using the apparatus in the gym may cause difficulties and games or sports involving a ball may cause inordinate difficulties.
- Dancing, particularly that which involves sequence and set 'steps' and oral instructions, such as in Scottish country dancing, may cause confusion or difficulties.

Occupational therapy or physiotherapy can help these pupils to acquire and improve these skills, and therefore help with the physical aspects of handwriting, but it will probably not help the dyslexic child to read or spell.

Critchley (1970) said 'personally, I do not think that there exists any close correlation between dyslexia and what paediatricians sometimes call "the clumsy child"'. Many dyslexics are outstanding sportsmen and ball players, others are highly artistic and skilled craftsmen.

Handwriting is an explicit skill

It is important for parents and teachers to be aware that some dyslexic children never succeed in developing a legible hand and that modern technology, for example word processors, may have to come to their aid. Chasty (1995) reminded us that 'dyslexia is a learning difficulty which affects the motor skills necessary to control the pencil in writing'. Some pupils make some improvements to their handwriting as a result of intensive practice and tuition, but when this ends there is a regression because the skill has not become instinctive. This is not usually due to a lack of motivation; often it is due to a neurological dysfunction because the writing never becomes an automatic skill, unlike the majority of motor skills do for most people. Some years ago, Professor Peter Fellgett (1986) wrote a very touching 'open' letter to the BDA in which he chronicled his dyslexic difficulties. He wrote: 'Writing for me has always remained laborious; I simply do not go onto auto-pilot. I believe it is essential that teachers should understand that what is just a reflex to some people is an explicit task for the dyslexic, and requires specific time for its execution.'

The essentials for writing

Handwriting is a physical skill which needs to be taught in a structured way and it has to be practised. The pupil needs to develop hand/eye co-ordination as well as gross and fine motor control. According to Johnson (1976), 'like any acquired motor skill with neurological responses, the more the subject is taught, the better the results'.

Developing motor control

Motor control skills should be developed over a period of time in the pre-school child, using activities such as tracing, colouring, drawing, doing dot-to-dot exercises and copying patterns. According to Beery (1982), 'a child needs the verbal language of the average four year old to learn geometric shapes and he should master drawing horizontal and diagonal lines, circles, squares, triangles, before he is taught to write'. Once these skills have been developed sufficiently, the pupil can begin to learn to write.

Cox (1992) reminded us that it is essential to 'develop the student's motor control by training his large muscles first and then carefully reducing the size of the letters until he can control the finer muscle movements of his lower arm, hand, and fingers'. Her work was developed with children in the paediatric neurology department at the Scottish Rite Hospital in Dallas.

She devised a number of practical ways to develop motor control and motor memory in a pupil with fine or gross motor problems. She advocated the following strategies:

- Learn to write in a large form, for example on newspaper. The financial pages of newspapers carrying Stock Market results are ideal because they provide lines to guide the pupil's hand. The pages can be used horizontally and the spaces provide excellent material on which to practise.

- Work on a blackboard to help develop motor memory.

- Trace over velour paper, a piece of carpet or denim fabric to help the pupil to develop and reinforce an automatic recall of the letter by using tactile methods.

- Use skywriting, which is the tracing of the letters in the air using fingers and arms, to help develop a memory trace for the letter and to help pattern letter shapes. The paediatric neurologist Lucius Waites (1982) of the Scottish Rite Hospital in Dallas said that the best memory traces are in the muscles of the upper arm and furthermore motor memory is one of the strongest senses. The pupil and teacher stand side by side. The teacher simultaneously gives verbal instructions and a demonstration, For example: point the index finger on a level with the waist and 'write' the letter in the air; it should be written two feet high. The pupil then copies the teacher's action. The pupil should then go back to his desk and write the letter on the page (or he may write it on the blackboard).

- The teacher can make models of the letter about three inches high and put these on lined A4 paper which can then be put in a plastic see-through sheet. The pupil can then trace over these on a daily basis using a washable felt pen.

Tools of the trade

The writing tool
The pupil should use a standard shape pencil, about 15 cm long. If it is too short, it will not balance in the hand. Do not give the pupil a thick barrel pencil or a triangular shaped pencil because these do not develop the correct 'feel' of the writing. Cox (1992) said that 'thick pencils should be avoided from the beginning, even for young children [because] thick chunky pens with broad points cannot make accurate letter shapes'. The pencil should have a sharp point so that the writing can easily be seen and so that it moves easily across the page. The pencil should be an 'HB'. An 'H' is too hard and resistant and can produce writing which is too faint.

When all the letters have been taught and mastered, then the pupil can progress to using an ink pen, probably at about the age of seven or eight, and depending on school policy.

Paper
Use lined paper. There is much debate about whether or not lined paper should be used, and if so, when it should be used. The use of lined paper has many advantages, and as many adults do not feel comfortable writing unless using lined paper it seems illogical to insist that a child cannot do so. Lined paper helps the pupil to write

along the line. It also helps to develop an awareness of the size and height of the letters. This is extremely important when teaching particular punctuation skills such as upper case (capital) 'C' or lower case (little) 'c'. Teach the pupil that all lower case letters begin on the line, then he knows where to start each letter. Research has shown that stories written on lined paper were found to be more legible than those written on unlined paper.

Use good quality paper. Don't use coarse or recycled paper. The rough surface on such paper can cause resistance to the pencil and prevent the pencil gliding across the page.

When beginning to learn to write, paper printed with double parallel lines should be used.

Example of parallel lined paper.

Pencil grip

How often does one hear a pupil complain after an examination, 'My hand is tired and my arm aches.' Is it because he is not holding his pen or pencil correctly? The pupil needs to be taught how to hold the pencil properly. Correct pencil hold is a life-long habit. Incorrect pencil hold is very difficult to remedy. Johnson (1976) said that 'by the age of ten pen grip will have been pretty well established'. Teach the right-handed child to hold the pen between the pads of the first finger and thumb and to rest it on the side of the middle finger. The fingers should flex slightly outwards. The side of the hand and the little finger should touch the page and flow across the paper in smooth continuous movements. The end of the pencil should sit on the crook of the hand and should lean slightly backwards towards the body.

The left-handed pupil should hold the pencil a little higher up the barrel so he can see what he is writing.

The pencil, if it is correctly held, should be easily removed from the pupil's fingers by the teacher. If it is held too tightly, the muscles are strained and become tired more easily. If the fingers are white, it shows that the grip is too tense. If the pencil is held too near the point, the pupil cannot see what he is writing; it lessens his control and prevents good letter formation.

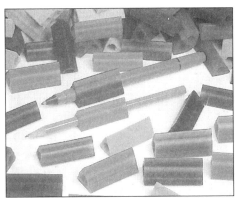

Triangular-shaped pencil grips.

Finger-mould pencil grips.

Pencil grips are devices which are fitted to the barrel of the pencil and which help the pupil to hold his pencil correctly. Some teachers give the pupil a triangular-shaped plastic mould upon which the pupil rests the fingers he is using to hold the pencil. The disadvantage is that the pupil often moves his fingers below the grip, counteracting its purpose. The finger-mould grip (both grips are available from Learning Development Aids) is one of the best on the market. It can be fitted to the end of the pupil's pencil. The pupil's fingers fit into the moulds on the rubber grip which helps to establish a correct pencil hold. It also prevents the pupil from holding the pencil too near to the lead. The pencil grip should be used at all times, both at home and in school. Some pupils dislike using them, but are encouraged if they are referred to as pencil 'rests' – little cushions to make your fingers more comfortable.

Position of the paper

The teacher must show the pupil where to place the paper on his desk. Researchers say that the paper should be tilted to the left of the body and at about an angle of 20–35 degrees for the right-handed pupil. For the left-handed pupil, it should be slanted to the right and be at a slightly greater angle.

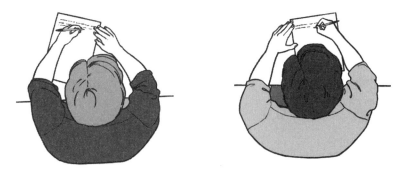

How to position the paper for the right hander and the left hander.

Writing position

To achieve a good writing position the pupil should rest his elbows on the edge of the desk with the palms of his hands against his cheeks. He should then drop his arms so that the forearms are on the desk and the thumbs are together. The non-writing hand and arm are now in the correct position to anchor the page and the pupil's writing hand should be below the line of writing so that he will be able to see what he is writing. It should not be hooked above the line on the page. It is very important that the pupil is encouraged to sit up straight rather than adopting a crouched or slouched position. It helps if he keeps his feet on the ground. He must be taught to anchor the page with his free hand. Remember to teach him to move the writing paper up the surface of the desk as he works down the page otherwise his arm becomes unsupported.

Teaching the dyslexic pupil to write

Why dyslexic pupils should be taught cursive handwriting

Hickey (1977) argued that all children should be taught cursive handwriting to avoid having to learn two systems. 'It is much easier for them to learn the letters initially, with the connecting strokes [approach and exit strokes] attached in readiness for joining them as soon as possible.' Cox (1992) said that 'cursive writing discourages reversal and transposition of letters and promotes speed and ease in handwriting'.

Cursive handwriting is an essential element of the multi-sensory training for dyslexic pupils and should be the automatic choice. The arguments for the exclusive use of cursive handwriting are:

- To eliminate the need to have to decide where each letter begins and the direction it should go.
- To provide directional left-to-right emphasis.
- To lessen the chance of reversing letters by eliminating the need to lift the pencil between letters and words.
- To provide unique letter shapes which are not mirror image of other letters, for example:

To illustrate how the cursive style makes letters that are not mirror images of themselves.

- To promote a flowing rhythmical movement. This ultimately leads to greater speed and fluency rather than stilted stop-and-go movements. Cox (1992) demonstrated this to the pupil by blindfolding him and then asking him to write his name. People who have strokes or receive head injuries can sometimes still retain the ability to write despite being unable to read or understand what they have written. Motor memory can be very strong.
- To avoid the need for the pupil to learn two different styles of writing. Once the individual cursive letters have been taught, most pupils begin to use 'joined up' writing spontaneously. 'Young children have great difficulty unlearning one habit and forming another' (Hickey, 1977). 'Furthermore, the work of Cruickshank et al (1961) and Bannatyne (1968) found that in special education classes young children learned cursive writing more easily than manuscript.' (Phelps and Stempel, 1987)

Teaching individual letter shapes

The process of learning to write 'initially depends on memorizing the graphic forms of every letter' (Luria, 1973). Dyslexic pupils should be taught to write using multi-sensory methods. There are three main strokes to learn which are:

1   The **entry stroke** which indicates where to *begin* the letter. Cox (1992) described this stroke as a 'swing-under-and-up' stroke. Taylor (1994) disagreed with this shape and said that 'it is very important that the entry stroke is a diagonal line and not moon shaped' and observed that 'this is a fault in many of the writing schemes produced in the dyslexic world'. The entry stroke is important because all lower case letters begin with it and it helps to differentiate between the upper case letter, for example:

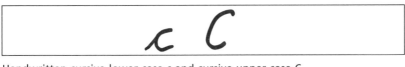

Handwritten cursive lower case c and cursive upper case C.

The entry stroke helps to establish where the letter begins and the direction on the page. The emphasis is on rounded gliding continuous strokes rather than series of individual movements.

The entry stroke.

2   The **drop stroke** which brings the letter back to the base line.

The drop stroke.

3   The **exit stroke** which finishes off the letter, helps to leave equal space between each letter and develops rhythmic writing.

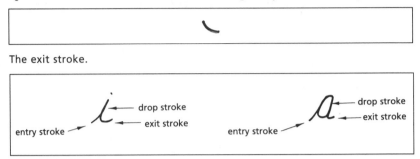

The exit stroke.

entry stroke — drop stroke — exit stroke

entry stroke — drop stroke — exit stroke

A full letter with the entry stroke, drop stroke and exit stroke labelled.

Three rules for lower case letters

1   All the lower case letters begin on the line. It is sometimes useful to put a red dot on the line initially to help establish where the letter begins. Some teachers prefer to use green because of its associations with 'go'.

2   The pupil must hold his pencil correctly and firmly anchor the page with his other hand. It is important to try to establish this habit otherwise the page wobbles or shifts and this can result in even further distortions in the writing.

3   The pupil must not lift his pencil until the letter or word is completed.

To teach the individual letters

Once the pupil has mastered the entry stroke, the drop stroke and the exit stroke he can go on to learn the individual letters. Two letters a week should be practised, first the lower case letters and then the upper case letters, until the pupil has mastered the whole alphabet. Use multi-sensory teaching methods:

- The teacher writes a letter on the page as a model.
- The pupil says the letter name.
- Then he traces over it with a fine felt tip pen.
- Then he makes his own copy with his pencil.
- The teacher gives the verbal instruction at the same time as the child is writing the letter. This seems to help many pupils in the initial stages of learning. Eventually these oral instructions are not necessary, but they help to 'pattern' the letter.

Research shows that 'mental rehearsal of a movement pattern improves performance by two or three times compared with performance without rehearsal' (Haskell, Barrett and Taylor, 1977).

The full cursive alphabet for the lower case letters

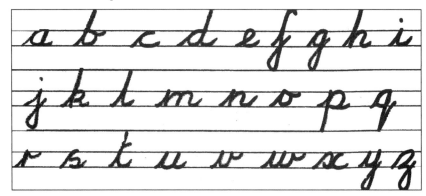

Full lower case handwritten cursive alphabet on parallel lined paper.

The letters should be taught in the following order:

I	i l	*i l*
2	c a	*c a*
3	n h	*n h*
4	b o	*b o*
5	d e	*d e*
6	g t	*g t*
7	j m	*j m*
8	q u	*q u*
9	k v	*k v*
10	y r	*y r*
11	s f	*s f*
12	x p	*x p*
13	z w	*z w*

The full cursive alphabet for the upper case letters

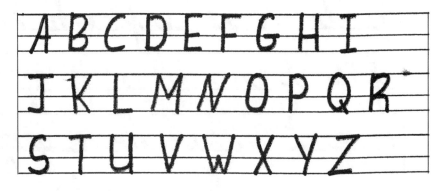

Full upper case handwritten cursive alphabet on parallel lined paper.

Most pupils will already have some knowledge of how to write capital letters as this is what they will have used when they first started to write at the age of three or four. A child of three can copy a circle and a straight line, and he can therefore be taught how to make capital letters, which are all variations of straight lines and circles.

Three rules for capital letters

1   Capital letters begin at the top of the line. This helps to differentiate between the upper case and the lower case letter. Many dyslexic pupils have great difficulty in remembering when and how to use this most basic form of punctuation.

2   Capital letters are not joined to the next letter. This helps to differentiate between them and the lower case letters.

3   The pencil may be lifted when writing capital letters.

To teach cursive writing

Cursive handwriting practice should be treated as a separate activity, and the pupil should not be expected or asked to use cursive writing in his spelling or dictation exercises until he has been taught and mastered all the letters. Neither should the pupil be required to use it when doing 'free' writing as the pupil with poor literacy skills will be overloaded. Faludy and Faludy (1996) reminded us that 'there is a difference between copy-book writing, where all you have to do is concentrate on the act of transcribing, and work where your brain is supposed to be thinking of a topic, and not of what your hands are doing'.

Many pupils start to use 'joined up' handwriting spontaneously, and quickly begin to use it for all their written work, which is the ultimate objective. Others need constant reminding to encourage them to use 'joined up' handwriting.

Cursive lower case alphabet 'joined up'

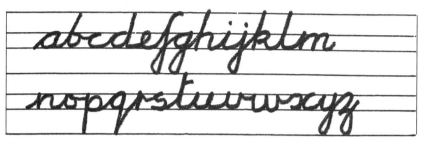

Cursive lower case handwritten alphabet joined up on parallel lined paper.

Where to begin the entry stroke

A way to remind the pupil to join up his writing seems to be to say 'pencil on the line'. It may be necessary for the teacher to keep echoing this to help establish it so that the pupil does it spontaneously. This prompt seems to act as a trigger and helps him to join up all his writing. Cox (1992) insisted that '[the] student use an approach [entry] stroke for every letter, even when it is initial [at the beginning] in a word. In this way he avoids confusing his starting point or his direction' or forgetting to join the letters.

Space between words

Some pupils have difficulty remembering to leave space between the words, which makes their work untidy and difficult to read. Teach the pupil to use his index finger as a space marker between the words. If he does do this for a short while, it helps. A continuous aural prompt 'space' from the teacher seems to be more easily assimilated by the pupil.

Margin

Always use a margin. Pupils should be reminded to begin the sentences at the margin. For a pupil who continually indents (and some do), put a red or green spot on the page and get them to put their pencil on that to help them establish the correct starting position.

Practice sentences

Holoalphabetic sentences are useful to practice because they contain the 26 letters of the alphabet:

'The quick brown fox jumps over the lazy dog.'

'The five boxing wizards jumped quickly.'

'Pack my box with five dozen liquor jugs.'

The older pupil

Cox (1992) conceded that 'writing retraining is more difficult and lengthy for most students than reading remediation. Reading is interpretation of printed symbols, while writing requires the student to visualize the symbols mentally before he translates the symbols into cursive slopes. Writing involves eye-hand co-ordination and motor control, as well as the visual modality'. Smith (1979) said 'try threading a needle with a pair of extra thick gloves on and you will come close to the feeling of the child whose hands don't work well for him when he tries to hold a pencil to write'. The experts disagree about the age limits on remediating handwriting. Johnson (1976) argued that a student cannot successfully change from hand printing [manuscript] to connected [cursive] handwriting after the age of ten. Alston (1989) cited evidence from the French researchers Athènes and Guiard which shows that 'right handers have developed a consistent posture for handwriting from the time they leave primary school. However, even at the age of eleven or twelve, the left hander may remain confused'. Cox (1992) disagreed and gave a more optimistic view when she said that 'it is never too late to change pencil grip, slant, or letter shapes if [the] student sustains motivation and perseveres diligently'.

To identify the errors

The pupil's errors should be classified, using a checklist such as the one below, and discussed so that they can be used as a basis for an individualized remedial programme. Some pupils may need help with just a few individual letters to improve radically the appearance of their work, for example the letter 's'. The older pupil must be motivated to improve. Researchers who worked with university undergraduates in the USA decided to assess their writing under the following headings:

Checklist of handwriting errors

Check a sample piece of writing and establish whether the following criteria are followed:

1   Is there a consistent use of margins? Is it on the correct side of the page?

2   Is there adequate space between the letters and words?

3   Is the letter placed correctly on the line?

4   Are the letters of uniform height?

5   Are the letters of uniform size?

6   Are the letter sizes too small?

7   Are the letter sizes too large?

8   Is the pencil pressure too heavy?

9   Is the pencil pressure too light?

10   Can the rubber/eraser be used correctly?

11   Are the letters inverted or reversed?

12   Are the letters correctly joined in cursive writing?

13   Is there a consistent slant to the letters?

Source: Alston J. and Taylor J. (1987) *Handwriting: Theory, Research and Practice.* Routledge, London: 190–1.

Left-handed pupils

There is a widespread perception that left-handed pupils particularly have problems with handwriting. There are more dialect words to describe left handedness than any other human condition. If one looks at the words for 'left-handed person' in different languages or different societies, one can immediately see the deep-seated prejudices and the stigma attached to the left hander. The Romans described them as 'sinister' and the French word is 'gauche'. The Irish call them 'citóg' which in Gaelic literally means 'awkward' or 'clumsy'. In certain parts of this country they are known variously as 'cuddy-wifties', 'keggy-fisties' or 'corrie-paws'. The Victorians tried to make the child change the dominant hand and used to tie the left hand behind the pupil's back to encourage the pupil to use the right hand for writing. This practice persisted until well into the twentieth century. Burt (1937) acquiesced with this policy when he commented that 'obstinate introverts and their old-fashioned teacher were not wholly unjustified in assuming that, when his left-handed pupils declined to use their right hands it wasn't because they couldn't, but because they wouldn't'. What seems now to be a draconian attitude prevailed almost universally. King George VI was left handed and commentators attribute the onset of his stutter to his being forced to write with his right hand against his natural inclination.

In 1982 further emphasis was placed on left handedness and its associations with dyslexia as a result of research by Geschwind and Behan (1982). Their findings are now referred to as 'The Geschwind Hypothesis'. Their key findings were that there is 'a three part association between left handedness, some learning disabilities –

particularly dyslexia – and certain immune disorders' (Galaburda, 1990). It is well established that there is a higher incidence of left handedness amongst the dyslexic population.

Incidence of left handedness

Geschwind (1983) reminded us that 'we know that at least in northern European populations left handedness is present in about 8 per cent of all individuals'. A survey conducted by Bentley and Stainthorpe in 1993 to discover the incidence of left handedness in a sample of 6,300 five- to seven-year-old pupils showed that 12 per cent of girls were left handed and 14 per cent of boys were left handed. Even more significantly, 24 per cent (in Buckinghamshire) and 18 per cent (in Berkshire) of those children receiving specialist help in school aged between seven and nine years were left handed. Paul (1990) stated that 'in the average state school class of thirty, three children will be left handed'.

Handwriting and the left-handed pupil

The left-handed pupil needs to be treated differently from other pupils, but this does not always happen. A survey conducted for the Centre for Left-Handed Studies in Manchester found that 'although 63 per cent of teachers were aware of left handers in their class, few offered practical help' (Paul, 1996).

Left-handed pupils fall into two categories. In the first the pupil has very severe grapho-motor problems, often including a very awkward pencil grip with the hand inverted and hooked above the line of writing. He often works very slowly and with difficulty, but Johnson (1976) was of the opinion that 'if the student writes easily and effectively he should be allowed to maintain it' and he added that 'violent and disruptive change of positions of paper and pen grips do not necessarily create better handwriting'. In the second category are those pupils who write neatly, fluently and legibly, although they may initially be slower at developing speed.

Sassoon (1983), an authority in Britain on the teaching of handwriting, berated the DfEE because 'there is no mention [of left handers] and their needs in the National Curriculum which puts handwriting on the agenda after decades of absence'. She insisted that 'all left-handed children deserve individual help in handwriting'. Alston and Taylor (1987), who specialize in teaching handwriting techniques, strengthen the argument in favour of the importance and awareness of the needs of left-handed pupils and stated that 'because writing is a complex task that has to be learned and because the conventions of teaching tend to favour the right-handed writer, left-handed writers may, in general, be predisposed to greater difficulties than their right-handed counterparts'.

Practical suggestions
for helping left-handed pupils

Never attempt to change the hand the pupil uses for handwriting without adequate dominance tests, which should be carried out by a qualified and experienced diagnostician.

Handwriting movements should be modelled with the left hand for left-handed pupils.

The literature on dyslexia records much evidence of a lack of a firmly established dominant hand. Waites (1982) stated that 'the development of the preferred hand for manual dexterity is usually completed by the [child's] fifth birthday. The establishment of the preferred hand is not to be confused with learning right and left ... as these are quite different functions'.

The writing tool

The left hander needs to hold the pencil about 4 cm rather than 2.5 ·cm from the tip so that he can see what he is writing. Encourage the pupil to keep his hand below the line at all times so that he can see what he is writing. Ensure that the pupil has a sharply pointed pencil and a pencil sharpener to hand. When the transition comes to using an ink pen, the rollerball or fibre tip pen are a great help as they do not blot or smudge (unlike the ink pen). There are also special nibs available for the left hander (available from the The Left-Handed Company). Sassoon (Tyrer, 1992) said 'there is no reason why left handers should have difficulty developing a fast and legible handwriting – provided they are given practical help and encouragement'.

Paper

The best advice that can be given to a left hander is to angle the paper correctly. Tilt the paper in a clockwise position, at about 20–30 degrees angle to the right. This helps to prevent the adoption of the 'hooked' held grip with its attendant problems. This advice is backed up by the research of Enstrom (1962) who concluded that it is better 'to turn his paper in the clockwise direction but certain degrees of turn are more efficient than others' and also that 'the hand below the line is best'. Ensure that the pupil holds the page with the other hand.

Alston (1989) divides adult left handers into two groups: 'those who rotate the paper clockwise, and hold the pencil pointing towards the top of the page [and] those who rotate the paper anti-clockwise, placing the pencil towards the body and generally adopt a hooked writing position'.

Tool grip

Some hold their pencil too tightly.

- Drawing their attention to this can help.

- Finger and hand relaxation exercises can help.

- In severe or persistent cases, put a sheet of carbon paper under the page and compare the pressure used with a sample copied simultaneously by the teacher. This heightens awareness of the error.

Seating

The table or desk should have a flat surface. The chair should be at the correct height for the pupil. If it is too low it will necessitate the pupil raising his shoulders which can often result in the his using a 'hooked' position to hold his pencil. If the pupil is sharing a desk with another pupil, he should be seated at the left side of the desk. When seated, the pupil's feet should be firmly on the ground. The left-handed pupil should not be seated in a position where he has to turn around or is at an angle to the blackboard. If his feet don't touch the ground an inverted wooden box can be used for him to rest his feet.

Speed

Some dyslexic pupils remain slow writers and frequently complain that they do not have enough time to finish off work, for example in an examination. According to Thomson and Watkins (1990), 'many dyslexics are daunted by the thought of writing and often will only write a few lines'. They suggest that speed can be improved by the use of timing and dictation, and advocate using Bramley's (1996) Speed Test idea to develop speed and an awareness of this:

- Write ten words at the top of the page.

- Ask the pupil to write ten separate sentences for the words provided.

- Give the pupil ten minutes to complete the task.

- Add up all the words used. Divide the total by ten to find out how many words per minute the pupil produces. Keep a record of this and encourage the pupil to beat his own record. This also helps motivation.

Source: Bramley W. (1996) *Units of Sound: Teachers' Notes.* The Dyslexia Institute, Staines.

Summary and conclusions

1   The teaching of handwriting has regained a place in the classroom curriculum with the advent of the National Curriculum. At Key Stage 2 (seven to eleven) pupils 'should be given opportunities to continue to develop legible handwriting in joined up and printed styles'.

2   There are many different styles of handwriting. The teaching of cursive (joined-up) handwriting has been shown to result in writing that is easy to read and good to look at. It also leads to speedy and fluent writing.

3   Handwriting has to be taught. This should be done in a systematic and structured fashion with much practice.

4   Schools should adopt a 'whole school handwriting policy'. This should apply to letter shapes, height of the letters and where the letters should begin and end on the page as well as directions on the correct pencil hold and hand position.

5   Dyslexic pupils need to be taught using multi-sensory methods. Cursive handwriting is best and easiest for such pupils.

6   It is necessary to teach letters individually rather than using whole sentences. This should help to prevent or eliminate the '85 per cent of the illegibility caused by the misuse of one or all of three of the control strokes' (Johnson, 1976).

7   There are many (dyslexic) left-handed pupils whose specific difficulties in the classroom and in the home need to be addressed.

Chapter 6

Spelling

- classification and analysis of spelling errors as a means of detection
- structured approaches to teaching spelling

Introduction

Spelling is a subject that generates universal interest and often heated debate among the public, politicians, employers, the literati and, most frequently, the teaching profession. As long ago as 1750 Lord Chesterfield berated his son for his poor spelling and wrote to his son about the fate of 'that man of quality who never recovered from the ignominy of spelling "wholesome" without the "w"'.

The press is quick to target the spelling mistakes made by well-known people. In the US run-up to the vice-presidential election in 1988 Dan Quayle was dealt a severe blow when he added an 'e' to the spelling of the word 'potato' on a classroom black board. His *faux-pas* will continue to be cited by teachers in English-speaking countries for many years. In the UK, John Patten, when Secretary for Education, drew howls of derisive laughter because of his misspelling of 'sincerely'. Undoubtedly 'society condemns those who cannot spell' (Scragg, 1974). The view of many employers was summed up by Russel (1993) when she said 'for applicants, such poor spelling will jeopardise their chances of a job'. The National Curriculum (1995) puts great emphasis on the importance of spelling at each of the Key Stages, and states that pupils should be helped to increase their knowledge of regular patterns of spelling, word families, root words and their derivations. Good spelling is a passport to educational opportunities and employment for the majority of the population.

How does the good speller spell?

The problem of how to teach spelling is often tackled by examining the methods that good spellers use. Sloboda (1980) did a series of experiments with proficient adult spellers and concluded 'that people who spell well, although they do know the rules governing spelling, probably do not know how to spell by virtue of these rules; they spell well by a rote memory process'. They are what some people would call 'natural spellers'.

Strategies good spellers use to spell

- They learn and remember words as part of their reading experience.

- They have met similar words and remember them. They have been taught lists of words or 'word families'. This method is useful for the good speller and has long been in use in classrooms throughout the world.

- They have good phonemic awareness, that is, they can pick out the sounds in the words and they can then relate a letter to these sounds when they meet an unfamiliar word.

- They use the meaning or [semantic] knowledge of the derivation of words to spell, for example Latin and Greek prefixes and suffixes – 'century', centenary', 'centurion'.

- They can remember the origin of the words – 'mutton' comes from the French *'mouton'* for sheep.

- They remember spelling rules – 'i' before 'e' except after 'c'.

- They have been taught grammatical constraints (rules) and can remember these – plurals of nouns ending in 'y' change 'y' to 'i' and add 'es' except when there is a vowel before the 'y'.

- They seem to absorb the everyday words that are not spelt the way they sound – 'done', 'none'. The origins and idiosyncratic spelling of many of these words, some of which come from Anglo Saxon or Old and Middle English do not present a problem for the competent speller. But because many of these words are not spelt phonetically they can cause great difficulties to the poor speller.

- The good speller can often remember a word because it is unusual – 'diarrhoea' or 'onomatopoeia'; because it is exotic – 'pharaoh'; or because it is weird – 'Eschscholtzia' (a type of Californian poppy!).

'English has from the beginning followed the practice of begging, borrowing and stealing [from many languages]' (Calfee, 1984) and this goes some way to explain some of its 'strange' spelling.

The complexities of spelling

Bernard Shaw had firm views about English spelling and punctuation. He campaigned for its simplification and pointed out that even a sound knowledge of phonics does not always ensure accurate spelling. He illustrated this with the phonetic representation of the word 'fish' which he said should be spelled as 'ghoti' and demonstrated its spelling as follows.

/gh/ = 'f' as in laugh

/o/ = 'i' as in women

/ti/ = 'sh' as in nation

A structured approach to teaching spelling

Many people argue that all pupils should have some formal instruction in spelling and not the random methods used in many classrooms. The 'lucky dip' approach whereby the teacher gives a haphazard selection of words to take home 'to learn' does not produce a lasting knowledge of how to spell them. Often parents and pupil will spend considerable amounts of time copying the list out and rehearsing a hotchpotch of spelling which may be linked to a specific subject or task currently being studied in the classroom. This is not the way to teach spelling. All children can benefit from a structured and systematic exposure to the rules and patterns that underpin a language. The principles and methods used to teach pupils with a specific learning difficulty can be adapted for use with all pupils in a class. At the same time the dyslexic pupil will be able to overlearn and reinforce that which he may be learning with his specialist teacher.

Some suggestions

on how to incorporate multi-sensory teaching methods into a spelling lesson for the whole class

The lesson might be organized as follows when teaching, for example, the Doubling Rule:

- Revise the concept of consonants and vowels orally.
- Write the word 'bell' on the blackboard and colour the double 'll'.
- Invite the pupils to comment on the double 'll'.
- Ask the class to contribute other examples of words with a similar spelling (the principles of self-discovery are important).
- Individual pupils could be invited to come and write their 'word' on the blackboard while being encouraged to say the letter names aloud as they write it.

- Rehearse verbally the concept of a short vowel.
- Write the rule on the blackboard that words with short vowel endings in 'l' take double 'll'.
- Pupils then copy this into a spelling notebook.
- Pupils write ten more words in their notebooks that follow the rule, preferably words with different short vowel sounds. They will have heard the examples given by other pupils. Simultaneously they should be encouraged to vocalize the letters as they write them in cursive writing in their spelling notebooks thus using ears, lips and hands to reinforce the spelling.
- Finally pupils turn over the page and the teacher dictates a short passage incorporating the words written on the board to reinforce the rule.
- Pupils exchange notebooks and mark each other's work.
- Ask pupils to spend some time learning the rule and the words at home. Perhaps ask the pupil to make sentences for each of the words.
- The following week, test pupils using dictation to check their retention of the spelling pattern that was taught.

Spelling is a complex task and it presents problems for many, not just dyslexic people. Furthermore we know that 'poor spelling is an inevitable concomitant of dyslexia' (Cook, 1981) and she postulated that 'it is difficult to remediate even in those dyslexic persons who are able to profit from intensive instruction in reading'.

The research findings of Thomson (1981) showed that 'in their spontaneous writing, dyslexics make one spelling error in five, whereas the ratio for normal readers is one in thirty five'. Many dyslexics retain the hallmarks of dyslexia in their spelling even when they are adults.

Spelling tests

The Graded Word Spelling Test (Vernon, 1983) is widely used. It is a short test which diagnostically is a disadvantage as the tester needs as much evidence as possible if she is to be able to analyse it and look for a particular pattern of errors. The WRAT–3 (Wilkinson, 1993) spelling test is also becoming more widely used. Its norms cover the ages 5 to 75.

What is distinctive about a dyslexic's spelling and how can it be recognized?

Cook (1981) said that 'misspellings are regarded as a better source of information than correctly spelled words' and that they are 'a potentially fruitful assessment device'. Many authors such as Goodman (1969) and Peters (1967) have suggested ways of analysing spelling errors. Miles carried out research for over twenty years, and kept a record of the spelling errors of the dyslexic people he assessed (Miles, 1993). A detailed examination of their spelling mistakes showed that the spelling of dyslexics is 'qualitatively different from those of normal learners' (Cook and Moats, 1983). Miles said that 'bizarre spelling is a common characteristic of younger dyslexic subjects' (Miles and Miles, 1983). But it is important to remember that 'such spelling is not in fact limited to dyslexic subjects but is characteristic of anyone who is 'out of his depth' in the sense that he needs to spell words that are too hard or sophisticated for him' (Miles and Miles, 1983). He said that the spelling of some dyslexic individuals is 'plausible' and bears some relationship to the sound–letter correspondence.

There can be little argument about the persistence and uniqueness of each dyslexic pupil's spelling. There are underlying features that send signals to the trained and experienced eye – some errors are so idiosyncratic that it would be difficult to invent them. There are certain characteristics in a dyslexic pupil's spelling that can be identified, classified and then used to make a diagnosis of dyslexia. Miles refined and collated these characteristics. In some cases these errors are resistant to all forms of remedy and for many this is a lifelong handicap. The dyslexic is likely to remain a weak speller throughout life.

Classification of the dyslexic speller's errors (Professor T. Miles' '13 millstones')

These examples of spelling errors can be used to analyse the errors made in a standardized spelling test and in the exercise books and creative writing of anyone who is thought to be dyslexic, be they aged 7 or 70. It is not enough to know the pupil's spelling age as calculated on a standardized spelling test. Pollock and Waller (1994) stated that 'spelling ages on spelling tests may vary from one test to another, and, indeed, so does a person's performance'. A careful record and analysis of the particular pattern of errors made is one of the simplest and most effective methods of screening for dyslexia. In the experience of Kline and Kline (1975) 'a written spelling test is the most sensitive of all tests in indicating the presence of a language problem'.

Miles' '13 millstones'

1 **The impossible trigram**

   This is the use of a cluster or combination of letters that are impossible in English spellings:

   – 'lqu' for liquid; 'cwiyatly' for quietly

2 **The misrepresentation of the sound**

   – 'cet' for get
   – 'pad' for pat } of consonants

   – 'cot' for 'cut'
   – 'mat' for 'met' } of the short vowels

   Miles argued that this is not an auditory difficulty but that 'they are memory errors resulting from auditory confusability'. Parents or teachers sometimes think that the child has a hearing loss and his spelling difficulties have been attributed to this. During the late 1970s and early 1980s glue ear 'otitis media', an infection in the middle ear that often results in intermittent hearing loss, was often given as a cause of a child's difficulty with spelling. Sometimes this was indeed the case, but sometimes the 'temporary' improvement made when defective hearing was treated resulted in a further delay before the problems of a dyslexic child were identified. Kibel and Miles (1994) pointed out that 'children with spelling ages as high as nine years sometimes made phonological [awareness of sounds] errors in regular one-syllable words. It was also noticed that if children were afterwards asked to re-spell their incorrect words they tended to get them right. Thus it seems that their phonological skills were not yet automatized'.

3 **When wrong boundaries are used**

   This can be either a single word written with a space between the parts:

   – 'a-nother'

   or words written together without a space:

   – 'firstones' for 'first ones' or 'halfanhour' for 'half an hour'

4 **Wrong syllabification**

   Either too many syllables or too few:

   – 'sundly' for 'suddenly', 'rember' for 'remember'

5 **Inconsistent spelling**

   The same word is spelt in different ways on the same page:

   – 'schule', 'skchool', 'school'

6 **Wrong letter doubled**
 – 'eeg' for 'egg'
 – 'beel' for 'bell'

7 **Mistaken recall of order**
 All the letters in the word are present but in the incorrect order. This is sometimes attributed to poor visual sequential memory:
 – 'tow' for 'two'
 – 'pakr' for 'park'

8 **There is false match for order**
 The letters in the word are the wrong way round:
 – 'sitesr' for 'sister'
 – 'poelpe' for 'people'
 This is similar to **7** but Miles (1993) said that the ordering of the letters occurs for different reasons.

9 **Omission of one or more sounding letters**
 – 'amt' for 'amount'

10 **Duplication of one or more sounding letters**
 – 'piyole' for 'pile'

11 **Phonetic attempt misfired**
 – 'yuwer' for 'your'
 – 'yoos' for 'use'

12 **The intrusive vowel**
 – 'miy-yils' for 'miles'
 – 'tewenty' for 'twenty'

13 **'b-d' substitution**
 – 'bady' for 'baby'
 – 'decos' for 'because'

Source: Miles T. R. (1993) *Dyslexia: The Pattern of Difficulties* (2nd edition). Whurr Publishers Ltd, London: 75–85.

Other common mistakes

A number of other mistakes commonly found in the writing of a dyslexic could be added to Miles' 'millstones':

• Letters are sometimes reversed.
 – 'gip' for 'pig'

Many children reverse letters when first beginning to spell but most have overcome this by the age of seven or eight. For others it remains a persistent feature of their spelling.

- The use of upper case 'B' or 'D' in the middle of words or middle of sentences. Miles (1993) and Vellutino (1979) attribute this to 'left–right confusions of verbal labelling [...] and not to visual perception alone'.
  - 'daDDy' for 'daddy'

- Misspelling of the past tense of the verb that requires 'ed'. The poor speller does not remember this and when he hears /t/ or /d/ or /id/ at the end of the word, he writes:
  - 'walkt' for 'walked'
  - 'playd' for 'played'
  - 'mendid' for 'mended'

- Letters are inverted.
  - 'frout' for 'front'
  - 'dot' for 'got'

Persisting errors

These spelling errors are a summary of the possible mistakes a dyslexic speller might make. Rarely, if ever, would they all be found in one dyslexic pupil's work. It is the cluster of these errors that is diagnostically significant and the fact that they have been made consistently over a period of months and years. As the pupil gets older, or if there has been specialist teaching, it becomes more difficult to diagnose these difficulties purely from the results of a spelling test.

What are the underlying principles of teaching spelling to dyslexic pupils?

The revival of teaching phonics in many classrooms since the 1980s has undoubtedly helped many pupils to spell, but in some instances this masks some of the obvious errors made by pupils and can make the diagnosis of dyslexia more complex. Some pupils seem to be able to spell a word correctly when their attention is focused on spelling, but when they are doing 'creative' writing they may misspell many of these same words. Miles (1993) refused 'to go along with those who say that all the spelling problems of the allegedly dyslexic child would disappear if the teaching methods used in the early stages were adequate'.

Almost all the research evidence points to the benefits to be derived from teaching the relationship between the letter name (grapheme) and sound (phoneme). The work of Hornsby and Miles (1980) and

Frith (1985) provided evidence of this. Thomson (1990) reiterated Gillingham and Stillman's advice that the teaching of spelling should be done using multi-sensory methods 'because the child hears (auditory), says (follows speech/motor articulation), writes (kinesthetic/motor), says as written (speech/auditory linked to motor) and reads out loud (visual/auditory feed back)' (Gillingham and Stillman, 1956). This is sometimes called the VAKT method because it refers to the Visual, Auditory, Kinesthetic and Tactile approach used to teach spelling by Gillingham and her disciples.

Multi-sensory teaching of spelling

The dyslexic child should always be taught spelling by the use of multi-sensory methods.
a) The pupil looks at the word using his eyes.
b) He says the word aloud using his lips.
c) He writes the word using his hands while at the same time he says the letter names.
d) Then he reads the word he has written.

The pupil needs to reinforce all he does daily using this method so that his response becomes automatic by practising spelling, and reading and writing whatever sound or pattern he is learning.

Simultaneous Oral Spelling method (SOS)

Like so much else involved in the teaching of dyslexic pupils this method too has its roots in the work of Gillingham and Stillman (1956). There are two forms of this method. One method requires the pupils to sound out the letters in the word, the other asks the pupil to give the letter names as he spells the word. Orton believed that the pupil should 'sound the phonograms while writing [because that was what he heard]. The muscles of the mouth moved along with the muscles of the hand' (Sheffield, 1991). The sounding out method is essential in the early stages of learning to spell, but older pupils tend to make the transformation to spelling using the letter names spontaneously.

Fernald method

Cotterell (1970) summarized the procedure as follows:

1 The word should be written on a piece of A4 by the teacher – using a cursive script.

2 The teacher pronounces the word very slowly and clearly. Then the pupil repeats it.

3 The pupil examines the word carefully, noting any particular difficulty or 'tricky' letters.

4 He then traces over the letters with his fingers, saying the letter names aloud as he traces them.

5   Then he folds the paper over.

6   He writes the word from memory.

7   He then turns over the piece of paper and checks that he has written it correctly.

8   He then uses the word in a sentence – or a story.

Cotterell suggested storing these in a shoe box for easy reference, for example when writing a story. A card index box is probably more appropriate nowadays.

The Fernald method is based on the methods devised by Grace Fernald (1943). It is useful and it works with some children, particularly those with good visual skills; others don't remember the words in the long term. It is another crutch for the speller who cannot remember what the letters are in a word or for the many words that cannot be spelt by sounding them out. It is useful for teaching irregular spellings to some pupils. According to Cotterell (1970), 'the system is often referred to as kinesthetic [muscle memory], it is really a look, say and do method. Phonics are not involved'.

Other visual approaches to spelling

'The purely visual inspection approach to spelling has been shown "to give" very poor results in dyslexics', according to Thomson (1991). This includes the traditional classroom technique of the spelling list given to pupils to learn for the weekly test. Schonell's *Essentials in Teaching and Testing Spelling* (first published in 1932) is still being used in many classrooms. For the dyslexic pupil the use of its word lists can be an unmitigated disaster and a source of frustration and futility as he tries to remember a hotchpotch of spellings. Some dyslexic pupils may be able to remember the spelling for the day of the test. They will often have forgotten them a week later. Likewise, they often forget words they may have been asked to correct in their exercise or essay if they have copied them out six times. Other teachers, according to Pollock and Waller (1994), give 'words for class spelling tests [that] are often topic based rather than grouped for structure and the dyslexic child is at sea and anchorless with words such as "kitchen" "cooker" "fridge"'.

Brand (1992) stated that 'too much emphasis has been placed on learning to spell through visual methods. The ears and the mouth have been forgotten and power of the hand ignored'. Researchers such as Aaron (1993) showed that 'memory for orthography (spelling patterns) is not purely visual in nature but is supported by semantic and phonological features of words. Visual memory in isolation, as compared to phonology and semantics, plays a relatively limited role in word recognition'.

'Look/Cover/Check' method

The pupil is often encouraged to use the 'Look/Cover/Check' method to learn a new spelling. Its success depends on the pupil having a visual perceptual and a visual sequential memory. Advocates of this method often suggest that the pupil's spelling can be improved by reading experience.The pupil is asked to:

a) Look at the word carefully and note anything unusual about it, such as a silent letter or a prefix.
b) Close his eyes and try to remember the letters.
c) Write the word down.
d) Check to see that what he has written is correct.

The procedure is repeated if he has made an error. The underlying principle is the same as that used by the teacher who asks the child to copy out his spelling corrections ten times. For many dyslexic pupils this is an utter waste of time – often he won't be able to read the word correctly; some even copy out the spelling 'correction' incorrectly.

Books for teaching dyslexic pupils spelling

- Books suitable for day-to-day use in the classroom and by parents:
  Signposts to Spelling (Pollock, 1980)
  Spelling Made Easy (Brand, 1992)

- Comprehensive teaching programmes for reference and resource purposes. These fall into three categories and are suitable for:

  1 Classroom teachers
  Dyslexia: A Teaching Handbook (Thomson and Watkins, 1990)
  The Bangor Dyslexia Teaching System (Miles, 1993)
  Units of Sound (Bramley, 1996)

  2 Specialist teachers and requiring basic training
  Alpha-to-Omega (Hornsby and Shear, 1994)
  The Hickey Multi-sensory Language Course (Augur and Briggs, 1992)

  3 Restricted to specialist teachers trained by the Dyslexia Institute
  The Dyslexia Institute Literacy Programme (Dyslexia Institute, 1993)

Spelling step by step

The pupil must never be asked to spell words unless he has been taught them. This eliminates failure and builds confidence. If the programme of spelling remediation has been followed correctly the pupil should be getting 99.9 per cent correct of what he is asked to write. Each step must be fully mastered before moving on to the next. Brand (1992) argued that 'only one word family should be taught a week, irrespective of the age of the student'.

The researchers Bryant and Bradley (1985) have shown that phonological awareness and skills are an important component in learning to spell. This means that it is important to be aware of sounds of words and how they are represented in writing. Everything is taught by using multi-sensory methods.

Workbooks are useful for reinforcing spelling rules and concepts being taught and as part of the particular spelling programme being followed. The dyslexic pupil will derive little benefit from being asked simply to fill in missing letters.

Suggestions for workbooks
Key stages 1–4
Stages 1, 2 and 3 Alpha-to-Omega Activity Packs (Hornsby and Pool, 1990/1991/1992)

Key Stages 3–4
Solving Language Difficulties: Remedial Routines (Steere, Peck and Kahn, 1971)
Spellbound: Phonic Reading and Spelling (Workbook) (Rak, 1972)
Spelling Made Easy. Books 0–3 (Brand, 1992)
Exercise Your Spelling. Workbooks I, II, III (Wood, 1982)

Step 1 The letters
Before the pupil begins to study the spelling rules he must know that a letter has four properties:
a) a name – 'a' for 'acorn'
b) a sound – /a/ for 'ant'
c) a shape (or symbol) – A a *a*
d) a feel – how to write A a *a*

'When children learn to spell they must analyse the sounds in the words that they wish to write, and then decide how to represent these sounds in print.' (Goswami, 1991)

Step 2 The alphabet
• Check that the pupil can identify the four properties of a letter by getting him to write down the alphabet in lower case, then in capital letters.

- Ensure that he knows the initial sound of each of the letters of the alphabet otherwise he will find it very difficult to spell the word correctly, because if he cannot immediately recall from his visual memory what a word looks like, his next strategy has to be to sound it out. If he cannot immediately write 'pig' he should then say the word and then attempt to sound it out. He will hear the sounds /p/ /i/ /g/ but if he does not know what letter to write for the 'g' sound, for example, he has a problem. The letter 'g' can be difficult because it sometimes says 'j' – 'gin' or 'gym'.

- He should know that there are 26 letters in the alphabet and he must know their names. It is also useful to tell him that there are approximately 44 different sounds that can be made from the letters. He does not need to remember this but it alerts him to the fact that a letter or a group or letters can have a number of different sounds.

- He needs to work on the alphabet in its spoken and written forms. He must practise saying the alphabet letter by letter, then saying it in pairs and triplets alternately with another person. He needs to practise writing the alphabet in capital and lower case in tandem while simultaneously saying the letter names. He needs to develop an awareness of what letter goes after, before and between the other letters when he both says and writes the alphabet. This can be reinforced by using workbooks, arranging plastic or wooden letters in sequences and by playing various games.

Step 3 Vowels and consonants

The pupil must be taught that there are two different kinds of letters, vowels and consonants. The vowels are 'a', 'e', 'i', 'o', 'u'. The letter 'y' is sometimes a vowel, such as in words like 'my' and 'try'. The letter 'y' is sometimes referred to as a semi-vowel.

Step 4 Short vowels

Short vowels say their sound:

$\breve{a}$ = $\breve{a}$pple

$\breve{e}$ = $\breve{e}$lephant

$\breve{i}$ = $\breve{i}$ndian

$\breve{o}$ = $\breve{o}$range

$\breve{u}$ = $\breve{u}$mbrella

Step 5 Long vowels

Long vowels say their names.

$\bar{a}$ = $\bar{a}$corn

$\bar{e}$ = $\bar{e}$mu

$\bar{\text{i}}$ = $\bar{\text{i}}$ron

$\bar{\text{o}}$ = $\bar{\text{o}}$pen

$\bar{\text{u}}$ = $\bar{\text{u}}$niform

It is important that the pupils realize that 'getting the vowel sound right depends on taking into account the letters that follow the vowel' (Stanback, 1992).

It is necessary to use worksheets and exercises to reinforce this concept such as those found in *Alpha-to-Omega Activity Packs* (Hornsby and Pool, 1990/1991/1992). It is important that excercises include coding and reading the word and that the ultimate objective of teaching syllables is kept in mind. It will help with reading and spelling long or unknown words.

Step 6 Consonant digraphs – 'sh', 'ch', 'wh', etc.
Consonant digraphs are often confused, particularly at the ends of words.

/sh/ – 'ship' or 'rush'

/ch/ – 'chap' or 'much'

/wh/ – 'whip'

/th/ – 'thin'

/ph/ – 'phone'

/gh/ – at the end of the word such as 'laugh' or 'cough'

(The last two are not to be given as spellings yet because they contain long vowel sounds which have not been taught).

Step 7 Consonant blends – 'cl', 'gl', 'pr', etc.
Teach these and reinforce them using multi-sensory learning methods and SOS (Simultaneous Oral Spelling), as well as dictation.

Step 8 Assimilations
These are sounds made down the nose and contain 'm' or 'n' at the end of words:

/ng/ /nd/ /mp/ /nch/ /nt/ as in 'bang', 'sand', 'jump', 'lunch', 'mint'

Spelling rules

Many teachers and learners are overwhelmed by the task of teaching and learning to spell. One of the most important things is to analyse the task and to have a strategy and a structure for the teaching of spelling. The National Curriculum leaves no doubt that at Key Stage 2 pupils should be taught to:

- spell complex, polysyllabic words that conform to regular

patterns [spelling rules], and to break long and complex words into more manageable units [syllable division], by using their knowledge of meaning and word structure [prefix and suffixes]

- memorize the usual patterns of words, including those that are irregular
- recognize silent letters
- use the apostrophe to spell shortened forms of words
- use appropriate terminology, including vowel and consonant.

The most encouraging piece of information to give to poor spellers is to tell them that, despite what they might think, many words are regular and follow a spelling rule or pattern which can be learned. According to Crystal (1987), 'a computer analysis of some 17,000 English words showed that 84 per cent of words were spelt according to a regular pattern' (Thomson and Watkins, 1990).

There are about twenty spelling rules that need to be taught, although the word 'rule' (when applied to English spelling) is somewhat misleading because it implies universal application. Almost every spelling 'rule' has attendant 'rule breakers'. 'Yet, the fact remains that without the crutch, *aide memoir* or spelling rule, the dyslexic child would be floundering.' (Thomson and Watkins, 1990)

Top spelling rules

Farrer (1993) made some crucial comments about rules when she said 'It is extremely important that the rules are not taught in isolation. They must be backed up by visual materials, worksheets, games, dictation. The aim of teaching spelling rules is not to expect the student to use them for the rest of his life but to help him to learn spelling patterns and, eventually to be able to spell words automatically'. Learning rules is not an infallible way to teach spelling but it puts down markers, charts unknown territory and can prevent the dyslexic child floundering in the quagmire of English spelling. Breaking the task into manageable, logical steps is a lifeline for many poor spellers. Spelling rules should be taught step by step. The rule itself should be put on the pupil's card index and reinforced daily by using spelling, dictation, worksheets or games as a stimulus. Teaching too much too quickly is a disservice to a dyslexic pupil.

This list of spelling rules is not complete. The teacher and pupil can add to them. Keep these on separate index cards to be revised and revisited frequently.

1 Doubling Rule

A good rule to begin with is the Doubling Rule. Words with a short vowel ending in 'f', 'l', 's' or 'z' double the final consonant:

stiff, bell, miss, fuzz

Don't forget to teach the exceptions – yes, gas, if, of, pal.

Some teachers call this 'The Flossy Rule'.

2 'y' has three different sounds

Brand (1992) reminded us that 'the consonant "y" can cause problems from infant school to adult-hood'. Revise the concept of long and short vowels and ensure that vowels and consonants are easily identified.

'y' can be a consonant as in 'yes', 'yet', 'yen'.

'y' when it is a vowel sometimes says /i/ as in 'my', 'by', 'try'. No English word ends in 'i'. English uses 'y' instead – spy, shy. 'taxi', 'semi' are abbreviations. Words like 'ski' (from Norwegian) and 'spaghetti' (from Italian) are not English words.

'y' when it is a vowel can also say /ē/ as in 'lady', 'copy', 'daddy', 'sunny'.

3 The 'w' Rules I, II, and III

These are called 'Wanda the Wicked Witch's Rules' by some.

* Rule I states that the /o/ sound after 'w' is spelt with 'a':

  wash, swan

* Rule II states that the /or/ sound after 'w' is spelt with 'ar':

  ward, warm

* Rule III states that the /er/ sound after 'w' is spelt with 'or':

  world, word

4 The 'v' Rules

* Rule I says no English word ends in 'v' except 'spiv'. There is always an 'e' after 'v' at the end of a word:

  have, serve

* Rule II says there is no such spelling as 'uv', English uses 'ov' instead:

  love, shove, glove

5 Magic 'e'

Having established that the pupil can tell the difference between long and short vowels, tackle the Magic 'e', or the lengthening 'e' rule as it is sometimes called. When 'e' is added to the end of a word it makes the directly preceding vowel into a long vowel which says its name. The following illustration is helpful:

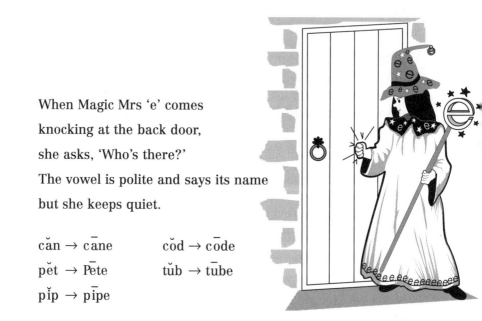

When Magic Mrs 'e' comes

knocking at the back door,

she asks, 'Who's there?'

The vowel is polite and says its name

but she keeps quiet.

căn → cāne   cŏd → cōde

pĕt → Pēte   tŭb → tūbe

pĭp → pīpe

Each of these long vowels should be worked on separately, maybe one a week for the very poor speller, and should be reinforced daily. Don't ask the pupil to spell the homophones (words with the same sound but a different spelling – 'ate' and 'eight', 'pair', 'pear' and 'pare') because he has not been taught them yet, but do alert him to their existence and tell him the meanings of them.

6 Teach when to use 'c' or 'k'

- When teaching the /k/ sound, point out that the majority of words starting with the /k/ sound are spelt with a 'c':
  cat, cot, cup

- However, there are some useful rules to help the pupil remember when he should use 'k' instead.
  'k' before the letters 'e', 'i' and 'y' keep the /k/ sound:
  kettle, king, key
  A useful mnemonic for this is as follows:
  'You can put the kettle on and make a cup of coffee for the King.'

- Use 'k' after another consonant at the end of a word:
  ask, walk, ink

7   How to spell /k/ sound at the end of a word

- Words with a short vowel take 'ck':
  back, pick, duck
- If there is a consonant before the /k/ sound it takes 'k':
  bank, milk, desk
- If there is a long vowel and Magic 'e' it takes 'ke':
  make, bike, duke
- If there is a vowel digraph (two vowels making one sound), it takes 'k':
  oak, leak, cheek

Rule Breakers! take 'c'
panic, picnic, music, Arctic, fabric, attic, Atlantic

8   Hard and soft 'c'

- Hard 'c' says /k/:
  cap, cop, cup
- Soft 'c' says /s/ when the next letter is 'e', 'i' or 'y':
  cent, city, cycle

  This applies whether the 'c' is at the beginning, middle or end of a word:
  circle, recent, entrance

9   Hard and soft 'g'

- Hard 'g' says /g/:
  game, god, gun
- Soft 'g' says /j/ when the next letter is 'e', 'i' or 'y':
  gem, gin, gym

  This applies whether 'g' is at the beginning, middle or end of a word:
  gypsy, energy

10 How to spell /j/ sound at the end of a word

- Words with a short vowel take 'dge':
  edge, lodge, judge
- If there is a consonant before the /j/ sound it takes 'ge':
  bulge, hinge, large
- If there is a long vowel and Magic 'e' it takes 'ge':
  cage, rage, stage
- If there is a vowel digraph (two vowels making one sound) it takes 'ge':
  stooge, gouge

11 How to spell /ch/ sound at the end of a word

- If there is a short vowel it takes 'tch':
  match, fetch, ditch
- If there is a consonant before the /ch/ sound it takes 'ch':
  bench, lunch, church
- If there is a vowel digraph it takes 'ch':
  coach, touch, teach

Rule Breakers!

such, much, rich, which, sandwich, duchess, bachelor, attach, ostrich

12 Long vowels and their spelling

Vowels are long:

- At the end of an open syllable:
  mē, gō
- With a Magic 'e':
  hat → hāte
  pet → Pēte
  rip → rīpe

As noted in the tables on pages 119–20.

The different ways to spell long vowel sounds

There is a little ditty which may be helpful for remembering that vowel digraphs are long. It is not always true and should not be taken too literally:

When two vowels go out walking

the first vowel does the talking

and usually says its name

This means that when there are two vowels side by side in a word, the first vowel is the one that says something and this is usually its name:

'train'. It does not say 'tran' or 'trin', it does say 'train'.

Each of the long vowels needs to be taught individually. Miles (1994) advised caution and urged parents and teachers to 'do them gradually with Primary School children and never to introduce another pattern for the same sound immediately'.

Alternative ways for spelling long /ā/ sound

a	a-e	ay	ai	ea	ei	e
baby	spade	play	sail	great	reign	they
gravy	plate	tray	fail	break	eight	grey
table	tape	day	rail	steak	their	prey
paper	date	way	wait	bear		obey
used at the end of an open syllable	*used in Magic 'e' words*	*used at the end of a word*	*used in the middle of a word*			

Rule breakers! Words that say /ā/ but which are spelt 'ei':
neighbour, veil, weight, rein, reign, heir, eight, eighty, eighteen, heir, vein
Names never follow spelling rules! Just to prove it, think about Neil, Keith and Sheila.

Alternative ways for spelling long /ē/ sound

e	ea	ee	e-e	ie	ei	y	ey
evil	neat	speech	mete	chief	ceiling	baby	money
emu	eat	weed	athlete	thief	receive	lady	honey
legal	each	three		niece	deceit	copy	donkey
Venus	speak	teeth		field	receipt	pony	valley
used at the end of an open syllable				*use 'i' before 'e' except after 'c'*	*used after 'c'*		

Alternative ways for spelling long /ī/ sound

i	i-e	y	igh	y-e	ie	i
iris	five	fly	might	rye	pie	child
Irene	hive	dry	tight	lyre	tie	mild
iron	nine	cry	night	type	lie	kind
Simon	wine	why	fight	thyme	die	wild
used at the end of an open syllable	*used in Magic 'e' words*	*used because in English words do not end in 'i'*	*used in the middle of words*			*used in words that have a short vowel spelling but a long vowel sound*

Alternative ways for spelling long /ō/ sound

o	o-e	ow	oa	oe	ough	o
open	rope	snow	coat	toe	dough	gold
Roman	pope	slow	boat	foe	though	sold
polo	note	grow	goal	hoe	although	fold
used at the end of an open syllable	*used in Magic 'e' words*	*used at the end of words*	*used in the middle of words*			*used in words with short vowel spelling but a long vowel sound*

Alternative ways for spelling /ū/ sound

u	u-e	ue	ew	eu	ui	oo
Una	tune	true	stew	Europe	suit	food
music	cube	clue	chew	queue	fruit	school
pupil	rude	value	grew	Eucharist	juice	fool
student	pure	avenue	flew	Eureka	cruise	tooth
used at the end of an open syllable	*used in Magic 'e' words*		*used at the end of a word*			*used in the middle of words*

13 'q' and 'u' always go together
quick, queen, quiet

14 'all'
When followed by another syllable, 'all' has only one 'l':
also, always, altogether

15 'ful', 'wel' or 'til'
'ful' or 'wel' at the beginning of a word have one 'l':
fulfil, welfare

At the end of a word 'ful' and 'til' have only one 'l':
hopeful, helpful, useful, until

16 Prefixes and suffixes
The pupil must learn the spelling and meanings of Latin and Greek prefixes and suffixes. According to Cox and Hutcheson (1988), 'Latin roots can be identified in 50–60 per cent of the words in any English Dictionary'. This knowledge can help with spelling and reading. It also widens the vocabulary. The snag for the poor speller is that he needs to be taught the suffixing rules. They are among the most important rules any pupil can be taught and a great source of help to many spellers, not just dyslexics.

Root
The root is the main part or the stem of a word. It can take a prefix or a suffix or even both. For example the root word 'form' can take the following prefixes:
(re)form, (de)form, (per)form, (in)form (uni)form

It can take the following suffixes:
form(ed), form(ing), form(er)

It can use both a prefix and a suffix:
(per)form(ance)
(in)form(er)

Prefix
A prefix is a letter or a group of letters that go at the beginning of a word and usually changes the meaning of a word. (Many of these words are derived from Latin or Greek.) Commonly used ones are:
'il' **il**legal
'in' **in**correct
're' **re**take
'mis' **mis**take
'de' **de**form
'per' **per**form

121

Suffix

A suffix is a letter or a group of letters used at the end of a word which changes the use of the word. Frequently used ones are:

'ed' form**ed**

'er' form**er**

'ing' form**ing**

'able' formid**able**

To reinforce these concepts Stirling (1990) suggests picking out ten words from the daily newspaper, with the pupil, and then asking him to identify the root word, prefix and/or suffix.

- **The One-One-One Rule**
  Words that have one syllable, one short vowel and end with one consonant double the consonant before adding a suffix beginning with a vowel:
  run (root word) → runn**er** runn**ing**
  wet (root word) → wett**er** wett**est**

- **The Lazy 'e' Rule I says:**
  Drop the 'e' before adding a suffix beginning with a vowel:
  like (root word) → lik**ed** lik**ing** lik**en**

- **The Lazy 'e' Rule II**
  Keep the 'e' before adding a suffix beginning with a consonant:
  hope (root word) → hope**ful** hope**less**

- **The Lazy 'e' Rule III**
  Keep the 'e' in words ending in 'ce' or 'ge' when adding the suffixes 'ade', 'able' and 'ous':
  orange (root word) → orange**ade**
  service (root word) → service**able**
  advantage (root word) → advantage**ous**

- **The 'y' Rule I**
  Change the 'y' to an 'i' when adding a suffix:
  rely (root word) → rel**ied** rel**iable**

- **The 'y' Rule II**
  Keep the 'y' when adding the suffixes 'ing', 'ish' and 'ist':
  copy (root word) → copy**ing** copy**ist**
  baby (root word) → baby**ish**

- **The 'y' Rule III**
  Keep 'y' if there is a vowel before the 'y' when adding a suffix:
  employ (root word) → employ**ed** employ**er** employ**ing**

17 'shun'

There are four different ways to spell 'shun' but none are spelt like that sound. They are:

'ssion' – progression, profession, discussion, session, mission
'tion' – prevention, protection, detention, station, information
'cian' – politician, musician, electrician, physician, technician
'sion' – decision, precision, incision, confusion, revision

Rule Breakers!
cushion, suspicion, coercion

18 Rules for making nouns plural

- **Add 's'**

  The most common way to make a noun plural is to add 's'.
  (Check that pupils can differentiate between 's' or 'x' at the end
  of a word – fox, box, bus, gas):
  cat → cats
  pin → pins

- **Add 'es'**

  Nouns ending in 'ch', 'sh', 's', 'x' or 'z' add 'es' in the plural:
  church → churches
  wish → wishes
  bus → buses
  fox → foxes
  buzz → buzzes

- **Nouns ending in 'f' change 'f' to 'v' and add 'es' in the plural:**
  wife → wives
  leaf → leaves
  shelf → shelves

  Rule Breakers! Some just add 's'
  roofs, cliffs, chiefs, hoofs, reefs, dwarfs, gulfs, chefs, waifs,
  handkerchiefs

- **Nouns ending in 'y' change 'y' to 'i' and add 'es' in the plural:**
  lady → ladies
  copy → copies
  penny → pennies

  Rule Breakers! If there is a vowel before the 'y' just add 's':
  donkeys, toys, keys, valleys

- **Nouns ending in 'o'**
  Some add 's' and others add 'es' in the plural:
  Add 's':
  piano → pianos
  solo → solos
  banjo → banjos
  Eskimo → Eskimos
  soprano → sopranos
  curio → curios
  dynamo → dynamos

Add 'es':

negro → negroes
potato → potatoes
hero → heroes
cargo → cargoes
tomato → tomatoes
volcano → volcanoes
echo → echoes

- **'en'**

  Some 'Old English' words add 'en' in the plural:

  ox → oxen

- **Foreign words**

  Words derived from foreign languages often follow the rules of their own language:

  gâteau → gâteaux (French)
  alga → algae (Latin)
  phenomenon → phenonema (Greek)

- **Compound nouns**

  These have to be learned:

  man-of-war → men-of-war
  passer-by → passers-by
  man-servant → men-servants
  brother-in-law → brothers-in-law

- **Some nouns are the same in the plural:**

  deer
  sheep
  salmon
  trout

- **Some nouns are always plural:**

  braces
  scissors
  shorts
  tongs
  pants
  measles
  trousers
  suds

- **'Oddbods'**

  mouse → mice
  tooth → teeth
  foot → feet
  goose → geese (but mongooses)
  man → men

19 'i' before 'e' except after 'c' when it rhymes with me
field
priest

Rule Breakers! seize, protein, leisure
When it says /ay/, it is spelt 'ei' – 'neighbour' and 'weight'.

What else can be taught to help spelling?

Silent letters

Silent letters can be difficult but they need to be taught. To draw attention to the silent letter, it helps to brand them as The Stealthy Robbers (i.e. the letters that try to steal away so that you do not hear them).

Silent 'b'

bomb	doubt	subtle
comb	lamb	thumb
crumb	numb	tomb
debt	plumber	

Silent 'k'

knapsack	knight	knot
knave	knit	know
knead	knob	knowledge
knee	knock	
knife	knoll	

Here's a tongue twister to reinforce the silent 'k':

'The knight knocked a knave on his knuckle with a knotted knob, he knew when he knelt on his knees he had a knife in his knitted knickers.'

Silent 'c'

descent	discipline	science

Silent 'h'

heir	honest	honour	hour

A mnemonic can help to reinforce the silent 'h': 'it will be an honour to meet the honest heir in an hour's time'

Silent 'p'

pneumatic	pneumonia	psalm	psychology

Silent 'i'

business	marriage	parliament

Silent 'l'

chalk	folk	walk	yolk

Silent 'w'

wrong	wrap	wrath	write	
wrench	wriggle	wrinkle	wrist	wreck

Silent 'g'

gnat	gnome	gnash	gnaw
campaign	design	neighbour	sign

Silent 'n'

autumn	column	damn	solemn

Silent 't'

castle	listen

The horrible homophones!

Introduce the homophones gradually and practise them constantly. They are a constant source of grief. The essential ones are given below with a few suggestions to help spell them and to remember 'which is witch'.

to – two – too
I go to school.
We have two cars.
He is too tired.

here – hear
Remember! You hear with an ear.
I can hear the dog bark.
She sat here on the floor.

their – there – they're
Remember! If there can be a 'my', spell 'their' with an 'i'.
You can say 'My house is big.' You can say 'Their house is big.'
You can't say 'He lives my.' But you can say 'He lives there.'
You can't say 'My in the garden.' But you can say 'They're in the garden.'

herd – heard
Remember! You hear with an ear.
I heard the phone.
The farmer has a herd of cattle.

one – won
Remember! If you can win it then it has to have a 'w'. 'They win a prize' could be 'They won a prize'.

I have one sister.
They won a prize.

by – buy – bye
I go by car to school.
I must buy a new pen.
He waved goodbye.

sea – see
I can swim in the sea.
Did you see the boy?

meet – meat – mete
Remember! We eat meat.
I will meet you in London.
We had to eat the meat.
The bully will mete out blows to the other boys.

(The word 'mete' is of academic interest as it is a slightly archaic word and the dyslexic pupil has enough spelling to master without burdening him with this.)

beach – beech
Remember! The tree is a beech.
The beach was sandy.
We have a copper beech tree in our garden.

past – passed
Remember! Passed is a verb – a doing word.
Mary passed her driving test.
In the past we lived in France.

no – know
The answer is no.
She and I know the answer.

made – maid
Mummy made a cake.
The maid served lunch.

fair – fare
That is a fair price and he must also remember that he could go to Beaconsfield Fair.
Peter paid his bus fare.

wait – weight
I can wait for my friend at the bus stop.
Guess the weight of the cake.

pair – pear – pare
I have a pair of shoes.
The ripe pear was delicious.
I can pare the skin off the apple.

peace – piece
I had a piece of pie.
We signed a peace treaty after the war.

Tackling the 'odd-bods' (irregular words)

The irregular words are those that cause most trouble to dyslexic spellers. Forgetting to double a consonant in a multi-syllabic word may be forgivable but teachers, employers and examiners get quite irate when common words, such as 'four', 'fourteen', 'forty', 'fourth' and 'fortieth' are spelt incorrectly. Unfortunately these common words can often be among the most difficult for a dyslexic pupil because they are often not spelt as they are sounded.

A list of the 100 most commonly misspelt words is helpful (see Appendix V). Work through these in a systematic way, and review and revise frequently using the SOS method (see page 108). Some pupils find it helpful to use the Fernald method (see page 108) to memorize the 'odd-bods'.

Teach mnemonics

The dictionary definition of mnemonic is:

a device or a system for improving memory

Source: Sykes J. B. (ed) (1982) *Concise Oxford Dictionary* (7th edition). Clarendon Press, Oxford.

It is derived from the Greek word for 'remember'. Thomson and Watkins (1990) told us that 'mnemonics can be a very useful tool for the spelling of those difficult words that are resistant to learning any other way'. The pupil and the teacher should make up a sentence containing all or parts of the word that the pupil finds difficult to spell, for example the sentence 'Have a piece of pie' helps to highlight that the word 'piece' contains the letters 'pie'. Write these out and highlight the relevant letters. The pupil remembers them better if he makes up his own sentences. The pupil's personal mnemonics should be put on a card index and reviewed constantly.

are 'are rhinos elegant?'

beautiful 'boys eat apples under trees in France until lunch'

because (there are two different ones for this but it does not still guarantee that they will be learned for automatic recall!)

'**b**aby **e**ats **c**ake **a**nd **u**ncle sells **e**ggs'

'**b**ig **e**lephants **c**an **a**lways **u**pset **s**maller **e**lephants'

believe 'never believe a **lie**'

build '**u** and **i** will build a house'

business 'Do your **bus**iness in the **bus**'

busy 'a **bus** is **busy**'

cemetery 'we **met** in the cemetery'

come 'come **on my** elephants'

could 'could old uncle lie down?'

does 'Does Oliver eat sausages?'

double/trouble '**o**, **u** be Mrs Ott's double trouble'

forty 'The Lord fasted **for** forty days and nights'

fourth 'the **four**th number is **four**'

friend '**i** to the end will be your friend'

'I have **fri**ends round on **Fri**day'

great 'it's great to **eat**'

intelligent 'Tell the **gent** to come in'

island 'an island **is land**'

lieutenants '**lie** under **ten ants**'

many 'there is one **man** too **many**'

mother '**Moth**er has a **moth**'

parallel 'parallel has three lines'

piece 'eat a **pie**ce of **pie**'

present 'She **sent** a present'

said '**s**aid Aggie **I**'m dizzy'

should 'should old uncle lie down?'

some 'some **of my** elephants are fun'

special 'a **special** agent is someone in the **CIA**'

sure 'save up red elephants'

Tuesday 'u eat sweets day'

Thursday 'This is the u r sick day'

turn 'Do not do a u turn'

Wednesday 'Nes was wed on Wednesday'

'We do not eat sweets day'

whether 'I wonder whether he will marry her?'

would 'would old uncle lie down?'

Syllables and syllable division techniques

Syllables and syllable division techniques are a great boost to dyslexic spellers. Miles (1993) said that 'it is a skill which they sometimes do not acquire unless they are explicitly shown how to do so'. These techniques take away the fear of long words and can help to boost the confidence of the weakest spellers. According to Thomson and Watkins (1990), 'this breaking up of the words into smaller units draws attention to the fact that each syllable is in fact easy to spell'.

Teaching syllable division techniques is slow and time consuming. Like the teaching of all other skills to dyslexic pupils, it must be taught in a structured and sequential manner with many opportunities for overlearning and reinforcing. Cox and Hutcheson (1988) said that 'practice in reading at least 50 words (while meticulously employing each step multi-sensorially) was found to be necessary in order to build the procedures into students' reflexes – which was the ultimate goal'.

Suggestions for teaching syllables and syllable division techniques

1 What is a syllable?
A simple definition is that it is a beat. A syllable can be a word or part of a word:

'pup' or 'a | bout'

Every syllable must have one vowel sound but sometimes that can be two vowels making one sound:

train

Teach this fact very early on.

2 Introduce and heighten awareness of syllables

- Ask the pupil to put his hand (with the back of the palm) flat under his chin. Then ask him to say a word. Then ask him what happened to his hand. Then ask him how many times his chin touched his hand:
  once when he said Bob
  twice when he said Pip | pa
  three times when he said Re | bec | ca

- Clap out the number of syllables in a word.

- The pupil counts the number of syllables while the teacher says longer words aloud. He uses the thumb of the non-writing hand, then the index finger and middle finger to count the first, second and third syllable.

- 'Lap-Slap' spelling (Koontz, 1994) helps to spell two-syllable words. The teacher says the word, the pupil echoes the word and then spells it aloud while slapping out its letters on the left knee with the left hand (if he is right handed).

3 Teach each kind of syllable

There are six different kinds of syllable: closed, open, vowel–consonant–e, diphthong, consonant–'l–e' and 'r'–combination.

Thomson and Watkins (1990) advised that 'approximately one week needs to be spent on each type of syllable'. Revision of long and short vowels is also helpful at this stage.

a) Closed syllables

A closed syllable ends in a consonant and the vowel is short. It can be encouraging to tell the pupil that 'closed syllables account for 43 per cent of all syllables' (Stanback, 1992). A visual aid, story and/or physical demonstration can help.

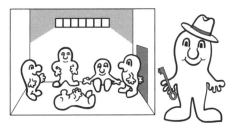

CLOSED SYLLABLE ROOM
The door is closed by Mr Consonant.
Vowel Men are shut in, we can only
hear their sound.

Ask the pupil to go outside the classroom door. Then tell him to close it. Whisper quietly. Then ask the pupil to come back into the room. Ask him if he could hear the whispering. He should answer no because the door has been closed, so he could not hear what had been said. This is what Mr Consonant does.

b) Open syllables

Open syllables end in a vowel and the vowel is long. Again, a visual aid and story can help.

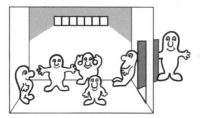

OPEN SYLLABLE ROOM
Mr Long Vowel opens the door.
When the door is open you can see the Long Vowel Men and you can call them by their names.

Ask the pupil to go outside the door. Ask him to leave the door open and call him by his name. This is what Mr Long Vowel does to the vowels.

Before proceeding to the next step, use a worksheet with a mixture of closed and open syllables to ensure that they are clearly recognizable and easily differentiated by the pupil.

c) Syllable division

Before teaching syllable division, rehearse and check that the pupil can recognize, read and spell the consonant digraphs, the blends and the assimilations:

- underline the digraphs: ship, dash, rich, chum
- code the vowels: shĭp, dăsh, rĭch, chŭm
- read the word: ship, dash, rich, chum

This awareness that certain letter clusters go together is important when the pupils needs to divide multi-syllabic words. There are four important steps in syllable division.

- Underline the vowels:
  combat, convent

  Remember! Each syllable will have only one vowel sound.

- Put the index finger of each hand on the lines under the marked vowels:

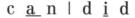

c a n | d i d

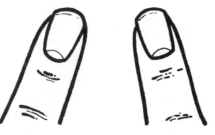

- Divide the word with a syllable division line between the two consonants:
  pup | pet
  rab | bit
- Read the word.
  Remember! A syllable division line usually comes between two consonants.

The pupil needs to work on words as follows:
- underline the vowel:
         magnet   velvet   fantastic   indignant
- divide the word:
         mag | net   vel | vet   fan | tas | tic   in | dig | nant
- code the vowels:
         măg | nĕt   vĕl | vĕt   făn | tăs | tĭc   ĭn | dĭg | nănt
- read the word:
         magnet   velvet   fantastic   indignant

It is very important that the pupil is encouraged to use his fingers as shown above.

- He then can work on words with open and closed syllables:
  sī | lĕnt
  ē | vĭl

- He can proceed to words with closed–open–closed syllables:
  dĭp | lō | măt
  ŏc | tō | pŭs

d) Vowel–consonant–'e' syllables

Revise Magic 'e'.
hăt → hāte
pĕt → Pēte
pĭp → pīpe
cŏd → cōde
tŭb → tūbe

Work on mixed closed syllables and vowel–consonant–e syllables.
cŭt   fĭll   dōle   spīne

Then introduce closed syllables with Magic 'e' syllables.
mĕm | brāne   ĭm | pēde

e) Diphthong syllables

Two vowels making one vowel sound.

Remember the ditty 'When two vowels go out walking, the first vowel does the talking and often says its name'.
trāin   hēel

f) Consonant–'l–e' syllables

This syllable is at the end of the word. The 'e' at the end is silent.

ple – ăp ǀ ple	tle – whĭt ǀ tle
fle – rī ǀ fle	ble – bŭb ǀ ble
gle – shĭn ǀ gle	zle – mŭz ǀ zle
cle – cȳ ǀ cle	kle – wrĭn ǀ kle

To work out the syllable division cross out the 'e' then count back two letters and this is where the syllable division line should come.

g) 'r'–combination syllables

'r'–combination syllables are sometimes endings of words:

ar   er   or

But they each say /ĕr/.

cŏl ǀ lăr   cŏr ǀ nĕr   dŏc ǀ tŏr

Source: Steere A., Peck C. Z., and Kahn L. (1971) *Solving Language Difficulties: Remedial Routines.* Educators Publishing Service Inc., Cambridge MA.

Proof reading

Some authorities, such as Thomson and Watkins (1990), say that 'expecting dyslexics to proof read their own spelling is an unrealistic goal'. Unlike the average speller, dyslexics seem to be unable to correct their errors spontaneously as they write the word but they can be trained to look out for errors that are particular to them. The National Curriculum (1995) requires pupils at Key Stages 3 and 4 to proof read their writing and states that 'they should be taught to spell increasingly complex polysyllabic words that do not conform to regular patterns, and to proof read their writing carefully to check for errors, using dictionaries where appropriate'.

'b – d'

Miles (1993), like many who work with dyslexic children and adults, reported that there are persistent difficulties with remedying the reversal of 'b – d'. 'Where the dyslexic person has difficulty because of his weakness at verbal labelling, is with symbols. This means that in the one case of symbols which are also mirror images, one complication may aggravate the other'. Vellutino (1979) also argued that 'left-right confusions are functions of verbal labelling'. Denckla and Rudel (1976) agreed that 'there is evidence that dyslexic children have difficulty in providing a verbal label or name for visually presented material.'

Two illustrations can help the pupil remember which is which:

Mr bed

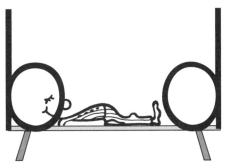

Mr bed can't lie down if the bed posts are on the wrong side.

Mrs BeD

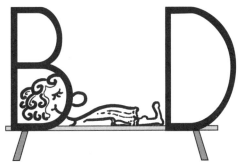

Mrs BeD can't lie down if the bed posts are on the wrong side.

Other teachers teach the pupil to remember which way 'b – d' go by training him to hold up his fingers as illustrated below. Ensure that the pupil puts his forearms on the table in front of him and that he turns his hands so that the knuckles touch each other when he holds up the thumbs.

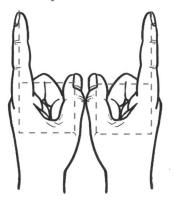

A useful way to remember how 'b–d' go, using fingers and thumbs.

Summary and conclusions

1 There are few absolute statements that can be made about spelling and dyslexics but many would agree with Snowling (1987) that 'most dyslexics fail to learn to spell effectively' and 'are also much slower, even when retrieving familiar word spellings'.

2 Dyslexic people's spelling errors have certain features which can be categorized and '[by] classifying errors in this way one is calling attention to dyslexic weaknesses which can be put right by teaching' (Miles, 1993). These features should help the teacher when assessing a pupil who has special educational needs.

3 Many of the normal classroom techniques used to teach spelling do not help dyslexics. Most people forget how they learned to spell and many have automatic recall of a word either through visual recall or phonological awareness.

4 Dyslexics need to be taught to spell using multi-sensory methods. The Orton–Gillingham principles of Simultaneous Oral Spelling (SOS) seem to be most effective.

5 All pupils, but especially dyslexic pupils, benefit from being taught the underlying principles of spelling. Dyslexics need to be taught spelling rules, even if they cannot always recall these. The structure and patterns they impose provide a framework on which to build a working knowledge of English spelling.

6 Thomson and Watkins (1990) stressed that 'the problem for dyslexics is of course homophones, spelling choices and irregular words'. These have to be taught in a structured way and need frequent reinforcing.

7 'Accuracy cannot always be achieved. To expect perfection is unrealistic and unkind' (Stirling, 1990). Writing comments on a dyslexic child's report such as 'his spelling is still poor' or 'his spelling still lets him down' has been likened to writing on a visually impaired child's report 'What a pity, he can't see very well.' Miles (1993) reminded 'examiners, prospective employers and others, that very strange spelling mistakes are not necessarily evidence of lack of ability'.

8 The National Curriculum (1995) places great emphasis on teaching spelling.

9 Much can be done to improve the dyslexic pupil's spelling, for example by teaching him to use mnemonics, prefixes and suffixes, and syllable division techniques.

Chapter 7

Mathematics

- identification and assessment
- the problems encountered by the dyslexic mathematician
- strategies and techniques to help

Introduction

In 1970, Critchley postulated that 'arithmetical retardation may be associated with developmental dyslexia but not necessarily so'. Since then there has been a growing awareness of the problem and by 1992 Miles T. R. was declaring that 'all or most dyslexics have mathematical difficulties of some kind, but these can be overcome to varying degrees and in some cases dyslexics can become extremely successful mathematicians'.

Until fairly recently there was very little published material in the UK on the subject, either on the prevalence or the characteristics of the problems experienced by dyslexic pupils. O'Leary (1995) reported that 'research is said to be fifteen years behind that for language dyslexia, and those who cannot master the simplest arithmetic are simply dismissed as slow learners'. There were few specific maths programmes which were widely used or accepted as useful by those working in the dyslexia field. There has been a lack of training and little expert knowledge and experience in ways to teach the pupil who is dyslexic and has mathematical difficulties. The gap has been partially filled by the publication in 1992 of *Dyslexia and Mathematics,* edited by Miles and Miles, and by the publication in 1993 of *Mathematics for Dyslexics: A Teaching Handbook* by Chinn and Ashcroft. The latter contains straightforward advice and is set to become a classic text for those who teach mathematics to dyslexic pupils. The ignorance surrounding the problem of dyslexia and mathematics was encapsulated by a maths teacher who commented that 'in twenty years of teaching maths I have never been aware of any specific problems in maths among dyslexics, and I have taught many dyslexic pupils'. Yet Joffe's (1980) research findings showed that of '800 diagnosed dyslexics … the findings that 61 per cent of them are retarded in arithmetic to some extent, is noteworthy'.

Steeves (1983) pointed out that 'the highly intelligent dyslexic, already an under-achiever in the area of language, becomes doubly handicapped if his or her mathematical talent is not fostered or challenged'.

Inclusion of mathematical difficulties in the definition of dyslexia

Definitions of dyslexia did not include mathematical difficulties until fairly recently. In 1988 Kavanagh and Truss defined a learning disability to include 'significant difficulties in the acquisition of mathematical abilities'. The BDA included mathematics in its definitions of dyslexia and defined dyscalculia as 'a dysfunction in the ability to organize and manipulate symbols as needed for mathematical processes. In particular, the recording and computation of digits are unreliable, not because of weak concept development or weak mathematical knowledge, but rather the result of directional or sequencing difficulties, usually congenital in origin' (BDA, 1981).

The prevalence of mathematical difficulties in dyslexic pupils

Joffe (1980) found that while about 12.5 per cent of dyslexics are good mathematicians and 'performed 18 months or more above their chronological age' and showed no particular difficulties, the remainder have some of the typical difficulties associated with dyslexia. Miles and Miles (1992) found this a 'simplistic' explanation in view of the fact that dyslexic pupils rarely have the same cluster of symptoms. Waddon (1975) said 'it seems that mild arithmetical problems of one sort or another are to be found in the majority of cases of dyslexia'. Miles (1974) took a broader view and said that 'the majority of dyslexics have difficulty in recalling and repeating multiplication tables, the difficulty is so widespread it cannot be accidental'.

The severity of the language problems experienced by the dyslexic pupil and his level of IQ also need to be considered when assessing mathematical attainments and potential.

Identifying mathematical problems in a dyslexic

Another reason that the prevalence and awareness of the mathematical problems experienced by dyslexics has been slow to emerge was that professionals in the diagnostic field, such as the educational psychologist, did not readily identify them in the pupil. Psychometric testing was a lengthy process and because of time restraints a standardized, written mathematics test was often not given. The 'arithmetic sub-test' in the WISC–R was given orally. Miles (1992) pointed out that 'any child, including a dyslexic, who has learned the names of the numbers and has grasped how the number system works, will almost certainly be able to do the first seven items in the test'. Items later in the test depend on a knowledge of tables, but a young child is not expected to know these. The results of this test therefore are not reliable indicators of mathematical strengths or weaknesses in young children. It is important to carry out written tests, examine the errors made and try to identify the cause of those in order to understand the nature and the extent of the difficulty. Lever (1994) pointed out that many of the published and standardized maths tests do not pinpoint or identify the dyslexic learner's specific problems and said that the 'norms' are unreliable. Chinn (1992) said 'full diagnosis requires a closer look at how children (and for that matter adults) *actually do* mathematics – at the errors which they make, and at the background skills which they bring to each problem'.

Standardized maths tests

The following tests may be administered by the classroom teacher or SENCO. They can be administered individually or to groups.

Basic Number Diagnostic Test (Gillham, 1980). Age range 5–7 years.

Basic Number Screening Test (Gillham and Hesse, 1976). Age range 7–12 years.

The Staffordshire Mathematics Test (Barcham, Bushell, Lawson and McDonnell, 1986). Age range 7–8 years 7 months.

Graded Arithmetic – Mathematics Test: Junior Form (Vernon and Miller, 1986). Age range 6–12 years.

Mathematics Competency Test (Vernon and Miller, 1986) Age range 11 to adult.

Specialist help

As with the pupil with intractable reading and spelling difficulties, once the problem has been identified the next step is to give specialist help. According to Pollock and Waller (1994), 'extra lessons which consist of more of the same, can aggravate children's feelings of failure and convince them that they will never be able to do maths'. To avoid this, the teacher needs to have an understanding and knowledge of dyslexia and the mathematical implications.

Recommended texts
Mathematics for Dyslexics: A Teaching Handbook (Chinn and Ashcroft, 1993)

Dyslexia and Mathematics (Miles and Miles, 1992)

What specific difficulties do dyslexic pupils have with mathematics?

In 1980 Joffe did pioneering research. Miles, Chinn and Sharma have spearheaded more recent interest in the recognition and awareness of the difficulties that dyslexic pupils have with mathematics. The *Code of Practice 1994* includes mathematics when describing children's special educational needs and says that in most cases, they will have difficulty acquiring basic literacy and numeracy skills and many will have significant speech and language difficulties.

For some time, teachers of children with specific learning difficulties have been aware that dyslexic pupils may have specific strengths and weaknesses. Some dyslexics have been described as good mathematicians and poor arithmeticians. They seem to have difficulties with operations which involve short term memory, sequencing, directional and spatial awareness, and language aspects of mathematics. Their workings and their work often display a particular pattern of errors. Some of these pupils, after resolving their initial difficulties, often go on to become highly skilled mathematicians.

Some pupils may find difficulties with some of the problems described below but few pupils will exhibit all these problems – the distinguishing feature is the unusualness of a problem and its persistence. It is well established that many dyslexics have a problem with spoken and written language. According to Chinn and Ashcroft (1993), 'difficulties in mathematics go hand in hand with difficulties in language'. It is often assumed that oral language develops naturally and that only written language needs to be explicitly taught. This is often not true for the dyslexic pupil. He needs to be taught the meaning of many words and concepts that the average learner acquires easily and automatically.

The language of mathematics

The language of mathematics can be confusing. Miles E. (1992) highlighted this by giving examples of the colloquial uses of words which have different meanings when used in a mathematical context, making them ambiguous or confusing for the dyslexic pupil.

'take away'	*Chinese take-away*
'square'	*Meet me in the square*
'division'	*Liverpool is in the first division*
'set'	*Tea set (set the table)*
'dividend'	*What Dad hopes to get from the Pools*

Street (1976) said 'the worst word was "write/right", "Put it on right" or "right we'll do another one", "write it down", "do that sum right away", "put it in the right place"'.

The dyslexic pupil may also struggle with the written aspects of the language, not least if he is a poor reader, and, according to Henderson (1989), 'if students already have reading difficulties, then a written maths problem is double trouble, for not only does it require reading with understanding, but also means identifying a problem that needs to be solved'.

Mathematical symbols

plus	+
minus	–
multiply	x
divide	÷

The four core mathematical symbols (or operators) can cause many problems.

This is not surprising because, according to Joffe (1983), 'written language and school mathematics share a lot of common features: both are universal languages consisting of arbitrary representational systems which are symbolically mediated'. Henderson (1989) said 'because of the dyslexic's distinctive weaknesses, the symbol/language connection needs continually to be talked about'. This symbol/language connection may also account for the fact that some dyslexic pupils find algebra terribly confusing because they have to cope with letters being used along with numbers. The way language is used, either formally or informally, when talking about mathematics also needs to be considered. Formally worded 'Divide the product of nine fours by three' would be less challenging when informally worded 'times nine by four and share into threes.' However, Pollock and Waller (1994) pointed out that additional problems can arise if the teacher uses different words to those in the textbook being used. Thus dealing with mathematical terminology and symbols may be very demanding for the dyslexic pupil. The pupil has to be able to name the sign *and* understand the process.

Henderson (1989) pointed out that the five core mathematical symbols have 27 words which may be used about them in varying contexts, and that the equals symbol also needs to be thoroughly understood (see opposite). Some pupils also have a problem recognizing, identifying and differentiating between the shapes of the signs. A child with directional or spatial difficulties may rotate the + sign reading it as x and so multiply the sum instead of adding it. It helps if the symbols are placed on card indexes or in a maths notebook to be used for reinforcement and revision.

Numerical problems ('word sums')

Vocabulary used in word sums can be deceptively familiar, and many simple and frequently used words have different meanings when used in a mathematical context. Louisa, an eight year old with a Full Scale IQ of 128, demonstrated this when reading the story sum 'Farmer Brown grew 378 carrots, 149 were too small to sell. How many carrots could he sell?' She enthused 'Oh! that's easy! Take "too" away from 378!'.

Sharma (1989) argued that 80 per cent of all people have difficulties with word problems (story sums). It is not surprising that dyslexic pupils experience particular difficulty with them, often with the mechanical reading of the sum before they even attempt to solve the problem.

Another pitfall (Eade, 1995) is that subtraction and division may be described by both active and passive forms of the verb:

6 take away 5 is not the same as 6 from 5

7 divided into 14 is not the same as 7 divided by 14

This may confuse a dyslexic pupil who has directionality difficulties.

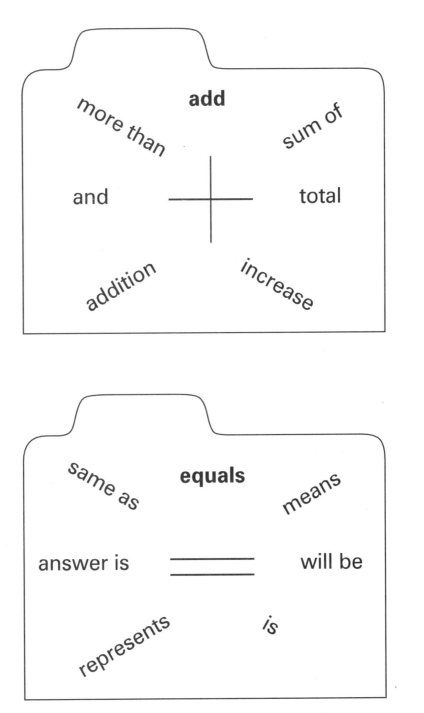

Source: Henderson A. (1989) *Maths and Dyslexics*. St David's College, Llandudno: 28–9.

Further information about Maths and Dyslexics may be found in *Maths for the Dyslexic: A Practical Approach* by Anne Henderson, published by David Fulton Publishers Ltd.

To establish abstract concepts

Multi-sensory teaching methods for mathematics are essential for dyslexics. The pupil needs to work with concrete objects, for example:

Dienes blocks

Cuisenaire rods

Matchsticks

Dried pulses

Map board pins

Straws

Lego bricks

Multi-sensory teaching methods

The pupil will need: Dienes blocks, including units and rods, a large piece of card with a place value grid drawn on it which has tens and units (T and U) marked on it (it is useful to laminate this with plastic so that the pupil can write on it again and again with a washable felt pen). (Nash, 1996)

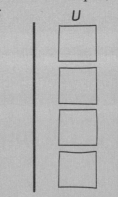

The teacher will need: a large + sign on a piece of card.

- The teacher says the following sum to the pupil: 'four add nine'.

- The pupil is then told to take four cubes of Dienes blocks and to place them in the units column of the grid and to count the blocks aloud at the same time as he places them on the grid.

- He counts out aloud nine further cubes and places these in the units column under the four cubes already there.

- He is told to put a plus sign at the left side of the grid (it is useful if the teacher has a large + sign on a piece of card for this purpose).

- He rules a line under the sum on the grid on the card so that the answer can be placed below it.

- He counts the total number of cubes in the units column of the grid and when he reaches ten he is told to exchange the ten cubes for one 'rod of ten' (which consists of ten cubes joined together).

- He places the 'rod of ten' in the tens column below the line which he has drawn.

- He leaves three cubes in the units column below the line.

- He then looks at the 'rod of ten' and the cubes sitting below the line and reads his answer.

- The teacher reinforces this by inspection of the cubes and points out that there is one ten and three units, making the total of thirteen.

- The pupil then opens his 1cm squared exercise book.

- He is instructed to write T and U in adjacent squares.

- The teacher repeats the sum, including the answer, to the pupil.

- The pupil repeats the sum and writes it down in the grid. He says that the answer is one ten, writing '1' in the tens column of the answer, and three, writing '3' in the units column of the answer.

- The teacher then asks him to read the sum and tell her the answer.

Money

Miles E. (1992) said that 'dyslexic children need to learn initially by operating with materials, only later should they be introduced to symbols'. Use plastic pieces of money which are available commercially. The practical operation should be carried out first.

Setting out money sums can be problematic. The pupil may be able to give the answer to a word sum which he does orally but writing down the answer to 'How much change will you have from five pounds if you spent three pounds 10p?' might result in the pupil writing down the answer as he would speak it – £190p.

Ensure the pupil uses multi-sensory techniques and verbalizes what he is doing.

When teaching about coins and signs, use a card index as follows:

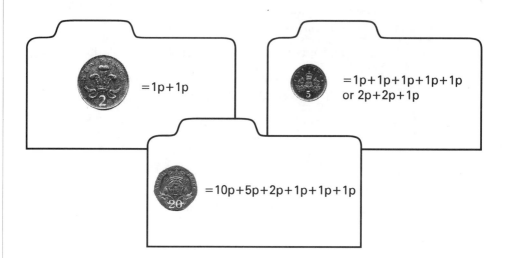

Source: Henderson A. (1989) *Maths and Dyslexics*. St David's College, Llandudno: 28–9.

Further information about Maths and Dyslexics may be found in *Maths for the Dyslexic: A Practical Approach* by Anne Henderson, published by David Fulton Publishers Ltd.

Times tables

'Almost all dyslexic pupils have difficulties in learning their tables and in reciting them, [they] may lose the place or become confused' (Miles T. R. 1992). Learning and saying tables is a continuous struggle because pupils may have auditory sequential memory deficits. Miles T. R. (1992) identified the main difficulties:

- Losing their place:

    $6 \times 2 = 12$
    $6 \times 3 = 18$
    $6 \times 4 = 24$
    $6 \times 7 = 30$

    'Where was I ?'

- Attempting to lessen the verbal load:
  Pupils might respond, 'seven, fourteen, twenty-one' instead of 'one seven is seven', etc.
- The 'consistent' error:
  6 x 3 = 20
  7 x 3 = 23
- Confusing the tables:
  7 x 3 = 21
  3 x 8 = 24
  4 x 8 = 32
  (when doing the three times table).
- Some lose their place and go back and repeat it:
  4 x 6 = 24
  6 x 6 = ?
  4 x 6 = 24
  5 x 6 = 30
  6 x 6 = 30
- Some will skip a few facts and finish with a great flourish having already got lost on the earlier part of the table:
  10 x 7 = 70
  11 x 7 = 77
  12 x 7 = 84

It is important to give the dyslexic pupil as many different aids to learning as possible. Each individual has a different cognitive style, meaning that it might be necessary to stimulate several different senses before the 'right' one is activated.

The work of Bath and Knox (1984) described the two different working methods and approaches that pupils have in mathematics. They dubbed these the 'grasshopper' and the 'inchworm' approach. The 'inchworm' follows processes step-by-step, for example when doing mental arithmetic he will work it out carefully in a linear fashion or will follow formulas. The 'grasshopper' takes a global view – even estimation – and will have devised some unorthodox strategies to arrive at the answer. For a full description see Chinn and Ashcroft (1993).

It is important for the teacher to be aware of the different cognitive styles of the individual pupil and to tailor the method of teaching to what best suits the individual pupil.

It is useful if there is a whole school policy on the method used when learning and reciting times tables to avoid the confusion and frustration that may arise when individual teachers use different methods.

Suggestions
to help with the times tables

- Use concrete materials to establish an understanding of the concepts. To teach the pupil the three times table, use map pins stuck into a cork pinboard. He should then copy the table into a maths notebook using the multi-sensory method – saying it aloud, for example 'one three is three', so that he hears it; writing it down using his muscles and memory; then reading it back using his eyes.

- Be consistent with the wording when repeating the times table. Always use the same format. There are two alternatives for reciting the times tables:

2 x 0 = 0	or	0 x 2 = 0
2 x 1 = 2		1 x 2 = 2
2 x 2 = 4		2 x 2 = 4
2 x 3 = 6		3 x 2 = 6

- Teach the times tables in the following order:

  2 x

  1 x

  0 x

  10 x

  11 x

  3 x

  4 x

  5 x

  9 x (with the 'trick' method first and then without it)

  6 x

  7 x

  8 x

  12 x

- A number of hints can be put on a card index to be used by the pupil for quick reference:

When you times 0 by a number, the answer is 0	**When you times 1 by a number the answer is that number**
0 x 8 = 0	1 x 7 = 7
16 x 0 = 0	1 x 259 = 259
421 x 0 = 0	

When you times 5 by an even number, the answer will be even and will end in 0

10   20   30

When you times 5 by an odd number the answer will be odd and will end in 5

5   15   25

The even number trick
For 5 times table
'What is half of 4, 8, 10?'
Then $4 \times 10 = 40$
$8 \times 10 = 80$
$10 \times 10 = 100$
So 5 x these numbers is half
$4 \times 5 = 20$
$8 \times 5 = 40$
$10 \times 5 = 50$

9 x trick method
$1 \times 9 = 9$
$2 \times 9 = *18$
$3 \times 9 = *27$
$4 \times 9 = *36$
$5 \times 9 = *45$
$6 \times 9 = *54$
$7 \times 9 = *63$
$8 \times 9 = *72$
$9 \times 9 = *81$

* the first number of the answer is 1 less than the number being multiplied by 9.

The two numbers in the answer should together add up to 9.

10 times table
When you x 10, add on 0
to the other number.
$4 \times 10 = 40$

11 times table
When you x 11
double the other number.
This works up to 99.

Multi-sensory teaching of times tables
- The pupil may make his own tape of the times tables and play it back. He should write down the answers and play back the tape listening to and reciting the tables as he checks his work.

  Times table tapes are available commercially on audio and video cassette.

Times table square
- Teach the pupil how to use the times table square and encourage him to say his workings out loud as he uses it. Make him his own copy to use. There are two forms of the times table square, as follows. Use one form consistently at home and throughout the school, otherwise existing directionality difficulties can be exacerbated.

x	0	1	2	3	4	5	6	7	8	9	10	11	12
0	0	0	0	0	0	0	0	0	0	0	0	0	0
1	0	1	2	3	4	5	6	7	8	9	10	11	12
2	0	2	4	6	8	10	12	14	16	18	20	22	24
3	0	3	6	9	12	15	18	21	24	27	30	33	36
4	0	4	8	12	16	20	24	28	32	36	40	44	48
5	0	5	10	15	20	25	30	35	40	45	50	55	60
6	0	6	12	18	24	30	36	42	48	54	60	66	72
7	0	7	14	21	28	35	42	49	56	63	70	77	84
8	0	8	16	24	32	40	48	56	64	72	80	88	96
9	0	9	18	27	36	45	54	63	72	81	90	99	108
10	0	10	20	30	40	50	60	70	80	90	100	110	120
11	0	11	22	33	44	55	66	77	88	99	110	121	132
12	0	12	24	36	48	60	72	84	96	108	120	132	144

12	12	24	36	48	60	72	84	96	108	120	132	144
11	11	22	33	44	55	66	77	88	99	110	121	132
10	10	20	30	40	50	60	70	80	90	100	110	120
9	9	18	27	36	45	54	63	72	81	90	99	108
8	8	16	24	32	40	48	56	64	72	80	88	96
7	7	14	21	28	35	42	49	56	63	70	77	84
6	6	12	18	24	30	36	42	48	54	60	66	72
5	5	10	15	20	25	30	35	40	45	50	55	60
4	4	8	12	16	20	24	28	32	36	40	44	48
3	3	6	9	12	15	18	21	24	27	30	33	36
2	2	4	6	8	10	12	14	16	18	20	22	24
1	1	2	3	4	5	6	7	8	9	10	11	12
x	1	2	3	4	5	6	7	8	9	10	11	12

Initially it is helpful to point out that multiplication is a quick method of repeated addition.

The table square builds confidence, helps to build the concept of visual patterns and increases an awareness of their value in mathematics. Efficient use of the table square can lighten considerably the 'load' of material to be learned.

Encourage the pupil to look at the patterns:

10 times rises in tens: 10, 20, 30, 40 etc.

Colour in relevant numbers of the times table being tackled.

Make the pupil aware that 7×3 is the same as 3×7.

Draw the pupil's attention to the patterns/tables he already knows – 2, 4, 6, 8 etc. of the 2 times table.

Point out to the pupil that if he already knows his ten times table, then he can then do his five times table using the 'even number trick', outlined on page 149.

The gypsy method

- There are different tactics that can be used to teach the times tables, such as the Gypsy method. Some authorities frown on the use of these tactics as they fear that the pupil will not have understood the processes involved or the pattern but it is important to give the dyslexic pupil any crutches that may help him.

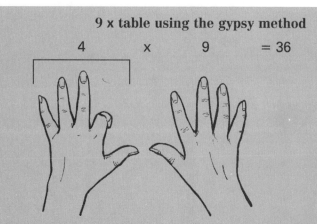

9 x table using the gypsy method

4   x   9   = 36

Hold both hands out in front, palms facing downwards. Tuck away the number finger that is to be multiplied by nine (in the example illustrated this is the fourth finger). The number of the fingers to the left of this finger stands for the tens. In the example given, there are three fingers to the left, therefore the answer will be thirty-something. To find the 'something' (or the units), count the number of fingers to the right of the tucked away finger. In the example given, there are six fingers to the right. Therefore, the answer to 9 x 4 is 36.

Calculators

The calculator is a godsend to the dyslexic pupil but it does not answer all his problems. To be most useful, it should have a large, bold display. Coloured calculators are very helpful. Teach the pupil how to use it and ensure that he *fully understands* how to use it. Make sure he brings it to all his lessons and practises using it. Also ensure that the pupil has been taught and uses estimation to check his calculations. It is vital to teach him to do this as a way of 'proof reading' what he does. The dyslexic who has a problem with sequencing may press the wrong buttons and in the wrong order. If the pupil is to sit an examination or test, it is important to discover well in advance whether or not the use of a calculator is allowed.

Multi-sensory teaching methods are helpful when using the calculator. Encourage the pupil to read the numbers aloud. Henderson (1989) gave a useful hint and said 'if the answer is constantly read incorrectly from the calculator, read on to a tape and play back to check'. This heightens awareness of the difficulties. A pupil who has difficulty transferring a column of he may *say* three times seven is twenty one but then reverse numbers and *write* 12, giving the incorrect answer:

$$\begin{array}{r} {}^{1}27 \\ \times \quad 3 \\ \hline 72 \end{array}$$

A lack of understanding of the propositions 'before/after' and 'past/to' cause great difficulties. Dyslexics find sums such as the following very challenging:

Underline the correct answer for 8 years after 869 from the following:

795, 848, 935, 877, 1008.

Underline the correct answer for 50 years before the year 1655 from the following:

1495, 1605, 1753, 1381.

Re-order the digits in each of these numbers to make the highest number possible: 29534, 35890, 17852.

Decimals

Dyslexic pupils often fail to understand the significance of the decimal point. This is hardly surprising as the same pupil may be struggling with full stops when reading. If asked to do the following sum:

1.9 + .93 + 19.2

the pupils may set it down as follows:

$$\begin{array}{l} 1.9 \\ .93 \\ 19.2 \end{array}$$

and attempt to work out the answer accordingly.

Further problems can arise with the multiplication of decimals. The pupil may have a tendency to line up the decimal point as when he is doing an addition or a subtraction sum rather than counting the appropriate number of decimal places and then inserting the decimal point.

$$\begin{array}{r} 21.4 \\ \times \quad .22 \\ \hline 428 \\ 4280 \\ \hline 47.08 \end{array}$$

figures accurately will be helped if he realizes that 'C' on a calculator clears the *last* item. If he pushes 'AC' he clears all the figures and he has to repeat the whole process again with its inherent risk of errors. (This does not apply to all makes of calculator, even though it is the method most frequently used, so check in the handbook for the alternatives.)

Directionality and sequencing

The orientation and directional confusion that dyslexics make when they reverse words or alphabetical symbols such as:

'b'   'd'

'p'   'q'

is very similar to the errors that they make with mathematical symbols:

2 may be written as 5

6 and 9 confused

3 may be written as 8

4 may be written as 4 which can be confused with 9

Left-to-right confusions in mathematics are not helped by the fact that the usual way of working in mathematics is in the opposite direction to that when reading.

Some children have difficulty when it comes to setting out sums. For example:

19 + 302 + 9

When the pupil writes it vertically in his book, it may be written

```
  19
 302
+  9
-----
 501
```

thus resulting in an incorrect answer.

Sequencing difficulty (putting letters in the right order) may also apply to numbers. When asked to add 24 and 8, the pupil may orally give the correct answer 32, but may write it down as 23.

Likewise, when asked to multiply:

```
  27
x  3
----
```

Subtraction

Subtraction creates great difficulties and 'dyslexics remain weak at subtraction' (Miles and Miles, 1983). A dilemma is which number goes at the top and which goes at the bottom, for example in the sum 9 from 12. They often find decomposition (borrowing) difficult to remember, sometimes forgetting to borrow, for example:

$$
\begin{array}{r}
4\ 3 \\
-\ \ \ 9 \\
\hline
4\ 6
\end{array}
$$

This shows that he has subtracted the 3 from the 9 instead of doing it the other way around. At other times they may borrow but forget to write it down, for example:

$$
\begin{array}{r}
4^{1}3 \\
-\ \ \ 9 \\
\hline
4\ 4
\end{array}
$$

Multiplication

Dyslexics have difficulty remembering that when doing a multiplication sum, they should go from right to left on the page.

Division

The pupil has to go from left to right on the page. Some forget this, as can be seen from the following example. When asked to do this sum:

$$27 \div 3$$

the pupil copied it down as:

$$
\begin{array}{r}
2\ 7 \\
\div\ \ \ 3 \\
\hline

\end{array}
$$

and calculated his answer by using a combination of addition and division methods and this was the result:

$$
\begin{array}{r}
^{1}27 \\
\div\ \ \ 3 \\
\hline
4\ 2
\end{array}
$$

He said:

- 'Start with the units
- 7 divided by 3 is 2 and 1 left over
- Put 2 down and carry the 1
- Now go to the 10s
- 12 divided by 3 is 4
- The answer is 42.'

The division symbol can also cause problems for dyslexics. A gifted dyslexic pupil persistently used ÷ sign incorrectly. He reversed it thus ⁒ so that it looked like a percentage sign: a significant error because a percentage relates to a fraction, for example 25 % = 1/4, therefore the '1' has to go at the top of the line and the '4' at the bottom of the line to give the correct value.

Long division, where you start at the left and work right, can be a nightmare because it involves multiplication and subtraction in specific sequence, with the overall operation of division.

Time

Chinn and Ashcroft (1993) reported that 'being unable to tell the time is a classic weakness for dyslexics'. They often need considerable practice in saying and writing the time. Confusion is caused because time is written and spoken differently:

'twenty-five past eleven' is written '11.25'.

Dyslexic pupils often have difficulty understanding words connected to time and dates: 'last week', 'next week' and 'the week before last' perplex them. It can take much longer than average to establish that there are 60 minutes in an hour and 24 hours in a day, as well as all the practical conclusions that are drawn from that.

Anecdotal evidence suggests that many dyslexics are over nine before they can read an analogue watch and that they find a digital watch less difficult. Chinn and Ashcroft (1993) commented that 'the advent of the digital watch has enabled more children to say the time, but it has not necessarily enabled them to have a concept of time'. This lack of awareness of time, as distinct from saying the time, can have lifelong repercussions, for example constantly being late for appointments or missing deadlines for completing assignments. Professor Fellgett (1986) recalled that he was constantly being chided for his lack of punctuality and was given a watch. He continued to be late, and, on being asked why he did not look at his watch, replied 'How did I know when to look at my watch?' Some have little concept of time, for example a teenager may not be able to calculate whether it is break time or lunch time. Many cannot remember when their own birthday is. Another possible difficulty for the left-handed pupil is that his natural inclination is to turn the hands of the clock in the anti-clockwise direction when he is asked to move the hours forward.

Short term memory

Poor short term memory causes many problems for the dyslexic pupil and mathematician. Some are excellent at mental arithmetic and some make fewer errors than when they write it down, but others find it impossible to remember the process of the instructions. 'Mathematics is easy, only writing it down is hard.' (Chinn and Ashcroft, 1993)

It is often said of a dyslexic pupil that 'B does not listen, he needs to concentrate.' A stream of verbal instructions, of the sort commonly used in classrooms, will totally confuse the dyslexic pupil who may not remember anything beyond the first command. The pupil may quickly forget or confuse methods when they have not been used recently and even with reinforcement tasks set for homework he may sometimes forget how to do work he was handling competently in his lesson earlier in the day. Some pupils cannot even recall the method from the time it takes them to return to their own desk after the demonstration at the teacher's desk, often much to the irritation of their parents and teacher. Perhaps this is why dyslexic children are often described as 'disorganized' or 'inattentive'.

Hand–eye co-ordination

Some pupils have difficulty drawing lines, including margins, angles, axes and graphs, because of their poor hand–eye co-ordination. They cannot measure accurately from a diagram unless the diagram has been accurately constructed.

Fractions

Fractions cause enormous difficulties for dyslexic pupils. The language can be a major stumbling block (vulgar, denominator, improper). Establish basic concepts, such as a fraction is a part of a whole thing and that it is less than one. Reinforce these with practical demonstrations, such as cutting a cake into quarters.

The most difficult concepts to teach are the words used to describe how a fraction is written. The numerator tells how many pieces the cake has been cut into, for example, and the denominator tells how many equal pieces in the cake altogether. The following mnemonic is useful:

$$\frac{\text{Numerator}}{\text{Denominator}} = \frac{\text{North}}{\text{Down}}$$

Directionality difficulties can become an additional problem – $2/3$ of six. The use of mechanical or concrete symbols is essential. Again, concrete examples are best.

A chocolate bar can be broken up and shared out. A 100 g Cadbury's Dairy Milk Bar has eighteen squares. Do lots of work with it, breaking it up and sharing it. There is an inbuilt incentive at the end of the lesson that some may be eaten as a reward. Some teachers use a pizza to teach fractions.

Pollock and Waller (1994) said that 'fraction strips are far clearer than circles to demonstrate the understanding of an equivalent fraction'.

1 whole				
	$\frac{1}{2}$ half			
		$\frac{1}{3}$ third		
			$\frac{1}{4}$ quarter	
				$\frac{1}{6}$ sixth

Fraction strips

Chinn and Ashcroft (1993) recommend that the pupil learns about fractions by folding paper squares, and folding various fractions to establish the concept. They stress its multi-sensory implications by using paper, written and spoken versions:

Paper version	Written version	Spoken version
	1/5	one fifth
	3/5	plus three fifths
	4/5	four fifths

Suggestions

for teaching mathematics to dyslexic pupils

- Pay particular attention to teaching the pupils how to write the numbers and insist that they always begin at the top of the line.

- Check that the pupil can count backwards as well as forwards. It is often very difficult for them to count backwards.

- Put keywords on a card index system or in a maths notebook to be used for reference and revision.

- Rehearse mathematical vocabulary constantly, using multi-sensory methods.

- Use and encourage the use of estimation. Joffe (1980) noted that 'probably the best indicator of numeracy is estimation and this should be encouraged from an early age'. Parents can do a lot of useful work on this when the pupil is in the supermarket or helping with the preparation of food.

- Use concrete examples:
  'If I owe you £4.80 pocket money, how much change will I get from a ten pound note?' Round the figure up to five pounds, so the answer will be five pounds, roughly. Chinn and Ashcroft (1993) confirmed that 'the knowledge of money is a survival skill'.

- Use margins and a ruler. Use squared paper for as long as possible. Use a square for each figure. Paper with larger squares can be helpful.

- Encourage the pupil to use and show his 'rough' working on the page.

- Use concrete materials for as long as is necessary to establish a concept. A jar of sweets helps with addition or subtraction and can help to stimulate the most reluctant learner. Even teenage pupils may still require concrete materials to work with.

- Encourage the pupil to use an arrow to help him remember in which direction the sum goes.

- Put the decimal point in red ink. It helps visual perception.

- Teach and practise using the calculator and encourage the pupil to estimate his answer, just as he should proof read a written exercise for spelling and punctuation errors. It can often help to alert him to some of his errors, such as reversing a number.

- Be aware that the pupil may have reading difficulties. Many mathematics books are workbooks and often involve much reading, even at a very early age. The pupil's neighbour should be allowed to tell him the word if he can't remember what it says.

- It is important to explain to a pupil from a very early age that numbers are a bit like shorthand or a secret code. Use a number line containing the numbers 0–10. It is important that the number line should start at zero. This helps to avoid a common error when using a ruler of placing the 1 of the ruler at the beginning of the line to be measured. Get the pupil to practise counting using the number line:

Using $2 + 3$ the pupil first puts his finger on the number 2, then he counts with the finger starting on 3 and arrives at the answer 5. Encourage him to say aloud what he is doing. Make sure the number is by the line, otherwise the child may use the mark on the left or right.

0   1   2   3   4   5   6   7   8   9   10

- Many dyslexics, because of their lack of cerebral dominance, often remain confused about left and right. Teach the pupil to map read. This presupposes a sound knowledge of left and right and he may need lots of practice on this. Use simple games:

Simple Simon Says put your right arm out.

Read the signposts while in the car and get the child to tell you which way to turn.

- Some dyslexic pupils have difficulties when doing work with co-ordinates, where they need to remember the difference between (1, 3) and (3, 1):

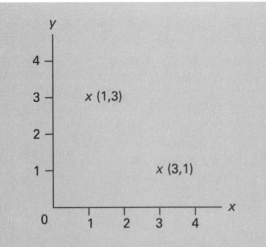

To remember that the x co-ordinate goes first, it may help to remember that the letter x is a cross. The following mnemonic is also helpful:

'go in the door, that is across; then up the stairs, that is upwards'. (Eade, 1995)

- Encourage the pupil to talk through a process. Multi-sensory techniques are very useful and important to the dyslexic learner.
- Use mnemonics as appropriate when teaching operations. The word:

B | ODM | AS

has been taught to generations of maths pupils to help them remember the order when doing the sum. The lines show the sequence of the operations, which is as follows:

1st	B	**B** rackets
	O	**O** f
2nd	D	**D** ivide
	M	**M** ultiply
3rd	A	**A** dd
	S	**S** ubtract

The lines are important as many dyslexics assume that the rule means they should do the operations in the order of the letters in the mnemonic, thus obtaining the wrong answer.

The following sum illustrates the point:

12 – 4 + 3

The pupil may do the adding before the subtraction, saying 3 + 4 = 7, then subtract it from 12 and the answer is 5.

The correct method is to take 4 from 12 which is 8, then add 3 and the answer is 11.

- To help pupils draw a line through two given points, for example to draw an axis or to draw part of the construction of a triangle:
  a) put the pencil on one of the given points
  b) put the ruler against the pencil
  c) holding the pencil fixed, turn the ruler so that it is next to the second point
  d) holding the ruler fixed, move the pencil on to the second point
  e) check that the ruler is touching the pencil at the second point
  f) move the pencil back to the first point and check that the ruler still touches it
  g) when the pencil touches the ruler at both points, rule the line.

- A number of mnemonics can help with teaching equations.

  Sin, Cos and Tan:

  'The Old American Sat On His Car And Hiccuped.'

  helps to recall:

  $$T = \frac{O}{A} \qquad S = \frac{O}{H} \qquad C = \frac{A}{H}$$

  Distance–Speed–Time calculations

$$D = S \times T$$

$$T = \frac{D}{S}$$

$$S = \frac{D}{T}$$

There is an unforgettable mnemonic to reinforce this:

'It's a Damn Silly Triangle.'

Some suggestions

to help the child aged beween four and seven

Number recognition

- The child can learn by counting the fish fingers on his plate. Then 'How many do we need altogether?' The next step could lead to counting the number in the packet. Montessori had many excellent ideas and much useful equipment for teaching number work, a lot of which could be used with all pupils to relate the numbers to everyday life.

- Put stickers or thimbles on the child's fingers. Number these one to ten. Number one is the small finger of the left hand. Get the child to keep his palms facing downwards on the table. Ask him to show you number 'three'. Get him to touch his fingers with his other hand. Then get him to count out loud as he puts three buttons on the table. The parent can write '3' for the child. The child can then draw three cats, balls, etc.

- Make numbers fun and a challenge. For the child who has difficulty remembering how to write a '3' for example, use a card index and put the number in a large bright colour on the card. Then get the child to draw three cats or dinosaurs beside it as a further cue. Encourage him to use this as he works and to keep it on the desk in front of him.

- Teach the child to begin to write the number from the top of the number.

1 2 3 4 5 6 7 8 9

- Play games with codes:
  A=1; B=2; C=3, etc.

  Then write secret messages and letters.

Counting

- Encourage the child to count the steps as he climbs the stairs. Paving stones or floor tiles can also be used for counting. Later he can skip every second step and count in odd and even numbers. Shopping trips to the supermarket can be useful: 'Get me three bags of crisps.'

- Board games such as snakes and ladders, ludo, as well as card games such as cribbage and rummy, or playing dominoes, are excellent ways to help teach counting. They also help to teach the concepts that many dyslexic children find difficult – up/down, backwards/forwards, in front/behind.

Sequencing and short term memory

• Use songs and nursery rhymes:

'Ten Green Bottles Standing on the Wall'

'One, Two, Three, Four, Five, Once I Caught a Fish Alive'

'Five Green and Speckled Frogs'

'One, Two, Buckle my Shoe, Three, Four, Knock at the Door'

Unfortunately, many of these traditional games and jingles are dying out and children have often missed out on these important early learning devices.

Fractions

These can be introduced by first baking a cake, then cutting it in half, then quarters, etc. Remember that fractions are equal parts of a whole. Another idea is to cut up an apple. Domino games may be used for fractions.

Place value

Children need plenty of practice with this, to help them understand the place value each number holds. Practice reading numbers 2, 21, 201, 2001. Read the numbers on buses, shops and houses. Reading car number plates also helps.

Height

The concept of height can be introduced by having a chart on the back of a door. Measure the child from time to time to keep a record. Doctor's surgeries often have commercially produced versions. A bar chart can be made and coloured in to compare the height of siblings in the family or pupils in the classroom.

Time

Being able to tell the time is a vital skill. Teach it by using an analogue clock. Use a working clock and practical examples: 'What time do you go to bed?' 'What time does a television programme start?'

• Use a paper plate as a clock when teaching the concept of 'half past' and 'quarter past'. Fold the 'clock' in half to demonstrate the before/after and half/quarter concepts.

Distance

Distance can be introduced by familiarizing the child with how the milometer on the car works. The child can then be shown and start to work out how many miles a particular journey has taken.

Money

Give pocket money from an early age. Encourage the child to see how many sweets he can buy for 20p if each one costs 5p.

Nought/zero/nothing

Ensure that the child understands the concept of nought, zero, nothing. Use plenty of concrete examples to emphasize and reinforce this because if not properly understood, it can cause problems later when writing or reading numbers.

Maths assessment report

Any assessment of a pupil's mathematical difficulties should include an analysis of his errors. This can then serve as the basis of the remedial programme. Remedying some basic errors can result in immediate, visible progress in the classroom.

Suggestions for
the format and layout of a maths assessment report

Name

Date of birth

Chronological age *8.3 years*

Verbal IQ *127*   **Performance IQ** *105*

Full Scale IQ *118*

Name of assessor

Date of assessment

Reason for assessment

'E' enjoyed number work and seemed quite good orally. This year he has begun to learn times tables and has great difficulties. He now says he 'hates maths and can't do it'.

A report from his classroom teacher said that he works well under her guidance but once he is left to continue alone at his desk he struggles and seems to forget how to carry out operations he had previously undertaken successfully (but with supervision). This also happens when he is doing homework. His teacher said that orally he appears to be bright and occasionally shows good understanding.

Background information

He was diagnosed as dyslexic 15 months ago and was tested on the WISC–R. The psychologist's report noted that 'he scored well above average on four of the six subjects which evaluate the spoken language skills. It indicated that he found it extraordinarily difficult to do the Similarities test which is a measure of verbal concepts. His lowest score which was well below average was on the Digit Span test, which is a test of auditory memory. He scored poorly on the Coding test which is indicative of a visual sequential memory problem. He has a specific learning disability of written language (sometimes referred to as dyslexia) which is expressed in the form of underachievement in reading and spelling.' It is of academic interest that 'he scored well above level on the WISC oral Arithmetic sub-test. This would give him an arithmetic age equivalent to 12–18 months ahead of his chronological age'. He subsequently had specialist teaching for his literacy problems and is reported to be making very good progress but his parents and teachers have recently become aware that he is struggling with mathematics and initiated the present testing.

Family history

Mr 'E' said he still cannot remember some of his times tables. He failed Maths 'O' Level six times. He now runs his own successful film production company. 'E' has an older sister who has also been diagnosed as dyslexic but she does not appear to have any mathematical difficulties.

Behaviour and attitude

'E' was anxious and had a tendency to bite his nails. Initially, he tended to say 'I don't know' when asked some questions. Often, with encouragement, he produced the correct response, but would not attempt questions without this because of his fear of failure. He often needed reassurance and would say, 'Am I doing this right?' Gradually he relaxed and there was no evidence of a lack of concentration during the lengthy testing process.

Testing

Formal and informal tests were used, including the Gillham and Hesse *Basic Number Screening Test*. This test examines some of the basic principles underlying the number system and some of the processes involved in computation. 'E' obtained a raw score of 8, which has an equivalent number age of 7.9 years. Test scores can be converted to give a number age but it is also used diagnostically as it is more revealing to know 'how' he found the answers, including the strategies he used to do so, rather than whether they were right or wrong. In order to see what he is capable of and where the breakdown of skill occurs, the following concepts and number skills were examined. An analysis of his errors in tests and from those in his school exercise books revealed the following:

Rote knowledge

His ability to rote count in ones, fives, and tens was good. When counting in ones, he seemed to hesitate when crossing over into a new set of tens, for example from 59 to 60. He did not know immediately how to count in odd or even numbers and he had some difficulty with this, even when the sequence was started for him. He had a problem counting in threes, he said for example '3, 6, 10'. When counting in fours, he said '4, 8, 10, 14, 19'. He was able to give 'one more' and 'one less' than a number. When asked to give 'ten more' than a number, he worked it out using his fingers but was obviously unaware of the pattern. This underlines the finding that his concept of 'tens' and 'units' is weak. (See Place value.) He found it difficult to give a number which was 'ten less' than a given number. He was able to recite the days of the week but he was unable to say the months of the year in the correct order, he said '... September, November, October, December'. He had difficulty counting backwards from 30 to 0. These are difficulties of short term auditory sequential memory.

Directionality

He does not seem to have any difficulties with directionality. He could identify his right and left at all times, he was able to carry out instructions such as 'Touch your left ear with your right hand' and he could identify the tester's right and left.

The Four Operations (+ - x ÷)
He did not always use the given symbol, for example he did addition in a subtraction sum.

Addition
He used his fingers (and other apparatus, such as lines on the page, when he needed more than ten) to do addition. This indicates that he has a need for concrete apparatus. He did not always reach the correct answer. When doing addition with exchange (carrying) sums, he appeared to be confused about which number to carry. For example, in the sum

$$
\begin{array}{r}
47 \\
+ \quad 204 \\
+ \quad 369 \\
\hline
= \quad 602
\end{array}
$$

he added the units and got 20. He then wrote the 2 in the units column and carried the 0. However, when adding the tens, he found that $6 + 4 = 10$ and he correctly carried the 1 to the hundreds column. This inconsistency seems to indicate that he is learning the mechanics of the operation but that they are not yet entirely established. It also seems to indicate that the concept has not been fully understood.

Subtraction
On the subtraction tests, he showed a misunderstanding of the language and used it incorrectly. When given the sum

$$10 - 6 =$$

he said '6 take away 10'. He did however, get the correct answer. He also did not understand the language in the question 'What is the difference between 8 and 12?', his response was that 12 is bigger than 8.

His solution to the sum

$$
\begin{array}{r}
240 \\
- \quad 186 \\
\hline
= \quad 066
\end{array}
$$

indicated uncertainty about subtracting from 0.

Multiplication

It appears that the concept of multiplication is not entirely established. For example, when asked to do the sum 3 x 2, he was unable to do this. It was also evident that he had difficulties with times tables and he appeared to be anxious about his performance here. He said, 'We've done them at school but I keep forgetting them.'

Division

He did not know what to do when faced with a division sum. He was unfamiliar with the mathematical notation:

$6 \div 2$ or $2/48$

The term 'sharing' did not help him. As yet he has not understood the concept of division. Division is often particularly difficult for a dyslexic child. A major complication is that three of the four basic operations (addition, subtraction and multiplication) have to be started from the right, whereas division has to be started from the left.

Place value

He had difficulty with this. He could not write a number in expanded notation ($165 = 100 + 60 + 5$) and he had difficulty in identifying the value of a number in a specific place. For example, when asked to identify which number stood for the 'hundreds' in 2370, he could not do this.

Fractions

His concept of fractions seems to be evolving but is not well established. He was sometimes able to shade in a given fraction of a shape, but he was unable to provide the answer for $1/2$ of 8, $1/4$ of 12, etc. He also had difficulty with the formal notation of fractions, for example he had difficulty in writing that $1/4$ of a shape was shaded.

Money

He had some difficulty with word sums involving money. This appears to be related to his general difficulty with basic addition and subtraction. He also had a problem with 'story sums', such as 'I have 7p, Paul gives me 6p more. Then I give 4p to Jill. How much do I have now?' Many dyslexic children have difficulty with story sums because they have to interpret the language and then carry out the mechanical operations of the sum at the same time. His dyslexic difficulties may also interfere with his ability to extract the salient information in order to carry out the mathematical operations.

Shapes

He was able to name most of the shapes that were presented to him, but was unable to name a pentagon, cuboid or prism. This seems to indicate that he is learning the shapes' names but that they are not yet firmly established. This may be accounted for by his word retrieval problem which was also seen in the WISC sub-test.

Summary and conclusions

From the above assessment it appears that many mathematical concepts are beginning to be established. However, there are definite gaps in his knowledge and he is not functioning at the level that he should be. There is evidence of the difficulties that are often observed in children with specific learning difficulties. He is clearly underfunctioning in mathematics. His results in his recent school examination highlight his continuing struggles. In view of these findings, it was recommended that he should receive some help from a specialist teacher to help him reach his potential. He needs to follow a multi-sensory teaching programme. He will also need considerable overlearning so that the concrete and abstract aspects of maths become linked.

Summary and conclusions

1   Until fairly recently little was known about and not much attention was given to the mathematical difficulties of dyslexic pupils. There was disagreement both in naming the problem and in establishing its features. Experts disapprove of the term 'dyscalculia' as being too limiting.

2   There is a dearth of suitable standardized tests to diagnose the specific mathematical difficulties of dyslexic pupils. Early identification of their problems depends upon the experience and the skills of the diagnostician.

3   Many pupils display some of the same difficulties as dyslexic pupils, but the mathematical difficulties experienced by dyslexic pupils tend to be idiosyncratic. Their problems with the language of mathematics is striking. Understanding the words used, remembering the function of the symbols and translating word sums into numbers is often a core concern for the dyslexic.

4   Times tables cause many difficulties both in learning and recall. Parents and teaching staff need to liaise about the wording used for reciting the times table to avoid confusion and complications for the dyslexic. A 'whole school policy' is desirable.

5   Modern technology, such as the calculator, provides many aids, not least in boosting confidence.

6   According to Joffe (1980), 'computation was a slow and laborious process, for a large proportion' of dyslexics. This should be taken into account and they should be allowed extra time, especially in examinations.

7   Many dyslexic pupils have difficulties which may include directional, sequential, visual, memory and organizational skills. It is also necessary to be aware that they have individual differences in their learning styles. Their difficulties must be identified and remedied using multi-sensory methods, and constant review and revision. Research has shown that once dyslexic pupils have grasped the basic concepts, those who have mathematical potential can succeed.

8   In 1982 Miles commented that, 'happily, about 10 per cent of dyslexics are likely to be really successful in mathematics and about 30 per cent exhibit no particular difficulty so it is just the 60 per cent you have to worry about.'

Chapter 8

Adolescence

- study skills and examination preparation
- hurdles, including modern foreign languages
- how to obtain concessions from examination boards

Introduction

The dyslexic child's problems are being identified at an earlier age. Since the end of the 1980s there has been a greater emphasis in schools on recording pupils' progress. An annual written school report is compulsory. More information showing how pupils are performing has become available. In some cases this has helped to identify pupils with special educational needs and triggered additional support for an individual pupil in the classroom and at home. The spotlight falls most frequently on the pupil who has a reading problem. Nicolson and Fawcett (1995) argued that 'if a dyslexic child is diagnosed (via reading problems) at say eight, and is then given structured reading support in small groups following established procedures, there is every chance that he or she will, within a year or two, have effectively overcome the reading difficulties'. Furthermore, technically, the pupil is therefore no longer dyslexic and no longer qualifies for support (according to the *Code of Practice 1994*). However, the pupil may well come across future difficulties.

Many dyslexic pupils may well learn to cope adequately with those skills required at primary school level but for some a new set of problems may arise when they enter adolescence and secondary school. These problems, coupled with those 'normally' associated with growing up, can make life very difficult. Denckla (1982) sounded a note of caution when she said 'we used to think if we brought kids up to par, we could fold our arms with satisfaction. But we've found almost all [dyslexic] kids will need help again'.

Study skills

One of the more reliable indications of success in education 'seems to be the student's degree of know-how, including how to study' (Greenwood, 1981). Any pupil needs to be able to cope adequately with the following: essay writing, proof reading, homework, note-taking, letter writing and examinations. Competence in these skills is important at school, in institutions of further education and later in life.

Many pupils acquire these skills almost by osmosis, but the dyslexic learner needs learning and overlearning to be able to work on equal terms in the classroom. According to Farrer (1990), 'teachers and schools are becoming increasingly aware of the importance of teaching study skills'.

Essay writing

Essay writing is arguably the most important accomplishment that a pupil must acquire if he is to succeed academically. 'The ability to pass any sort of English exam depends largely on competence in essay writing' (Stirling, 1985) and, according to Myklebust (1965), 'the writing process is said to be the most complex and sophisticated and the last of the language skills to be acquired'.

At various times in a pupil's education an essay will be called 'a story', 'a composition', 'essay' and ultimately a 'dissertation'. Northedge (1990) noted that 'the word essay originally meant a first attempt or practice, but it now has the more general meaning of a short piece of writing on a specific subject'. Whatever the age or standard of the pupil, the same basic skills are required to write a good essay: to answer the question or to discuss the subject of the title.

There are four main types of essay: narrative, descriptive, factual and argumentative.

The narrative essay
The word '*narro*' comes from the Latin and it means 'to tell' – a story. The story can be factual or fictional, for example 'A Trip to the Moon'.

The descriptive essay
This can describe a person, a place or an event, for example 'Burnham Beeches in the Autumn'. It has been compared to 'a picture in words'.

The factual essay
This gives all the main facts about a subject, including its history and its future development, for example 'Air Travel'.

The argumentative essay
This is usually a discussion and often poses a question which should be answered. Both sides of the argument should be discussed and it

should be concluded with the personal opinion of the writer, for example 'Should Blood Sports be Abolished?'

Essay planning

Some dyslexic pupils find essay writing a daunting task and there is much anecdotal evidence to support this view. It is not unusual to find such a pupil only producing about six or eight lines of writing despite a marathon effort and a long time spent in trying to write. According to Chinn (1994), 'children's awareness of their own spelling deficits often limits what they write. ... This results in a very limited vocabulary, which diminishes the quality and quantity of the children's work'. All pupils should plan their essays but it is imperative for the dyslexic pupil. 'To have a plan which allows the child to write following a structure without having recourse to stopping and thinking every few minutes helps no end.' (Thomson and Watkins, 1990)

Dyslexic pupils have difficulty in sequencing their ideas, leading to irrelevant and rambling writing. Gilroy and Miles (1996) said that their essays, 'even though they are full of good ideas, sometimes give the impression of lack of planning and structure'. According to Farrer (1990), 'the [dyslexic] student formulates in his mind what he is going to say but, due to difficulties with spelling and writing, gets half way through a sentence/paragraph and forgets what he was going to say next. This often results in stilted, ungrammatical sentences and a poor flow of ideas'.

Establishing the importance of an essay plan

The pupil's ideas and thinking processes can often be more apparent from examination of the plan than from the essay itself. To help establish the importance of making a detailed plan, teachers should encourage the pupil to write the plan at the top of the script, and perhaps award some of the marks for the plan, in the same way that the workings of a maths problem are awarded a number of marks.

Four approaches to essay planning

There are four main ways to approach planning an essay. The mode chosen should suit the individual's learning style and disposition. Pupils with good visual skills, sometimes described as 'right-brained' pupils, may find spider plans and mind maps the most helpful (Buzan, 1982). Those pupils described as left-brained may find linear family tree types more useful.

1 Master essay plan (linear plan)

The master essay plan is based on a framework of keywords which can be fleshed out with sentences and paragraphs. For example:

> **Lost in the woods**
> a) The introduction (Setting the scene)
>   *Tom White* – (always give the people and the place names as this makes the story more compelling and interesting) – *half term – walking dog*
> b) The people and the place (Introduction of characters)
>   *Blue Bell Wood – sinister character – mobile*
> c) Something happens (Event)
>   *Track – freshly dug hole – dog gets very excited*
> d) The exciting part (Reaction)
>   *Gold bullion bars – silverware*
> e) Sorts itself out (Resolution)
>   *Hides – observes gang – follows to hide-out*
> f) Conclusion (Consequences)
>   *Alert police – wood surrounded – helicopter – gang trapped – eligible for substantial insurance company reward*

This linear plan is a useful format for the narrative essay.

2 Spider plan (wheel chart plan)

As its name implies, this involves drawing a diagram, putting the title in the middle and adding the 'ideas' to be considered in the essay. This is very useful for the factual essay.

3 Mind maps (brainstorming)

All the ideas that the title of the essay brings to mind are written down. The page could be divided in half to list the arguments 'for' and 'against'.

4 The 'wh' plan

This is so called because it involves the 'wh' words (the question words): why? where? who? which? what? For example:

> **My dream house**
> **Why?** did you choose it – construction – design
> **Where?** is its location – convenience
> **Who?** did you buy it from – built it – will live in it
> **Which?** features you like – construction – luxury bathroom – swimming pool – sauna – panelled dining room
> **What?** do you intend to do with it – live in it – restore it – improve it – entertain in it

This is useful for the descriptive essay.

Suggestions
for essay writing

- The narrative title is often the easiest essay to tackle but beware of using clichés or common themes. The examiner is human and easily bored when the 56th of the 100 scripts to be marked ends with '...and when I opened my eyes, I realized it was all a dream'.

- The plan is the foundation stone – just as the poorly constructed house will fall down because of ill-prepared foundations, so too the badly planned composition.

- The beginning and ending should have been worked out before starting to write the essay. 'The planning stage is of crucial importance, since it is at this point that your argument acquires its central coherence.' (Northedge, 1990)

- The introduction of the essay is very important and should 'catch the eye' of the reader and court his interest. It should not be too long.

  Introductions can follow different formats:

  a) The dramatic statement

  'He pulled a huge hunk of beef from the pocket of his waxed jacket and hurled it at the jaws of the guard dog, a mean and vicious looking Rottweiler.'

  b) The exclamation

  'This is a hold up!' – impact and interest is aroused immediately.

  c) A suitable quotation

  'As he crawled through the tunnel, the words, "Oh bed! oh bed! Delicious bed! That heaven on earth to the weary head" kept surfacing in his mind.' This arouses interest and makes the reader want to find out what happened next.

  d) Direct speech

  This can be very effective if used correctly and judiciously – too much and it can be very boring and repetitious.

  'Jake's ready, the door is open, the engine is revving, let's make a dash for the Jag.'

- The conclusion needs careful consideration. It should draw together the main themes or arguments of the essay, and should not be too long-winded. 'The reader should be left in a satisfied frame of mind' (Charlton, undated).

- The factual essay can often be a safe choice of subject for the weak essay writer, but it is essential that the pupil knows something about the subject matter. Dyslexic pupils tend to panic in situations of stress and may choose an inappropriate title simply because they find it interesting or are curious about it.

- Descriptive essays are in many ways the most challenging. It is like painting a picture in words. A useful hint is to remember to use all five senses – and not just to describe the visual impact of a scene. Taste, touch, hearing and smell all complement what is seen and being described.

- The finished essay must be proof read by any writer, but especially if the writer is dyslexic.

Proof reading

Proof reading is one of the most important skills that dyslexic pupils need to learn. Their greatest problem is that they have a tendency to re-read what they wanted to say rather than what they have written on the page. Time must always be allocated to proof reading. Typically, dyslexics are weak at grammar, punctuation, omission and spelling and these all need careful attention when proof reading. Dyslexic pupils can be trained to be on the look-out for their own particular type of error.

Suggestions
for successful proof reading

Grammar
- Check that complete sentences have been used.
- Check that the personal pronoun has been used consistently. Don't talk about 'he' and then change to 'we'.
- Check that the use of tense is consistent.

Punctuation
Check that the following have been used correctly:

- Capital letters.
- Quotation marks.

- Paragraphing (indented correctly).
- Watch how the apostrophe has been used – check that it has not been used incorrectly, particularly in plurals of nouns.

Omissions

If the essay does not have to be handed in for a week, it is a good idea to leave it and then proof read later. Some pupils say it helps them if they read aloud what they have written, pointing at the words with a finger. This can often help them to notice that words have been omitted. Northedge (1990) agreed and said 'it gives you a new angle on how well the sense flows through the sentences'. Others find it helpful to read what they have written onto cassette so that they can listen back to what they have written.

Spelling

Many errors can be picked up by pupils at the 13+ age level, particularly if they have their own 'hit list' of words that they often misspell (see Chapter 6). A spell checker may also be used (see Chapter 10), but pupils must not become too dependent upon these because they are not allowed in the examinations.

Coursework

Continuous assessment is a great help to dyslexic pupils. Because the work is prepared throughout the year, pupils can prepare assignments that are accurate and error free. They can obtain higher marks because they are less reliant on a performance demanded during a short, stressful couple of hours in an examination room. The coursework folder must contain a specified number of pieces of work, which can be done throughout the year and during the previous academic year. This is a boon for the dyslexic pupil as he can draft and redraft his work, possibly on a word processor, until it is at a satisfactory standard. It is vital that each piece is dated, has proper headings and that the pages are correctly numbered, and that they are filed in a systematic way for easy recovery. It is essential to keep copies of essays and work which may later be used when the coursework is being compiled for the examination board. It is helpful to file them in see-through plastic covers.

Homework

The ability to study or to work by oneself is important both at school and in later life and, according to Hamblin (1986), 'homework is essential for academic success'.

Parental support and involvement is desirable, but not always possible. Some parents may be unable or unwilling to help because of their own commitments or learning difficulties. Others may find that their interventions or involvement lead to tensions in the home. Despite this, there are many discreet and subtle ways a parent can help a pupil, not least by giving support and encouragement, even simply bringing a cup of coffee to the door of the pupil while he studies.

Timetabling

Time is the pupil's most precious commodity. Budgeting time effectively is an important skill, and one which typically dyslexic pupils find hard, either because of an innate inability with the concept of time, or simply because certain tasks simply take them longer than the ordinary pupil. Careful time schedules are essential for the pupil who is a slow reader and/or has weak comprehension skills. He will probably need more time to write essays. He needs to check with his teacher how much time is recommended for spending on the homework for individual subjects. Some schools liaise carefully with the various departments within the school and have a written school policy for staff and pupils to try to ensure that the pupil is not overloaded with an unrealistic amount of work. This homework timetable, drawn up by mutual agreement with parents, teacher and pupil, should be displayed prominently:

- in the home (for parental information/support)
- inside the school bag, beside the pupil's lesson timetable (it is useful to put notes beside the lesson timetable: for example Monday – bring PE kit)

The homework timetable might look like this:

Monday – homework
5.00–5.45　History
Break
6.00–6.45　Maths
Break

7.15–7.45	Supper
7.45–8.30	English
Break	
8.45–9.00	Make revision notes for science

This approach can help to lessen family tensions that can arise over the timing of family meals or television viewing. It also emphasizes the importance of having regular breaks.

It is often best to get the most difficult assignment out of the way first while the pupil is least tired. Pupils should try to establish when they are most productive. Each individual has periods when he can work better. For many, a half-an-hour concentrated effort in the morning is equivalent to one-and-a-half hours' work in the evening.

Organization is crucial for the dyslexic pupil, and a lack of organizational skills is of course a classic feature of dyslexia.

Suggestions
for tackling homework

- Choose a suitable place to study. Ensure that it is organized and equipped for its purpose. It should include a work surface, a table or desk which is suitable for writing on (not the floor or the bed!).

- Have a comfortable upright chair which is at the correct height with the desk.

- There should be an adequate supply of stationery including pens, papers, file paper, rubbers, Tippex, ink eradicators, ruler, pencil sharpener, card index, files, dictionary and thesaurus to hand. 'Post-it' notes provide a quick and painless way of marking texts.

- Label files on the spine so that they are instantly accessible. Use subject dividers in files to keep information separate and easy to locate. Colour coding of files can also be helpful, for example green files for biology, red for history. Yellow 'post-it' notes are useful aide memoirs on the front covers of files. Tabulation on the side of the pages in the file is also useful, so that time is not wasted wading through piles of notes to locate a particular topic. The inside of the back cover of the file could contain a list of the twenty most important spellings for that subject.

The front cover could have a sticker that shows which days and times there is a lesson in that subject

- Many dyslexic pupils say that a card index box with alphabetic cards is of particular assistance to them. The cards should contain ready references, such as definitions, keywords and formulae. This information can be compiled throughout the year and should be readily retrievable. Some pupils put all their revision notes on these cards. Electronic notepads can also be used.

- Textbooks should be kept up-ended, if possible on a shelf so that they are readily to hand and clearly visible.

- A clock is essential to help organize and follow a working timetable. Some pupils like to use timers.

- A pinboard is useful for putting up such items as a list of keyword spellings, timetable and examination dates.

- Ensure that there is the least possible noise or interruption.

- Heating and ventilation need to be adequate, and good lighting is important. An anglepoise desk lamp is helpful.

- Plan the homework timetable carefully, clearly noting the time and day that the homework has to be handed in.

- Some pupils find it useful to count up and work out the number of hours and days they have until their exam. They can then do a daily countdown on a calendar.

It is prudent to put a sticker on the inside of the file cover to show important dates, such as half term, the first day of examinations and the date by which major assignments have to be completed.

Note-taking

Some pupils have poor short term memory, making it hard to follow lengthy explanations and to take notes, but with training they can improve and make good notes.

Diagrams

Some authorities advocate teaching the dyslexic pupil to take notes using diagrams rather than writing notes and often refer to these diagrams as mind maps. This seems sound advice for the pupils who have stronger visual memories. 'Many pupils learn better visually than through unsupported auditory recall' (Hamblin, 1981). Spider plans and linear plans similar to those used when planning essays can also be used to take effective notes.

Reading

It is very important to be able to study and take notes from a textbook.

For dyslexic pupils with weak reading skills, it is critical that they understand what they are reading. If the text is too difficult, they won't remember what they have read. This should not be regarded as laziness. Like all other pupils, the dyslexic pupil has only a certain number of hours to do his homework or prepare or revise for an examination. He cannot afford to waste some of this precious preparation time on an activity from which he is going to gain little. It might be appropriate for the pupil to use abridged versions of set texts, or to have texts on cassette, or even to have the book read aloud.

SQ3R method of studying a textbook

One method that is useful in organizing the way a pupil studies a text is the SQ3R method:

S   Survey – read the headings, subheadings, summaries

Q   Question – ask questions about what is being read, use the headings to do this

R   Read the whole chapter – underline the keywords

R   Recite the answers to the questions asked and write down the key points in note form

R   Review and go over what has been learned.

This is time-consuming but pays dividends in the long run. The notes can be reviewed and are ready for revision, perhaps once a week. They can eliminate the slog of going through a whole text before the exam.

Reducing the load is the key to successful learning for the dyslexic pupil. Using multi-sensory learning techniques, as the SQ3R method does, helps because it has involved the eyes, ears, lips and hands.

According to Northedge (1990), 'marking the text is a way of moderately increasing your time investment as you read, while considerably increasing the pay-off – both in terms of your immediate comprehension and in terms of your long-term recall'. When the pupil writes his own notes on the chapter, he is simultaneously learning the facts and compiling the information for revision later.

Listening

In school, the pupil spends 60 per cent of his time in listening, but very rarely is he taught how to listen. The pupil needs to be taught the following:

- to pick out the key points
- to follow the point of what is being said
- to follow the central sequence of ideas.

A useful way of teaching this is listening to news broadcasts.
A short passage can be recorded, played back and notes taken.

Summaries

Pupils need to learn how to summarize a passage. It is fundamental to all note-taking from either a lecture or a text. A summary should give as much information as possible using as few words as possible.

Letter writing

Examination papers often include letter writing and this is an important life skill. The setting out of the letter is something many dyslexic pupils have difficulty with. The pupil needs to practise writing formal and informal letters and to be familiar with the precise format for the display, punctuation and language used for them.

Business letters

It is especially important for the dyslexic pupil to understand the difference between formal and informal English and to know when and where to use which. 'Many dyslexic students tend to write as they would speak and find it very difficult to understand and use the subtle changes in language style required for different written situations.' (Farrer, 1990)

Written comprehension

Written comprehension skills involve reading a passage and then answering questions on the content of what has been read. Many lessons in the classroom also include this type of activity as an aid to learning a topic being studied, or sometimes as a skill in its own right. Dyslexic pupils, many of whom are very intelligent, can often do well here, so practice becomes even more important and it is essential for them to master the techniques involved. Obviously the ability to read the passage is a key factor, and it is the weak or inaccurate reading skills that hamper the more able dyslexic pupil. It is helpful to teach the pupil that there are essentially three different types of comprehension question. They can be answered as follows:

1   The literal answer – the answer is written in the text (cue words are: quote, evidence, facts, reasons, describe, define, information).

2   The inferential answer – needs searching for and sometimes requires reading between the lines (cue words are: opinion, compare, explain, suggest).

3   The evaluative answer – requires the writer to give his own interpretation or opinion (cue words are: imply, opinion, suggest).

Suggestions
for improving written comprehension

- Read the instructions and title carefully.

- Check the number of questions (in the case of an examination paper, there is sometimes a question written on the back of the page).

- Read the introduction. It may explain that the passage describes the scene when a secret agent during World War II sees his commanding officer before he goes on a mission. The passage does not refer to this. But it assumes that the introduction has been read. If it hasn't, it will be very difficult to answer the questions.

- Read the passage/questions quickly to get the general gist.

- Read the acknowledgement or source. This might provide further information on the contents of the passage.

- Re-read the question for meaning and understanding.
- Check how many marks each question has. If most questions carry two or three marks and one carries 15 marks it usually indicates its importance. This question will often require more information and a longer answer. It is important to be alert for these questions.
- Check the wording carefully – underline keywords such as 'quote', 'compare', 'contrast', 'evidence', 'give examples from the passage'.
- Work out the time allowance for each question.
- Answer in complete sentences, using your own words as far as possible.
- Attempt all the questions – marks are sometimes given for an attempt.
- If time starts to run out, outline the main points and answer the remaining questions in note form.
- Proof read carefully, checking for spelling, punctuation and omissions.

The GCSE examination has changed many of the traditional skills previously examined in 'comprehension' questions. The pupil may be asked to read a series of articles, including extracts from books and newspapers. He may then have to answer general questions on these which appertain to style, argument or comparison. This presupposes strong underlying critical skills, as well as powers of analysis, all of which may impose even greater demands on the dyslexic candidate with weak reading skills and poor short term memory.

To reinforce the importance of reading all the questions on an examination paper before beginning, it can be useful to use the following 'paper'. Ensure that the paper is face downwards on the desk. Then tell the pupil to turn it over and tell him that he is going to be timed to see how quickly he can finish it.

How fast can you finish?

Read all the questions through carefully before you start working.

1 Write your name in full.

2 Write the even numbers out in full from 2 to 20.

3 Write the days of the week in reverse order.

4 Name three football players.

5 Name the young of each of these animals:
   a) cat
   b) horse
   c) cow
   d) sheep.

6 Name the capital cities of:
   a) France
   b) Spain
   c) Italy
   d) Ireland.

7 What are the primary colours?

8 What are the names of the Queen's children in age order?

9 Where would you find:
   a) The Eiffel Tower
   b) Buckingham Palace
   c) EuroDisney.

10 What sports do you associate with:
   a) Wimbledon
   b) Twickenham
   c) Wembley.

11 Raise your hand for ten seconds.

12 Answer only question number one.

Source: Devised by William Perry. Known as the Harvard Experiment (Pauk, 1974).

There is anecdotal evidence of this being given to 80 teachers at a seminar. Only four of them followed the instructions.

Modern foreign languages

The National Curriculum (1995) states that pupils at Key Stage 3 and Key Stage 4 must be taught a modern foreign language. This includes listening, responding, speaking and writing which involves learning about and using the language. Foreign languages or second languages can often cause dyslexic pupils enormous difficulties. Sparks and Ganschow (1993) pointed out that, 'according to research findings, most students who experience foreign language learning problems are thought to have overt or subtle native language learning difficulties, primarily with phonological processing'. Some can cope with the oral skills but are defeated in their attempts to spell. Snowling (1985) said 'it is likely that a child who has difficulty in repeating unfamiliar words will be slow to learn "new" spoken vocabulary (foreign language learning would be particularly affected)'. 'They make stumbling attempts at gaining proficiency with a second language' according to Dinklage (1971). It is useful to know some of the problems that may face the dyslexic child when learning French and German.

French

The difficulties that dyslexic pupils may have when learning French are as follows.

Speaking
*   They find it difficult to produce unfamiliar vowel sounds such as the nasal vowels:
    '*une*' (one), '*lune*' (moon)

*   The intonation is totally different to English. The accent is placed on different words to that of English.

*   They have difficulty producing the words rapidly enough to build a sentence due to their word retrieval difficulties.

*   Learning and remembering new vocabulary is very difficult for many.

Listening
*   They confuse words that sound the same because of a lack of phonological skills:
    '*poisson*'/'*croissant*' (fish/croissant), '*tu*'/'*tout*' (you/all), '*tante*'/'*tente*' (aunt/tent)

*   They have difficulty equating what they hear with what they see on the page:
    '*Mademoiselle*' (Miss), '*Est-ce qu'il y a...?*' (Is there...?)

Spelling

- They have great difficulty with spelling because words are not spelt as they sound:

  words such as '*lundi*' (Monday) say 'e' but end in an 'i'

  This can cause further confusion for the pupil who may know the English spelling rule about not using 'i' at the end of words.

- Silent letters are another source of difficulty. In French they can come at the beginning or the end of words:

  'h' at the beginning of '*heure*' (hour)

  't' at the end of '*chocolat*' (chocolate)

  There is also a silent 'e' at the end of words like '*grande*' (big) and silent 's' at the end of '*souris*' (mouse).

- The letters used are often unexpectedly different to what they have learned in English. For example in English 'sh' says /sh/ as in 'ship' or 'dash' but /sh/ sound is spelt 'ch' in French:

  '*chèvre*' (goat), '*choisir*' (to choose)

- They find the concept of three vowels difficult. For someone with a poor visual sequential memory a further problem is to remember the order in which they occur in the word:

  '*sœur*' (sister), '*grenouille*' (frog), '*bouillant*' (boiling)

- They find the concept of conjugating the verbs difficult. The problem is exacerbated by the fact that they are pronounced the same way but are spelt differently:

  '*je donne, tu donnes, ils donnent*' (I/you/they give)

- The difference between the rules of English and French grammar cause confusion when they attempt to apply the rules of one language to the other. Some have a tendency to add 's' to the end of any verb used in the third person singular of the present tense. They may write '*il manges*' (he eats).

- The use of apostrophe 's' is another area of difficulty. They may write '*Monsieur Dupont's chien*' (Mr Dupont's dog) instead of '*le chien de Monsieur Dupont*'.

- Because one verb in the present tense in French represents the three versions of the present tense in English, pupils sometimes get confused:

  je mange   = I eat

  je mange   = I am eating

  je mange   = I do eat

  In an attempt to render 'I am eating' some pupils want to write 'Je *suis* mange'.

Reading
- Many letters are silent such as final consonants: '*ils travaillent*' (they work). It says /il travai/.
- Dyslexics find it difficult to remember what they have read because they have to pay so much attention to the mechanical aspects of pronunciation.

German

On the whole, English speakers find German pronunciation easier than French because the position of the lips, tongue and vocal chords are more relaxed.

- French can be difficult for English speakers because the lips and the vocal chords have to be tauter although some Scottish people find the pronunciation easier.

- Some pupils find the German multiple consonant combinations very difficult:

  '*Schweiz*' (Switzerland)

  '*ausschneiden*' (to cut out)

- Miles (1996) stated that the pronunciation can be challenging because of 'its use of long complicated polysyllabic words'. A classic example of this is the German word for a tank:

  '*Schützengrabenvernichtungspanzerkraftwagen*'

  The word has evolved from the German for the following series of words:

  'an earthwork you have constructed to protect yourself an armoured plated wagon for destroying trenches'

Word order

In French

There are some minor difficulties:

- Adjectives and adjectival phrases tend to go after the noun. This can be confusing for a pupil with a sequencing difficulty:

  '*le ballon rouge*' (the red balloon)
  '*des lunettes de soleil*' (the sunglasses)

- The possessive noun is placed in the reverse order to the order it is in English:

  '*la plume de ma tante*' (my aunt's pen)

In German
There are some major difficulties.

- Subordinating conjunctions cause the verb to be placed at the end of a sentence.
- Many verbs are 'separable', like English phrasal verbs such as 'to take off' or 'to give up', and result in the word being split up:

  'er *sieht* gern fern' (he likes watching television)
- All past participles go at the end of a sentence.

All this imposes great demands on the pupil who may have sequencing difficulties.

Which language to study

The best advice that can be given to a dyslexic pupil embarking upon learning a foreign language is to try one language, using multi-sensory learning techniques. Research has shown that this is the most successful method. If the written part of the syllabus is very difficult, the pupil should work even harder to pick up as many marks as possible in the oral and aural parts of the examination. In some instances this element can account for as much as 50 per cent of the final marks. A visit to the foreign country can be enormously beneficial to the pupil. Even if he does not return speaking fluently, his ability to listen and understand what is being said usually benefits.

As in all else relating to the dyslexia community there will be a wide variation in the aptitudes and skills of each pupil. There are dyslexic pupils who have obtained 'A' grades for modern languages at GCSE but for the severely dyslexic pupil who is unable to learn the conventions of his mother tongue, a foreign language can be an area of total confusion.

Preparation for examinations

Preparation, organization and reconnaissance skills are important for all examinees. These, rather than lack of study, could mean the difference between pass and failure for the dyslexic pupil.

All pupils, but especially dyslexic pupils, need to consider a number of things when preparing for examinations:

- carefully choose subjects for which there is an aptitude
- carefully choose subjects which are most suitable for the likely chosen career

- carefully choose the examination syllabus.

The pupil should practise study skills to enable him to:

- budget his time
- organize his notes and resources
- develop note-taking and examination preparation techniques
- make timetables for homework
- practise examination questions
- target his objectives to improve his motivation.

Subjects to study

The choice of subjects to study is very important. Five good GCSE grades are better than nine GCSEs with poor grades. Most of the schools regarded as being more academic only allow their pupils to take a maximum of eight subjects.

The pupil should choose subjects for which he has some aptitude. It is even better if he enjoys the subject. It is foolish to decide to take Spanish and German if he is already struggling with French. If suitable options exist, it is prudent not to choose subjects that require a heavy reading load, such as history, particularly for the pupil who is a slow reader.

Subject choice and career prospects

The pupil needs to consider career prospects. Choice of subjects at GCSE may determine what pupils can go on to study, should they choose to do so. It is prudent to try to keep the options open for as long as possible. It is important to remember that passes in English and mathematics are compulsory entry requirements for many university courses.

Examination syllabus

The pupil, his parents and teacher should study the examination syllabus carefully. Research showed that a third of students sitting Maths GCSE papers from two different boards did better on one board than on the other. It also pointed out that 'last year hundreds of schools changed exam boards in an effort to improve their grades and presumably improve their position on the league tables' (*The Times*, 1996).

The examinations set by some of the boards might be more suitable for the dyslexic pupil than others. This is particularly relevant in the English examination. Points to check and consider carefully are:

- What is the choice on the set texts?
- To what extent are writing skills tested in coursework and to what extent are they tested in the exam?

Timetabling and personal organization

Timetabling is very important. Thomson and Watkins (1990) said that 'it is surprising how the idea of chronological time causes many dyslexics confusion'. The pupil's personal organization system should be in place from the first day of term. For each subject it is helpful to break down the syllabus into its main components, and to be aware of how long a particular topic will be studied. It is also helpful to know how many topics will be covered in the term. This should help the pupil keep abreast of his studies. The teacher may have detailed lesson plans and may be willing to give a photocopy of these to the pupil. This will give the pupil the outline of the course.

Revision

Dyslexic pupils need to make three times the effort of the average pupil. The successful pupil will begin to prepare for his final or end of term examination from the first day of term. Thomson and Watkins (1990) commented that 'forward planning is vital for dyslexics, as experience tells us that cramming everything into the last few hours invariably results in chaos for them'.

Forward planning

One key to forward planning is to make revision notes. It is useful to condense the notes into brief summary sheets, perhaps putting keywords on a card index which can be reviewed the night before the test or examination. Numbering these is vital. Some pupils put these keywords on posters on the walls of their bedroom. The pupil with good auditory skills may want to put keywords onto an audio cassette and use this for revision purposes. Others prefer diagrams and mind maps. Some find cartoons with bubble captions helpful. Each pupil should find a method best suited to his own learning style.

Previous examination questions

Northedge (1990) pointed out that 'probably the single most useful revision activity of all is to attempt old exam questions'.

Back copies of previous examination question papers are available from the examination boards. Timing and technique can be improved with practice. Thomson and Watkins (1990) said that 'this preparation could take the form of practice in short, weekly sessions, in writing answers relevant to the subject being studied'. Some teachers are clever at predicting the questions that might be asked in examinations.

Suggestions
to improve motivation

- The carrot-and-stick theory works well. The pupil should set himself a target, for example to finish his maths homework, and his reward to himself for this may be, for example, to watch a television programme for half an hour.

- During study periods the pupil should stop for a break after a piece of work is finished, rather than in the middle.

- Parents can help by exempting the pupil from household chores when an important essay has to be completed on time.

- Targets and rewards should be realistic. They are not intended to put more pressure on the pupil.

- Recognition by the teacher of the pupil's progress can help to improve the effort of the most reluctant pupil, for example a poem published in the school magazine. Devlin (1995) said 'the common factor in all the successes, however minor, is the praise and encouragement that build up self-esteem and confidence. Without it, talent may never be discovered and children may grow up into adults with a sense of frustration and waste'.

- Do not compare the results of the dyslexic pupil with his siblings.

There are also the negative 'motivators': detentions, suspension of privileges, time restraints, suspension of pleasurable activities. These should be a last resort and should be avoided as far as possible. The teenage dyslexic pupil has so many pressures and demands made both on his time and on his emotions that it can be destructive and counter-productive to put him under further stress.

Suggestions
on how to tackle the examination paper

- Read the paper quickly to get the general gist of it.
- Read the whole of the question paper again, including the instructions, and check how many questions have to be answered.
- Decide which questions are going to be answered and mark them.
- Identify the type of answer required. It is important to distinguish between them.
- Check the wording of the question carefully. Newton and Thomson (1976) recommended that the candidate should:

  Read the question three times:
  a) *to check the actual words e.g. does it say 'quote', 'give examples from the passage'*
  b) *to find out what does it say*
  c) *to find out what does it ask.*

  Source: Newton M. P. and Thomson M. (1976) 'Dyslexia: A guide to examinations'. *Dyslexia Review*, 16: 16–19.

- The well-prepared pupil who has rehearsed questions and answers must still be aware of the dyslexic's innate tendency to misread words. This is exacerbated in examination conditions so this advice is even more important.
- Make a timetable. Jot it down and include adequate time allowance for the initial reading of the paper and for proof reading. Never spend too much time on any one question. Pupils seldom get full marks for an individual question and they cannot get marks for questions which have not been completed or attempted. If time is short, try answering the final question in note form. A few extra marks may be accrued in that manner. Note carefully the marks allowed for each question or part of a question (each part does not necessarily carry the same number of marks) and allocate time and effort accordingly.
- Underline the keywords in the question and answer that question. Marks are not given for writing down all that is known about the subject. Thus if asked to quote – quote. If asked to give examples from the passage then give the correct number of examples asked for from the passage.

- Jot down the key words or paragraph headings and number these if appropriate before beginning. Some pupils may benefit by writing a plan for the answer before commencing.

- Begin with the easiest question or favourite topic. This helps to quell the tension and boosts confidence. Questions do not have to be tackled in any particular order as long as they are carefully numbered.

- Help the examiners by labelling clearly and numbering the answers accurately. Write as neatly as possible and leave adequate space between the lines and answers.

- Write in clear, short sentences and use your own words as far as possible. Use paragraphs and watch punctuation.

- Write legibly. Leave a space between each line, particularly when doing an essay. When proof reading it is much easier to put in the corrected spelling or the omitted word in the space above the line.

- Before the question is completed and when reading the conclusion, check again that the question being asked has been answered.

- Proof read the whole paper once it has been completed, remembering to check particularly for:
  a) punctuation (capital letters) and the correct use of the apostrophe
  b) omissions
  c) spellings, particularly the past tense of the verb, the homophones 'their'/'there', 'of'/'off', personal 'difficult' words and 'because'/'was'/'were'/'where'
  d) check that tense is consistent and that the 'person' has not been muddled
  e) watch for and correct common errors of grammar such as:
  'must of' for 'must have'
  'bored of' for 'bored with'
  'He did it quick' for 'He did it quickly'
  'We was late for school' for 'We were late for school'
  'None have arrived' for 'None has arrived'
  'The team were winning' for 'The team was winning'
  (collective nouns should take a singular verb).

Up to 5 per cent of marks can be deducted in a GCSE examination for spelling, grammar and punctuation.

GCSE and 'A' Level Examinations: Concessions for the dyslexic candidate

The Joint Forum for the GCSE and GCE has produced a booklet, *Candidates with Special Assessment Needs: Special Arrangements and Special Consideration* to assist heads of centres and teachers to make requests for candidates who have special assessment needs. The booklet describes both the principles and procedures for requests for special arrangements (arrangements made in advance of the examination) and for special consideration (action taken following the examination). Requests for special arrangements and special consideration must be submitted and supported by the Head of Centre. The Examining Bodies have responsibility for the consideration and approval of such requests. Specific enquiries, requests for advice and all completed application forms should be sent to the particular Examining Body conducting the examinations. Questions of a general nature may be sent to the Joint Forum for the GCSE and GCE.

In its section, **Specific Learning Difficulties including Neurological Dysfunction**, the Joint Forum gives the following guidelines for identifying candidates for whom special arrangements may be requested.

Candidates are likely to have experienced difficulties in at least one of the areas given below:

Reading Accuracy	*This would include candidates who are unlikely to be able to read the examination material with sufficient accuracy to avoid making mistakes which will affect the understanding of what they read.*
Reading Speed	*This will be a particular problem where the speed of reading is so slow that the candidate loses the sense of what he or she reads.*
Spelling	*This will include candidates with spelling difficulties which significantly slow their work rate and result in the use of alternative words which are easier to spell or who are unlikely to achieve any score in the marking of*

spelling. The extent to which spelling errors are likely to lead to unrecognizable words should be reported.

Handwriting Speed *Candidates whose handwriting speed is so slow that it presents a particular problem should be trained to communicate the information required by questions as briefly as possible wherever this is appropriate. Where such a strategy is not sufficient, special arrangements may need to be sought.*

Handwriting Legibility *This may relate to writing under time pressure and in such cases the previous section will apply. There are, however, candidates whose scripts are illegible despite their being allowed to write more slowly.*

Other Difficulties *As well as the preceding areas of difficulty, some candidates have other specific problems, e.g. attention and concentration, clumsiness and disorganization of such severity as to prevent a candidate from demonstrating attainment. Such difficulties as these and others are often found to be associated with neurological dysfunction.*

Source: Joint Forum for the GCSE and GCE (1997) *Candidates with Special Assessment Needs: Special Arrangements and Special Considerations.* Manchester.

Guidelines on making the appeal

- The candidate, his parents and teachers should decide whether the pupil needs and might be helped by a concession. This should be discussed when GCSE subjects and options are being decided upon.
- The head of centre is responsible for applying for, and recommending, the special examination arrangements which are considered to be necessary.
- The 1997 regulations state that a formal application to the appropriate Examining Body using the official application form must be submitted by 30 September for candidates sitting the examination in the Autumn/Winter term, and by 21 February for candidates sitting the examination in the Summer term (unless the request is for the provision of special question papers, in which case applications must be submitted by 15 January).
- Requests must be accompanied by evidence from a psychological assessment which has been carried out not more than two years before the examination.
- The assessment should include 'historical evidence of the candidate's needs and an indication of how the centre meets these needs. You will be expected to establish that the candidate's needs have been recognized over a period of time and that the arrangements requested for the examination reflect past and present needs'.

The concession and special examination arrangements will be determined according to what is stated in the assessment. It might include some of the following:

a) additional time, which could be up to 25 per cent of the total time allowed for the examination
b) the reading of the questions to the candidate
c) the use of a word processor (but this does not allow for the use of a spell checker, thesaurus or grammar checker)
d) an amanuensis may be allowed for English Literature examinations in exceptional cases, but not for English Language examinations.

Candidates with Statements of SEN do not automatically qualify for special concessions. In examinations where spelling, punctuation and grammar form part of the assessment, candidates will be assessed like all other candidates. An *additional* 5 per cent of the total available marks is given for the assessment of spelling, punctuation and grammar. Marks are not actually deducted from the candidate's 'subject' score for any weakness in linguistic skills.

Candidates are sometimes allowed to do their coursework on a word processor.

All Scottish Examination Boards use the same criteria as those applicable in England and Wales. The information is contained in *Scottish Certificate of Sixth Year Studies Examinations Arrangements for Candidates with Special Educational Needs* (Scottish Examination Board, 1996). Applications must be submitted on form EX1 (Supplement) Special Educational Needs.

How the classroom teacher can help her dyslexic pupils

The classroom teacher and the SENCO roles should be mutually supportive. They need to work closely to implement and fulfil their statutory duties as laid down by the *Code of Practice 1994*. The classroom teacher who is well-informed and sympathetic to the needs of the dyslexic pupil can single-handedly do more than almost anyone else to make the education of these pupils successful. They can change the course of their lives for better or worse depending on how they carry out their duties. Classroom teachers have been set enormous challenges in their professional lives to deal with the subject of SEN although often they have had little training. All over the country teachers have strived to meet this challenge and adapted to the changes and challenges that have occurred with great rapidity and frequency in all maintained schools as a result of the Education Acts of 1988, 1993, 1996 and the *Code of Practice 1994*. The teacher is expected to be a pedagogue, a matriarch and an expert to a fractious brood whose needs may be as diverse as the severely physically or emotionally handicapped to the gifted highflier with a learning difficulty. This one person has overall responsibility for each pupil in her classroom and is expected to know and understand their problems, teach them and monitor and review the child's progress so that each and every child is 'making satisfactory progress'.

Suggestions
for encouraging the dyslexic pupil

Importance of enhancing self-esteem

Set realistic targets for the pupil and enhance his confidence. 'Error-free work might be beyond his grasp', according to Thomson (1990). He also reminded us that 'if the child's self-esteem is poor he will continue to perform inadequately in school' and furthermore 'we do not learn by failure, only by success' (Glasser, 1969).

Be aware that, for example, his essay skills may remain weak. Gilroy and Miles (1996), when discussing guidelines for marking the scripts of dyslexic candidates, said that 'it is important to look for evidence of creativity, knowledge and reasoning powers which are not apparent at first glance'. Flippant or caustic comments at the bottom of an exercise book can shatter the confidence and sap the motivation of a pupil who may have slaved for an hour over a piece of work which, in the end, may still be full of spelling errors, with a lack of punctuation and perhaps barely legible writing. Allowances have to be made for his constitutional handicaps.

Reading

Be aware that the pupil's reading skills may still be poor. Don't ask him to read aloud in the class. Allow him to use abridged versions of set texts, or cassettes or videos. Do allow him and encourage him to ask for a word from the teacher or a fellow pupil. Don't expect him to remember the words on the page just because the teacher has read the passage at the beginning of the lesson. 'Keep required silent reading to a minimum. Only the visual channel is stimulated, and the time it requires for so many dyslexic pupils is generally not worth the small amount of learning (and even utter confusion) that often results [for some pupils]' (Greenwood, 1983). Be aware that the pupil may read a passage correctly but that he may not understand or remember what he has read because his comprehension of the contents is impaired by the mechanical aspects of decoding the words.

Examinations

Remember that the dyslexic candidate's learning disabilities may penalize him heavily in an examination. He may find it hard to read the question paper. He may misread or misinterpret the question. If the pupil's difficulties are sufficient to warrant the concessions of extra time, a reader, a tape recorder, a word processor or an amanuensis ensure that the candidate has had adequate practice and rehearsal in these skills. Candidates may sometimes be allowed to take their examination orally.

Spelling

Remember that poor spelling will continue to dog the dyslexic pupil almost every day of his life. Spelling tests put the pupil under great pressure, particularly the test with randomized words containing no pattern or structure. Ask the dyslexic pupil to learn eight of the twenty set for the other pupils. Divide the words into syllables – highlight the tricky letter. It is destructive and non-productive to underline every mistake in an essay. This can lead to the pupil becoming fixated on spelling accuracy, which may mean that the pupil writes less, or subconsciously writes in an inhibited and restricted fashion using only monosyllabic words.

. . . a student can be hindered by poor spelling in three ways:

1   *if his spelling is so bizarre that a reader is unable to figure out his meaning*

2   *if his teacher takes off [marks] for poor spelling, and so he fails despite a good understanding of the material*

3   *and if his anxiety over his spelling inhibits his expression of his ideas by limiting him to the use of words he feels he can spell.*

Source: Morris G. (1983) 'Adapting a college preparatory curriculum for dyslexic adolescents II: The focus. Confronting the problems of what to teach'. *Annals of Dyslexia*, 33: 243–50

- Don't correct every spelling error when he writes an essay.
- Never put sp. beside an error.
- If the word is incorrect and it is necessary to draw his attention to it, give him the correct spelling. A dyslexic speller does not learn from his own spelling errors.
- It is important to mark essays for content and information.
- A flexible grading and marking policy is essential, just as golfers have handicaps. Try to offer praise when it is appropriate, make criticism constructive and give encouragement whenever possible. Give credit for effort, not just attainment.

Whole-school marking policy

A whole-school marking policy is beneficial for teacher and pupil. The SENCO can prepare this and produce it as a policy document. This can be improved upon, adapted and revised at the beginning of each academic year as necessary. A resumé of the dyslexic pupil's specific weaknesses and difficulties would be helpful.

Homework

Homework may cause problems. Frequently the pupil may have copied down the instructions incorrectly, such as the number of sums he is supposed to do or that the sums are on page 28 instead of 82 of the textbook. In the case of a younger pupil, check his homework diary before he leaves the room. Give photocopied sheets of instructions or notes if possible. A useful suggestion is to form a Homework Helpline where a parent is available for telephone queries concerning the homework on a rota basis. It could be a project for the Parent Teachers' Association (PTA). Do remember that the dyslexic pupil often works very slowly – some may have to make three times the effort that the normal child makes. He will get very tired, so don't make his life more stressful by punishing him for not completing homework or giving him a detention to finish his class work. Never give a dyslexic pupil 'lines' to write as a punishment; choose a non-academic punishment if one is necessary. Don't keep him in at break either as he, more than most pupils, needs to rush around the playground to get some fresh air, or to retreat to the tuck shop to eat a bar of chocolate to help boost his energy levels. Free time and relaxation are vital.

Mathematics

Do allow the pupil to use a table square or calculator (see Chapter 7).

Writing

Don't ask the pupil to write an essay again. Writing lists of spelling corrections is a waste of time for most dyslexic pupils. Many of them even copy out the correction incorrectly.

Multi-sensory learning techniques

It is now proven that dyslexic pupils learn best when taught by multi-sensory methods and these are suitable for everyone. Priscilla Vail, who is recognized and acclaimed as one of the most talented and innovative teachers in the USA, said 'multi-sensory methods and materials, originally designed for dyslexic or learning disabled students, work beautifully for the general population'(1992).

Personal organization

Encourage the dyslexic pupil and help him to structure his daily life as well as his learning. The supportive classroom teacher will introduce new topics gradually, and will review them at the end of the lesson. She will encourage the pupil by giving him notes and review sheets when it comes to revision for tests and exams. She will liaise with the pupil's parents to ensure that someone at home has a copy of the school timetables and the dates and times of special events, such as examinations. She will allow the pupil to borrow others' notes to catch up on work at home.

Writing in textbooks

Have a flexible policy about textbooks which are lent to pupils and the strict rules about marking them. The dyslexic reader should be allowed and encouraged to highlight and underline the key words and to number the facts to be memorized. This cuts down on his workload when the time comes to revise. PTAs may be willing to raise funds to buy additional copies of texts so that pupils with special educational needs may be able to have their own copies.

Reports

When writing reports, comments such as 'Tom still can't spell and his use of punctuation is poor' can be destructive. It leaves the writer open to ridicule and accusations of ignorance about basic, but unfortunately often universal, difficulties that the dyslexic pupil may have. Be aware that there may be learning disabled yet gifted dyslexic pupils in the classroom.

A whole-school marking policy which includes allowances for pupils with SEN is helpful.

Emotional effects of dyslexia

The dyslexic teenager, like his classmates, has to cope with the problems of growing up, but for the pupil with a specific learning difficulty this may involve additional loss of self-esteem, self-doubt and sensitivity to criticism. There are often feelings of inadequacy and embarrassment about lack of the skills that most of his peers do not have to think about. Some react by denying the problems and often reject help. Others do not wish their teachers or friends to know that they are 'different'. They often feel isolated and become alienated from their peers.

Evidence is coming to light of the suffering and embarrassment that dyslexia may cause. A number of books and television programmes have brought the subject into the public domain. There are reports of pupils who developed behavioural problems and depression or who were suicidal as a result of classroom experiences, the ignorance of their teachers or the bullying by their peers, or when the pupil did not match parental expectation.

The pupil's wishes must always be respected. Some may warrant counselling and support, and others will need to have further specialist teaching to help them to build the skills to compete on an equal footing with their peers if they are to attain their potential, and to prevent a primary learning disability leading to secondary psychological symptoms.

Edwards (1994) argued that 'the emotional effects of our treatment of the dyslexic pupils in our schools are severely under-estimated'. Many of these young people require professional counselling to help them cope.

Summary and conclusions

1   Dyslexic pupils often need specific, structured help with study skills.

2   The type of essay plan used often will depend on the individual's learning style. Dyslexic pupils with good visual skills might find diagrams such as spider plans and mind maps to be the most helpful. Others will probably find linear, family tree type plans more useful.

3   Study skills which need to be taught should include:
   - essay writing
   - proof reading
   - writing letters
   - written comprehension
   - private study
   - note taking from a text or a lecture
   - writing summaries
   - preparation for examinations
   - revision techniques

4   Dyslexic pupils need help in organizing their personal lives and their belongings as well as learning how to study.

5   The study of a modern foreign language can present many difficulties, and bilingualism can create enormous problems. Some dyslexic pupils cope orally but are unable to manage the written and reading elements. One of the best approaches is to use multi-sensory techniques, which are now common in language courses. As with much else relating to dyslexia, the exception often (dis)proves the rule.

6   Examinations are a great hurdle and some pupils need additional help with the preparation for these.

7   Concessions may be given by the examination boards and can include:

•   additional time
•   use of a word processor
•   an amanuensis
•   a reader

Application and arrangement for these concessions must be made within strict time lines as laid down by the examination boards.

8   The classroom teacher and SENCO are key players in the education of the dyslexic pupil.

9   Some dyslexic adolescents develop secondary emotional, social and behavioural problems, as a result of their unrecognized and unresolved dyslexia.

Chapter 9

Further and higher education

- choosing the right college and course
- completing the UCAS form
- how to maximize the help available

Introduction

An increasing number of dyslexic people are fulfilling their potential at school, and as a result they are now gaining places at colleges and universities. The overall statistics show that, of applicants for places at university, 3,446 stated their dyslexia as a disability. Of applicants granted a place, 2,433 were known to be dyslexic (UCAS, 1995). In 1981 there were only about 200 recognized dyslexic students at university.

There are a number of possible explanations for the increase in the number of recognized dyslexics obtaining university places. According to Gilroy (1994), 'it is a direct result of having their problems identified at an earlier age and then receiving the appropriate help as a consequence of these pupils being Statemented, hence more and more pupils are reaching the standard to qualify for a university'. The training of teachers and the quality of teaching for dyslexic pupils has improved. Singleton (1995) did not take such an optimistic stance, however, when he said that 'figures reported by British universities suggest that at the present time between 1 per cent and 2 per cent of undergraduates are dyslexic. Many of these students, while aware of their problems, often do not receive the help or support that they are entitled to, provision is patchy and the standard of help varies from excellent to abysmal'.

Routes to further and higher education

There are currently two routes through 16–19 education: the vocational (practical) route and the academic route. Sir Ron Dearing (1993) sounded a note of caution about the traditional GCSE and 'A' Level route when he said that 'it is disturbing that the system is serving least well those pupils who are less academically gifted [and] at 'A' Level, only one in seven pupils achieved three passes'. This is particularly relevant to students with special educational needs. A significant feature of the vocational route is that pupils emerge from their studies with work skills as well as academic qualifications. In his *Review of Qualifications for 16–19 year olds* (March 1996) Sir Ron Dearing proposed bringing 'the present academic, applied and vocational pathways into a common framework covering all achievements'.

Pupils need to consider carefully the options available and match these to their skills, talents and academic strengths and weaknesses before choosing a course.

The academic route

Although the academic route may appear to be the more difficult route for the dyslexic student, many dyslexics succeed academically, particularly in certain areas.

Research by Zdzienski (1996) at Kingston University highlighted that some dyslexics do have certain underlying skills, including strong spatial and visual skills, which influence their choice of course to follow. She found that from 109 dyslexics examined, the percentages studying in the different faculties were as follows:

Business	17 per cent
Human sciences	17 per cent
Science	20 per cent
Technology	22 per cent
Design	24 per cent

These figures support the commonly held view that dyslexic students tend to choose technical or practical subjects that are not primarily dependent upon essay writing.

The vocational route

Vocational courses are becoming increasingly popular in response to employers in business and industry who are actively seeking people with practical skills. Vocational qualifications can be obtained from a variety of bodies, and their courses may be followed in many places as well as in institutions of further and higher education. A number of colleges of further education run one-year Access courses for people over the age of nineteen. These are designed for adults who wish to return to study and move on to higher education. The course usually includes study skills, academic work and practical experience. Upon completion the student receives an Access Certificate which is nationally recognized and which helps with an application to a higher education course.

Business and Technology Education Council (BTEC)

The Business and Technology Education Council (BTEC) 'raised the profile and status of vocational training in Britain by awarding qualifications at technician level in business and technological disciplines' (Fennell, 1993).

There are programmes at three levels: the BTEC First, National and Higher National qualifications. Universities and colleges, as well as over 150 professional bodies, accept students with National and Higher National qualifications for entry for further study or to membership.

The Royal Society of Arts (RSA) Examinations Board

The RSA runs courses and gives awards that are nationally accredited and recognized qualifications. As an awarding body it approves organizations to offer its qualifications. These can be either written or assessment schemes. According to Brand (1990), 'the strength of the RSA teacher training schemes is that the demands of theory and practice are balanced, leading to the development of appropriate teaching techniques'.

This same emphasis on learning by doing applies to many of the RSA certificates and diplomas.

City and Guilds

City and Guilds offers a wide range of courses, which include skills and training. City and Guilds is one of the UK's leading body awarding vocational qualifications. It has developed assessments and awards in over 500 subjects. Its vocational qualifications for 16–19 year olds include the full range of General National Vocational Qualifications (GNVQs), as well as GCSE Technology and a number of core skills certificates. The City and Guilds Senior Awards structure offers a progressive, employment-based route to higher level qualifications. The awards comprise Licentiateship (LCGI), Graduateship (GCGI), Membership (MCGI) and Fellowship (FCGI). Senior Awards are offered in most industrial and professional fields.

National Vocational Qualifications (NVQs)

The National Council for Vocational Qualifications (NCVQ) was established in 1986. The Training and Enterprise Council (TEC), which replaced the Manpower Services Commission, is responsible for NVQs. The TEC's express purpose is to create wider access to further education.

National Vocational Qualifications are designed to provide qualifications for particular jobs or professions. They enable people in work to study part-time. There are also college-based courses and some that combine work experience and college attendance. The qualifications are based on standards developed by industry and commerce. This guarantees that they are relevant to the needs of the industry for which they are designed, and are valued by the employers. The course is made up of 'units' which correspond to modules in other courses. These 'units' can be totalled up (like 'credits' are in some courses) and may be put towards the final award. There are five levels: Level 1 – foundation; Level 2 – good GCSEs; Level 3 – 'A' Levels; Level 4 – degree; Level 5 – post grad. BTEC, RSA and City and Guilds all offer these courses. They are ideal for the pupil with special educational needs as the success achieved at work boosts confidence and the structure of the courses enables students to develop skills step-by-step. Success and a belief in oneself are invaluable when tackling the more demanding theoretical aspects of a course.

General National Vocational Qualifications (GNVQs)

General National Vocational Qualifications were introduced in 1992 and are available at three levels: Foundation, Intermediate and Advanced. The Foundation level enables the student to go on to a higher level of qualifications. The Intermediate level is equivalent to five GCSEs at 'A'–'C' grades. The Advanced level is equivalent to two 'A' Levels. GNVQs are based on standards and measured outcomes in a similar way to NVQs, but they cover a much broader range of knowledge and understanding than NVQs. Their original purpose was to provide a 'middle way' between academic and work-based qualifications. The GNVQ method of assessment is regarded as less daunting than conventional examinations.

The Further Education Funding Council (FEFC)

The Further and Higher Education Act 1992 placed a range of duties on the Further Education Funding Council, which funds colleges in England to run further education courses. The Disability Discrimination Act 1995 amended the 1992 Act to ensure that there are places on those courses for young people and adults with learning difficulties or disabilities. Colleges have to produce a disability statement which describes the support they can give. This should include the following:

- help with personal care
- teaching in small groups

- special equipment to use at college
- a support teacher or worker to help with parts of the course or with college life
- help with writing and maths
- help with how best to learn.

Scotland

Since 1993 colleges have obtained funding from the Scottish Office. Colleges now have to take into consideration the needs of students with learning difficulties and obtain higher funding if they provide learning support to individual pupils. They do this by appointing a learning support tutor who is responsible for drawing up a Personal Learning Support Plan.

In 1994 the Scottish Higher Education Funding Council began to provide funding for the cost of employing co-ordinators/advisers for students with disabilities and specific learning difficulties.

Before applying for a place in further or higher education*

When considering or applying for further or higher education, there are three essential considerations:

a) choice of course   b) environment   c) support for students.

Choice of course

Course design

The design of certain courses can help the dyslexic student achieve his final degree. Courses that include work placements allow the dyslexic student the opportunity to demonstrate his practical skills and sometimes this can result in higher marks overall. Courses with a continuous assessment element, in which marks towards the final degree are given for essays or a dissertation prepared during the year, benefit the poor examinee. Some courses entail less essay writing than others. It is an advantage if the examination or coursework involves multiple choice answers. Modular courses can also be great morale boosters for dyslexic students. The Open University (OU) courses and the format of their tuition are particularly suited to the dyslexic student as he can study at his own pace. He can choose as many or as few options as he wishes and

---

* Further information on this subject may be found in *Applying to Higher Education for Dyslexic Students* and *Dyslexia and Higher Education* by Dorothy Gilroy, obtainable from the Dyslexia Unit, University of Wales, Bangor.

can gradually accumulate sufficient points to enable him to graduate. The materials for the course involve the use of textbooks, videos, cassettes and television programmes. These can be recorded and replayed as often as is necessary, providing suitable material for multi-sensory learning strategies.

Course content

The course chosen should provide the student with the opportunity to use his strengths and develop his aptitudes. It is important to consider all the subjects that will be examined during the full course of study to ensure that there are no major stumbling blocks that could prevent the student succeeding. Some employers develop contacts with colleges and universities, or particular departments within these institutions. They may provide undergraduates with opportunities for work experience. Employers often turn to these colleges when recruiting.

Environment

There are many issues to consider, including the following:

- the choice of urban or rural location
- the size of the student community
- facilities for chosen leisure or sport activities
- social life – many students put this high on their list of priorities
- sociological factors – the cost and availability of student accommodation can influence the decision of some students
- the availability of public transport is yet something else to consider, particularly if the campus is out of town and the student does not have private transport.

Provision for support of students with learning difficulties

College support

Many colleges are improving their learning support provision. Southwark College, for example, has initiated and runs a training course for Special Needs Support Tutors, and co-ordinates a national network of tutors, lecturers and learning support staff. It also produces a directory of institutions which provide appropriate advice and support for dyslexic students. Support for students with special educational needs varies. All institutions produce policy documents about their provisions.

How tutors and lecturers can help

It is essential for the dyslexic to have strong support from his tutor, so that if a problem arises he may have a spokesperson to liaise with the rest of the department on his behalf. Such a tutor may also help in the following ways:

- teach study skills
- make notes available
- write keywords or terminology on the board
- when providing reading lists, highlight essential reading to distinguish it from background reading
- ensure that specific instructions, such as deadlines for completion of work, are written rather than conveyed orally
- encourage the student to produce an essay outline for major assignments in parts of the course and to do a draft before writing the final version
- allow the student to *volunteer* to read in a seminar or tutorial
- encourage the student and help him to organize his timetable
- support and encourage the student to use the technology available to help – photocopier, Dictaphone, word processor, etc.
- make arrangements for students to be assessed
- help make arrangements for examination concessions (if required)
- provide counselling and emotional support
- arrange meetings with other dyslexic students
- act as a mediator
- help to make colleagues aware of the particular needs and difficulties experienced by the dyslexic student
- help and advise the student regarding financial entitlements, for example from the Disabled Students Allowance.

Practical suggestions
to help choose a university or college and course

- Allow plenty of time to research the most suitable college and course.
- Read the UCAS handbook carefully and underline any significant parts. The section entitled 'The Gateway to Higher Education' is thought provoking and offers practical advice.
- Make a short list of universities/colleges and mark the courses to be applied for.

- Look at copies of prospectuses. These are available in many school and public libraries. ECCTIS 2000 is a computer information database which is a useful source of information on courses for students including those with disabilities. The Dyslexia Archive at the University of Kent (accessible on the Internet) collects and maintains information on dyslexia including the type of information that sixth formers are very interested to know, such as detail on exam allowances, help with coursework, and general support within the institution (Welch and Bowman, 1996).

- Contact the institutions and request a copy of their prospectuses and information on the chosen course.

- Ask to be sent any information the institutions may have about help or support for dyslexic/special needs students. The FEFC has made it compulsory for colleges to publish a disability statement.

- Choose the course carefully. Look at the content and subjects to be studied in all years making up the course. It is important that the student is capable of tackling the subsidiary subjects which may have to be studied in years two or three of the course. The prospective psychology student may find that he has to pass an examination in statistics at the end of his second year, even though he could not pass GCSE Maths – should he choose another discipline? It is worth considering doing a Higher National Diploma (HND) course, particularly for those who have thrived on the BTEC style of learning. It is often possible to transfer to a degree course upon completion of an HND course. An aptitude for and interest in the subjects chosen are essential.

- Check on the format and content of the course and the mode of examination. Is the qualification dependent upon a written final exam alone or is continuous assessment part of the final award?

- Check on the number of assignments required and the method of assessment. Does it include work experience or a placement?

- Visit the institution on its Open Day (if it has one).

- *Establish what support system is in place for students with learning disabilities*. This could be a disabled students adviser, tutor responsible for special needs or a tutor with knowledge of dyslexics and their needs. It may be possible to meet the member of staff (if there is one) who is responsible for dyslexic students.

- Try to find an institution that is sympathetic towards candidates with specific learning difficulties and has a properly funded and established support system. A useful source of data about this is SKILL, a voluntary body that runs a helpline and produces useful publications. It also has an ECCTIS 2000 database.

- Check on the number of students taking the course. Some argue that individual attention may be given to a small number of students. Others argue that integration is easier if there is a large number of students on a course.

- Check the examination results of the previous two or three years. These may indicate the standards of the course.

Guidelines
to help complete the UCAS/ADAR form

- Read the instructions and the form well in advance and then think carefully about the contents over a period of time.
- Read the handbook and the instructions carefully and underline key points.
- Make several photocopies of the form.
- Use the correct code numbers and dates.
- Use a black ballpoint pen and print as neatly as possible. The form will have to be reduced in size for administrative purposes, so the writing must be legible and not too small.
- The Disability/Special Needs code needs to be filled in. Dyslexia is number one on the code and there is room to give a short indication of possible needs. Some students are nervous about disclosing their difficulties, arguing that the admissions officer may be prejudiced by their disclosure of a handicap. The Disability Discrimination Act 1995 now makes this illegal. If the student still has residual problems which will affect his future work during the course, it is unwise not to make these known before embarking on a three-year course of study. He has to sign a declaration to say that the 'information given in the form is correct and complete'. He may run into difficulties if his academic

referee refers to his dyslexia or if, when he arrives at university or college, he immediately has to seek help because of his dyslexia.

- Discuss the contents of the form with parents, tutor and careers adviser, if possible. Make draft notes of any suggestions they may offer on the way to word the form.

- The student and his record of past achievements should be presented in the best possible way, in order to capture the interest and attention of the admissions tutor. Include details of any relevant voluntary work, or membership of any organizations. Now is not the time for modesty. Anything exciting or unusual that warrants a mention should be included – including fund raising for a charity. Be brief! Be concise! Be specific!

- Proof read the completed form and have it checked very carefully, particularly for the accuracy of the course codes. Also remember to put the institutions in alphabetical order, as directed by UCAS.

- Make a final copy and check it again in case copying errors have been made.

- Take a few photocopies for reference and keep these at hand. They will be useful when preparing for an interview or when contacting the institution directly, for example if the grades made in the conditional offer of a place are not achieved when the 'A' Level results arrive in August.

- Complete and send off the form as early as possible. Do not wait until the closing date for applications.

- UCAS will acknowledge receipt of the form and send an application number. Keep this to hand as it will be required when any contact has to be made with UCAS or the university/college.

The interview

Some students are called for interview. There does not appear to be any hard and fast rules about which candidates are and are not. The dyslexic student needs to be better prepared than the average student because 'the anxiety caused by the testing exacerbates the expressive language deficit' (Burton, Diana and Gennosa, 1991). On the other hand some dyslexics have good communication skills and may do well at interview, provided they have prepared themselves properly for it. The student may have to prove to the admissions tutor or interviewer that their dyslexia will not be an insurmountable hindrance to their completing the course successfully.

Suggestions
to help prepare for the interview

- Be well versed in the contents and details of the following:
  a) UCAS/ADAR form. This will help when asked about academic achievements such as examination results or school activities and may save embarrassment for the student with short term memory problems.
  b) Dyslexia assessment for the candidate – obtain a copy and ensure that it is an up-to-date report.
- Ensure that coursework or relevant projects are available. ADAR students will be required to have their portfolios of their work with them.
- Dress neatly and be quietly conventional in appearance and manner. (This criterion might not apply to the fashion or design student.)
- Sit down when told to and organize any paperwork so it is accessible.
- Shake hands firmly and look the interviewer in the eye.
- Try to avoid personal mannerisms which tend to surface when under stress.
- Listen carefully and if the question is not heard or understood, ask for it to be repeated.
- Some interviewers use an adversarial type of approach: they may raise a controversial subject and watch to see how the candidate handles it. Do keep calm even while politely disagreeing with the speaker.
- Be well rehearsed on dyslexia. Cite successes and achievements not included on the UCAS form. Give an honest and open history of any learning difficulties. Be prepared to elaborate on the type of help or support that might be needed to complete the course.
- It is important to know how to get to the interview venue and to leave enough time for the complete journey. Take a map and write down clearly the directions to the meeting. Do not rely on memory.

- Invest in a discount card from the national transport companies. This will help to reduce travel costs.
- Practise and rehearse interviews.

Skills the dyslexic student needs to complete the course

The study skills required at school (see Chapter 8) are just as relevant in institutions of further and higher education. Aaron and Phillips (1986) found, as a result of a ten-year study of dyslexic college students, that 'four symptoms constitute the core of the developmental dyslexia syndrome':

1 slow reading speed

2 incorrect oral reading

3 poor spelling ability

4 grammatical errors in written language.

Most of the student's work and study will be affected by these weaknesses. There will obviously be individual differences, but the overall picture is of a student struggling against his multifaceted handicap. 'Know thyself' is probably not necessary advice at this stage. The dyslexic has lived with his difficulties all his life, but his tutor or lecturer may have little experience of dyslexia and may be totally perplexed by the student's erratic performance. It is important that they are made aware of the particular difficulties experienced by the individual student if he is to survive and enjoy his undergraduate study.

How to help the dyslexic student cope with his studies

Having chosen a course that best suits his aptitudes and skills and one for which he can fulfil the entry requirements, and having found an institution that has a properly funded and established support system, the student should make contact with his personal tutor.

The personal tutor should be given copies of reports which should highlight specific areas of difficulty such as poor writing skills or slow reading. Students who are about to enter college or university should have an updated assessment which will highlight their special needs. This will be required if special provision is needed in examinations, or if the student applies for the Disabled Students Allowance. Assessments usually need updating about every two years.

Other students are an important source of help. They may be prepared to lend their notes or permit them to be photocopied. A student dyslexia support group can provide invaluable support.

Reading

For the dyslexic student his (slow) reading speed may constitute a major handicap. Zdzienski (1996) found 'that reading speed for dyslexic students is 130 wpm compared to the average of 300 wpm'. Problems in reading fluency can result in lack of speed and loss of understanding, because the student may need to read material several times to understand the content of what he has read. The student needs to establish what is essential and what is background reading. He needs sophisticated reading skills, such as an ability to scan and a predictive understanding of the author's intention as well as a comprehension of the text.

The institution may have a facility for putting texts on tape (a service often available for students with sight problems). A useful resource for audio books is Talking Books for the Blind which has a catalogue of over 9,000 titles. The annual subscription includes the loan of the cassette player. All postage is free. LEAs will sometimes pay the annual subscription fee.

Spelling

The spelling of many dyslexic students remains poor. Tutors must be asked to make allowances and not deduct marks.

Writing

Essay writing suffers as a result of poor literacy skills.

Dyslexic students are often unable to express themselves coherently or concisely and their writing can be convoluted and imprecise. Punctuation may be used sparingly or incorrectly which sometimes makes it difficult for the reader to understand what is being said. The dyslexic student often has a poor sense of audience; what he is trying to say is perfectly clear to him, but he does not always succeed in getting this down on paper. He often presumes that the reader knows what he is thinking rather than what he has written. 'I know what I want to say but it's getting it down is the problem' is a frequently made comment of dyslexic students. Essay planning and the skills required must be taught. The type of plan used will ultimately depend upon the learning style of the individual student (see Chapter 8).

Proof reading

At university, the student often has quite generous time allowances for handing in essays. It is a good idea to allow a few days to elapse before proof reading. Some students report that it helps them if they read their work aloud and listen to what they have written as they proof read. Some 'self-help' student groups arrange to proof read each other's essays. The tutor in charge of students with special needs may also volunteer to undertake this chore (the tutor can help with the mechanical aspects of the assignment but it will not be in his brief to alter the factual content of the material).

The student who has learned to type has a great advantage. 'The use of the word processor frees the learning difficulty student from the cumbersome physical task of writing; energies are utilized instead on the organization and reasoning inherent in good writing and it easily allows for deletions, substitutions, additions, etc.' (Dreyer et al, 1991). He can edit, and use the spell checker and grammar check to proof read. He can do this as many times as he likes until he is satisfied with the final result.

Note taking

Note-taking is adversely affected by poor writing skills but can be improved. There are two aspects to note-taking:

- from a book (visual)
- from a lecture (auditory).

Pauk (1974), when talking about taking notes from a book, said 'the essence of genius is to know what to overlook'. Researchers have found that the average adult can usually not remember more than seven separate pieces of information. Miller (1974) named this 'The Magical Number Seven Plus or Minus Two Theory' and Pauk (1974) postulated that this is why we have seven days in the week, seven seas, seven wonders of the world and seven notes in a musical scale. It describes the amount of information that 'average' individuals can place in their short term memory. The dyslexic student needs to use multi-sensory methods when learning to maximize his efforts. It is not sufficient for him to read the text and write notes; he must also recite the information to himself to help him learn.

Suggestions
for taking notes

Before the lecture

- Preview the course or lecture. Read a summary in an encyclopaedia or an abridged version. Watch a video or obtain a print-out from a CD-Rom.
- Put keywords on a card index, with their meanings if necessary.
- Put basic definitions on a card index.
- Identify and learn specialist vocabulary.

During the lecture

- Write in simple sentences. It will be less disjointed and easier to understand later.
- Write down the main points – names, dates, keywords, etc.
- Number the key points.
- Use abbreviations (but not too many) and ones that are familiar or self-evident.
- Write legibly.
- Use double spacing.
- Use wide margins.

After the lecture

- Re-read the notes as soon as possible, while the information is still fresh. Fill in further details that can be remembered.
- Underline the keywords.
- Use colour coding to highlight the contents, but remember that underlining/highlighting loses its purpose when over-used. Then study the lecture notes and use them.

The Cornell University System of Note-taking

1) *Record the main facts and ideas during the lecture.*
2) *Reduce the load to be learned by summarizing, underlining and numbering the key words.*
3) *Recite the key words and the ideas and facts.*
4) *Reflect – ask questions on the content of what has been read and compare this with the student's opinions and views.*
5) *Review what has been written.*

Source: Pauk W. (1974) *How to Study in College*. Houghton Mifflin Co., Boston: 128–9.

Some students may be unable to take satisfactory notes during a lecture. They may be helped in some of the following ways:

- They may be allowed to tape the lecture.
- The lecturer may be prepared to give photocopied notes.
- A fellow student may lend his notes.
- Keywords or ideas may be typed directly onto a personal laptop computer.

Time management

The concept of time management is very important. Clayton (1996) reminded us that many dyslexics do not appreciate the passing of time. They find it difficult to predict how long an activity will take. Allocating time for revision, examinations, study, planning projects and meeting deadlines is difficult. It is important that 'the student is helped to set priorities which realistically reflect the time available to accomplish them' and to remember that 'time management makes academic life more predictable and less stressful' (Schneld, Haber and Vincent, 1991).

A good diary/Filofax/personal organizer which is constantly referred to and updated is crucial. It should include deadlines for essays, time and place of tutorials, seminars and examinations. A duplicate can be kept on a chart/calendar on the wall of the place of study.

Examination tactics

The student should try to establish how he will be examined at the end of the term/year, because this will affect the type of notes he should take and the way in which he should study them. There are three types of examination question:

- short factual
- essay
- multiple choice.

The SCORER Method provides a few tactics for examinations:

S   This denotes *strategies* used to work out the time allowances.

C   Denotes the *cue word* in the question which should be circled on the paper, for example 'describe', 'illustrate', 'evidence'.

O   This is a strategy to *omit* the difficult question, and tackle the easy ones first, then return to the difficult one.

R   Stands for careful *reading* of all the instructions and directions – not just surface skimming.

E   Is used to encourage the student to *estimate*, that is guess the answer in cases where he is unsure.

R   Admonishes the student to *review* what he has done and to check his time allowance, and then to proof read all of the paper.

Source: Carman R. A. and Adams W. R. Jr (1972) *Study Skills: A Student's Guide for Survival*. John Wiley and Sons Inc. New York.

Essay examinations require the following approach:

- Time allowance must be carefully worked out.
- The wording of the title must be carefully checked and the keywords should be underlined.
- A plan should be made (see Chapter 8).
- Plenty of time for proof reading should be allowed.

Suggestions

on how colleges and lecturers can support their students

- A named person on the staff with special training and a knowledge of dyslexia is advisable. This person should know where a student can be assessed and by whom. If an assessment has to be carried out privately it is helpful to be able to advise the student of costs. It is useful if the tutor has a list of organizations or individual specialist teachers who may be able to provide tuition.

Essential text
Dyslexia at College (Gilroy and Miles, 1996)

- There should be a statement of policy about admissions, provisions available to students while studying and what special arrangements can be made when taking examinations. The Disability Discrimination Act 1995 has made provision of a disability statement compulsory.

- Counselling should be available within the college. The dyslexic student faces much more pressure than the average student.

- All members of the faculty should be given a list of their students who have specific learning difficulties. It is essential to seek the individual student's prior permission if he wishes his name to be included. Tutors repeatedly point out that 'our students are very watchful of confidentiality' (Gilroy, 1994). They should then be prepared to make allowances for their pupils' weaknesses, especially in written work. Allowances might include:

a) extra time

b) a different format for writing essays (a tabulated, note form of essay with diagrams will demonstrate that the student has mastered the facts and understands what he is studying, even though he may not have the skills to write this down in coherent English prose)

c) not deducting marks for poor spelling and grammar.

- Librarians need to be more tolerant of dyslexic students and should be prepared to find the book on the shelf for the student who, because of his sequencing difficulties, may misread the Dewey Classification System numbers or, because of his poor alphabetical skills, may be very slow at finding references himself.

- Arrange meetings between dyslexic students on the old adage that a problem shared is a problem halved.

- Lecturers should be aware that dyslexics often find it difficult to follow lectures because of their poor auditory sequential memory skills. It is helpful therefore if they do not speak too quickly and if they do not use very long sentences.

- It is helpful if the tutor can identify the key texts on prescribed reading lists.

Support provided for dyslexic students

Institutions of further and higher education are becoming increasingly sympathetic towards the needs of students with special educational needs, including their needs in examination and course syllabuses, as well as individual support for the student. Many now provide guidelines for internal use on a marking policy for dyslexic students.

National changes in attitudes towards the provision for students with special educational needs

Competition for students and for government funding has meant that applications from students with special educational needs are being considered more favourably than in the past. The media has reported that 'it is believed that universities are accepting these students [with low intelligence] merely to fill out their courses' (*Sunday Times*, 1995) and that 'the vast majority of those receiving grants for dyslexia were not genuine cases' (*Sunday Times*, 1995). In response to this and other issues relating to dyslexia, the Higher Education Funding Councils for England and Scotland and the DfEE set up a National Working Party on Dyslexia in Higher Education under the Chairmanship of Chris Singleton to tackle:

- serious concerns about the lack of national standards
- identification
- assessment
- support for dyslexics in higher education
- the production of national guidelines on assessment and support.

Institutions reported that they needed help with the following:

- arrangements for assessment including the credentials for assessors, type of assessment, criteria for diagnosis and payment arrangements
- content of dyslexia assessment and report in the light of the difficulty in identifying the student's needs and the paucity of suitable diagnostic tests
- the operation and way the Disabled Students Allowance system works and the LEA's point of view.

What financial assistance is available for dyslexic students?

Funds are available to help pay for the extra costs incurred by the student in higher education as a result of a disability. They may be forthcoming from the Disabled Students Allowance which can be paid by Local Education Authorities (LEAs) to students who can prove they have a disability or medical condition which affects their ability to study. The LEA needs evidence of the disability from either an educational psychologist or another person with specialist experience. The funds are an addition to the maintenance grant and an element of the mandatory award. LEAs can also give discretionary awards to those who are not eligible for a mandatory award. These should be claimed from the LEA in England and Wales, the Scottish Office Education Department in Scotland, and from the Education and Library Board in Northern Ireland. The LEA responsible is that covering the area in which the student has his main residence. There is a huge demand for these grants. According to Singleton (1993), '80 per cent of all such applications for such allowances were from dyslexic students'.

General allowance

The maximum general allowance was up to £1,185 per year (1994–5). The general allowance may be used to cover additional costs, such as buying copies of textbooks so they can be underlined, highlighted or have notes written in the margin, and can be used to supplement the other two allowances.

Allowance for non-medical personal helpers

There was an allowance of £4,550 (1994–5) for a non-medical helper. This could pay for the assistance of a typist or an amanuensis to write examination papers. It is paid termly. Claims have to be reasonable (about £12–£15 per hour for the help provided).

Equipment allowance

There was a sum available up to a maximum in 1994–5 of £3,560 to cover the cost of specialist equipment needed for a complete course, for example to purchase a laptop computer and a word processor. The National Federation of Access Centres will provide, on payment of a fee, advice and an assessment of the equipment needed. 'LEAs are unlikely to accept, as a basis for your entitlement, assessments of your equipment needs by retailers or manufacturers' (DfEE, 1996). A quotation or a receipt for the goods will be required. The student is allowed to keep the goods after graduation. Some LEAs are lending computers to dyslexic students who are registered as disabled and who are green card holders.

Other sources of funding

- Local charities sometimes have funds available. Some churches or church bodies also have resources for charitable purposes. They often have precise requirements and restrictions, for example recipients must have been born within two miles of the parish church. With the decline in the numbers of people attending church, there may be less demand for the funds. SKILL has a list of such trusts prepared to make grants.

- Local branches of worldwide organizations such as the Lions and Round Table sometimes make donations to individuals with special educational needs. The Citizen's Advice Bureau or a local library may be able to help with the names and details of local contacts.

- The Education (Student Loans) Regulations 1996 help colleges to work out who can get a loan and if so, how much. Any disability-related benefits will be disregarded when the income is assessed. If additional costs have been incurred because of the disability, there may be additional time given to repay the loan.

- Access funds are intended for support for students in need. These are administered by individual universities and colleges and are discretionary. They may, for instance, pay the cost of a psychological assessment.

How and where to obtain an assessment
- Help with obtaining an assessment may be available from the County Educational Psychology Service, the university's own psychology department, the student health service, private organizations such as the Dyslexia Institute, the Hornsby International Dyslexia Centre, or a chartered educational psychologist working privately. 'Your LEA cannot meet the costs of diagnosing your disability for establishing your eligibility to the Disabled Students Allowance (DSA).' (DfEE, 1996)

Recommended text
Financial Assistance for Students with Disabilities in Higher Education (SKILL, 1990)
Guidance Notes for Disabled Students in Higher Education (DfEE, 1996)

Criteria used to qualify for a Disabled Students Allowance
- Students must be on courses that qualify for a mandatory grant.
- Eligibility is means tested, as is the grant system for accommodation and subsistence. It includes the student's own income and that of his parents or spouse.
- Part-time or correspondence (distance-learning) students do not qualify.
- Post-graduate students on a State Research Grant (SRG), or Central Council for Education and Training in Social Work (CCETSW) or from a health authority are also entitled to certain allowances if they have extra needs which are related to their disability.
- An updated assessment and psychologist's report will be required.
- The student cannot start a claim for the allowance until he has been accepted by the college and after he has registered.
- An official letter from the educational establishment is required by the LEA confirming the circumstances of the student.
- Students with disabilities are eligible to claim Income Support and Housing Benefit, if they qualify.

Further information can be obtained from
The Educational Grants Directory. 1996/7 Edition (Smyth and Wallace, 1996)

Examination provisions for candidates with special educational needs

Individual examining bodies provide information about the provisions they make for dyslexic candidates.

General guidelines
on concessions for college and university students in the UK

Colleges and universities do not have an overall policy on examinations. Each institution is autonomous. It will be necessary to approach the Examinations Officer and enquire about their policy. Enquiries should be made within the faculty concerning their policy. Special concessions or arrangements should be confirmed with the Examinations Officer.

• Special arrangements must not give the candidate an unfair advantage over other candidates.

• Arrangements must not mislead the user of the certificate, that is employer/university about the candidate's attainments.

• A certificate may be endorsed indicating the concession given.

• Most examining bodies insist on a psychological assessment which must have been carried out within two years of sitting the examination. The current exception to this is BTEC, who 'will not make the provision of an educational psychologist's report mandatory but if one exists, it should be provided' (BTEC, 1993). The cost of this assessment can be a problem for some students.

• There is general consensus that the individual institutions need to be approached on an individual basis for an update on the policies as these arrangements are frequently revised.

• The person responsible for the administration and documentation of the student's arrangements is usually the special educational needs tutor or, in some cases, the personal tutor.

- Extra time is perhaps the most frequently requested and most often granted concesion. Twenty-five per cent extra time seems to be the average time allowance granted – some candidates read more slowly, others need the extra time because of their slow rate of writing.

- A reader of the questions is a less frequently requested concession and is usually only allowed when the candidate has an extremely low reading age. The reader cannot be the examinee's own tutor but should have practised with the candidate before the examination. He can give no other help except reading the questions and the rubric (instructions).

- An amanuensis (a scribe who writes the dictated answers) is sometimes permitted. There are precise instructions on what she may or may not do. This also often warrants an extra time allowance. It needs practice and frequent rehearsal before the examination. No help can be given other than recording the answers exactly as they are dictated. The amanuensis may also draw maps and do diagrams, as dictated by the candidate.

- Sometimes the candidate's best interests may be served by having a transcript made of his script. If the candidate's writing is almost illegible, arrangements may be made to have someone copy it so that it can be read. It must be a 'verbatim copy of the original script. Any errors of grammar, spelling or punctuation should be transcribed as given by the candidate and must not be corrected' (Joint Forum for the GCSE and GCE, 1996).

- Mechanical devices such as tape recorders, typewriters, computers and word processors are sometimes permitted in the examination. The candidate is not allowed to have access to files or to use a spell checker or thesaurus during the examination. The candidate must use the device himself.

- An arrangement can be made to have the question paper type enlarged to magnify the print, and make reading easier.

- Some examinations may be undertaken orally (*viva voce*).

The Scottish Examination Board (1996) has published guidelines for arrangements for candidates with special educational needs.

Summary and conclusions

1   There have been profound changes in the ways and means of gaining access to further and higher education in the UK.

2   There are many different qualifications, some of which are more suited to a dyslexic student than the traditional, academic 'A' Level and university degree course.

3   The student needs to chose carefully both the institution where he wishes to study and the course.

4   The student needs to be mindful that some admission tutors and lecturers are more sympathetic towards, and better informed about, the needs and requirements of students with special educational needs. It is advisable to make a thorough investigation before seeking admission to a particular institution.

5   The specific needs of dyslexic students may vary. The personal tutor or the college's special needs tutor may be able to help with aspects of work that cause problems, such as essay writing or study skills.

6   The student needs to prepare carefully for the interview.

7   The most important study skills to focus on include: note-taking, essay writing, skimming and speed reading, proof reading and examination techniques.

8   Institutions of further and higher education are increasingly sympathetic towards the needs of students with special educational needs. The Disability Discrimination Act 1995 imposes statutory requirements on all such establishments.

9   Extra financial assistance from the Disabled Students Allowance may be available for dyslexic students to help cover the extra costs they may incur. Funding may be available from other sources, but it takes personal initiative to unearth some of this financial assistance.

10   Certain provisions may be allowed for in examinations, and concessions are also available depending on the needs of the student. These are at the discretion of the individual establishments and subject to the individual needs of the student.

11   The arrangements in the UK as regards the recognition and help available to students and undergraduates with specific learning difficulties varies.

Chapter 10

Computers

- technology to assist and empower the dyslexic
- guidelines on choosing the most appropriate technology
- use in examinations

Introduction

Technology and electronic devices are an integral part of our daily lives. It is not a question of whether or not educators should be using technology to help dyslexics learn. The main issues are what to use, how to use it and what are the best principles for its use? The National Curriculum (1995) states that at Key Stage 2 pupils should use Information Technology (IT) 'to help them generate and communicate ideas in different forms, such as text, tables, pictures and sounds' and with some help they should be able to 'retrieve and store work'.

In the past some educators saw Computer Assisted Learning (CAL) as a solution to the problems of the overcrowded classroom. With the financial cutbacks of the 1980s the 'plugging in' to a machine was seen as a possible solution to the lack of education funding. Many schools were given machines, some of which were used imaginatively and effectively, some of which were not used at all. Ten years ago in primary schools there was one computer for every 107 pupils. In 1993–4 there was one computer for every eighteen pupils. The figures for the same period in secondary schools were as follows:

- 1986   one for every 60 pupils
- 1993–4 one for every 10 pupils.

Pupils themselves have been responsible for generating much of the enthusiasm that surrounds computers. Those who play with the electronic games available have no intrinsic fear of the machine, in the way that many of their elders do. A survey by a PC manufacturer (Wentke, 1996) revealed that technophobia is evaporating: 70 per cent of children thought computers were brilliant, 29 per cent thought they were easy to use, and only 1 per cent found them boring or difficult. Many teachers have grasped the opportunities to capitalize on the computer to stimulate and generate enthusiasm through a new way of learning. In the same survey children whose homes had a PC said that they spent less time watching television and 31 per cent spent more time on educational pursuits [on their computer]. The National Curriculum (1995) has made the teaching of Information Technology (IT) compulsory in all schools. But, as was pointed out in *The Sunday Times* (Heppell, 1995), pupils 'should use a computer as a tool in their learning lives: not learning about a computer directly but learning with a computer'.

In the past, parents used to raise funds to buy additional books for the school library. Now parents want to see the money spent on ensuring that there are enough computers in every classroom.

It is difficult to keep up-to-date with computer technology. The Dyslexia Computer Resource Centre at the University of Hull can provide regular information and updates on developments in the field. The University of Kent has produced *The Dyslexia Archive,* accessible on the World Wide Web on the Internet, which provides up to the minute information on the following:

- software and learning packages for dyslexics
- contact addresses of experts and workers in the field
- conference and exhibition details
- provision for dyslexic students at universities
- research reports and updates
- links to information held at other sites.

(Welch and Bowman, 1996)

Computer support in the management of dyslexia

The computer is intrinsically versatile. In the skilled practitioner's hands it can replace the 'chalk and slate' of our forebears, but the same fundamental skills, such as reading and spelling, still need to be taught to underpin its use. Computers can be invaluable aids to learning for all pupils, but they can play an even more significant role in the lives and the education of dyslexic pupils:

- They improve the motivation of the learner and are perceived as fun to use.
- They are non-judgemental.
- They can be programmed to go at the student's own pace.

- They can be adapted to suit the specific needs of the individual student.
- They can improve the presentation of work produced by the student.

Computers cannot solve all the difficulties of the dyslexic pupil. They do have limitations but many of these are being eliminated as computer technology improves.

Personalized tuition

One of the computer's greatest strengths is that the pupil has a built-in, personalized 'teacher'. Programs, for example to teach or reinforce spelling skills, can be tailored to the individual pupil's needs. The computer can immediately identify mistakes and reward the correct responses. This is a positive reinforcer, particularly for the learner with short term memory problems. Seeing the correct spelling on the screen as soon as the error appears is far better than finding out about the mistake a week later when the exercise book is marked by the teacher. The pupil can use the software package at home to reinforce whatever he has been learning in the classroom or from his specialist teacher.

Time management for the pupil

The pupil is in control of his mode and method of learning. This is particularly important for older students and adults. Lecture notes can be made on computer, stored on disk and expanded, redrafted and edited later.

Personal organization

Dyslexics with poor organizational skills can use the computer to store copies of essays, notes on the syllabus, and timetables easily and efficiently. The computer's facilities for locating files can reduce the problem of 'lost' work.

Improving basic skills

The computer can eliminate or circumvent some of the basic skills that the dyslexic pupil finds difficult, such as handwriting, leaving him free to concentrate on the content of the writing. Pottage (1996) said that 'good writing almost inevitably involves revision and improvement until the text not only says what you want it to say, but also flows so that the reader does not have to struggle to follow the message'. The computer makes this work much simpler, and at the end of the work a clean copy which is neat and legible can be produced.

Multi-sensory methods

Dyslexic pupils should be taught by using multi-sensory methods to see, hear, say, write and type. In this way they can use their auditory and visual skills simultaneously to learn. Multimedia is ideal because it can include excellent graphics, stereo sound and video clips and text. As a result the pupil has the opportunity to use his senses in a co-ordinated way to maximize learning.

Personal tuition versus 'impersonal' learning

Many people constantly fear that they will be made redundant and replaced by a machine. Teachers are no exception. Terrell and his colleagues hypothesized that the 'failing' reader would prefer to work with a computer because his mistakes could be made and corrected in private, and because the machine would be infinitely patient. Their research showed that the dyslexic reader preferred to be taught by a 'live' teacher and that they cherished the personal interaction (Terrell, 1994). Human contact is important in many learning situations but more so for the dispirited dyslexic. A friendly word of encouragement can work wonders for the morale of the dispirited learner. A listener who responds or interacts may also provide advice and reassurance that cannot be surpassed, even by the cleverest machine.

The way computers deal with mistakes

Some teachers are concerned about the way the computer deals with mistakes. The remedying and correction of errors can be more exciting than obtaining a correct response. Constant and dispassionate correction can also be demotivating for the demoralized pupil.

The assumption that the pupil can read

A crucial and intrinsic part of most work with a computer assumes an ability to read. Many dyslexics are weak readers so programs that have a heavy reading content may be off-putting or prove more trouble than they are worth. Consequently it is imperative for the teacher to check that the pupil can read with relative ease what is on the screen, otherwise the content and comprehension elements of the task may be lost.

What type of help can computers give?

According to Ingram (1984) 'there are four main categories of program applicable to education':

1 The 'didactic' program, suitable for 'drill and practice'. This is regarded as of fundamental importance by many authorities on dyslexia.

2 The 'content free' programs, for example the word-processing package. This is a toolbox which can be used in whatever way is appropriate for the pupil's needs.

3   The 'recreation programs' (sometimes referred to as adventure programs). These can be used to develop visual-spatial skills and co-ordination as well as planning and prediction skills.
They are used to reinforce a particular principle or concept and may be used at home or in the classroom. Many educationalists feel that they should be used sparingly and carefully. Hutchins (1994a) said that 'if a learner is receiving good dyslexia tuition, computer programs must compliment that tuition and not interfere with it'. 'Dyslexics do not regard these programs as work, and get really absorbed in them, to such an extent that they do not want to stop when it is time to go home' (Hutchins, 1994b). She pointed out that 'these programs cannot usually be used within conventional dyslexia lessons, as you need perhaps half an hour on several occasions to get through them'.

4   The 'diagnostic and screening programs' such as CoPS 1. These can be used by health care professionals, classroom teachers or the school's SENCO who are responsible for identifying special educational needs. This in turn should result in the 'appropriate' teaching being given.

Common problems experienced by dyslexics

The University of Kent became aware that dyslexic students who were on Access courses had specific problems. This has important implications for educators and funding authorities because nationally there is a high remission rate among students on Access courses. Evans and Welch (1996) noted the most common problems:

- Coping with the reading load because dyslexics are slow readers and have poorly developed skipping and skimming skills.
- Understanding the text.
- Difficulties in organizing and extracting material from different sources, for example when writing essays.
- Difficulties in listening and writing simultaneously, for example in a lecture. Slow writing can create problems when note-taking from a blackboard or an Overhead Projector.
- Difficulty reading texts which use different fonts, such as an italicized font.
- Some have difficulty with reading using certain colour combinations.

HyperStudy

Evans and Welch designed a program called HyperStudy to help the student overcome some of the problems listed above. It uses hypermedia and contains multimedia and hypertext features. Hypertext allows the user to access on screen pages of information, including text, graphics and diagrams. The reader can click a button to choose which information to concentrate on. It can be used to slow down, overlearn, go back and return to pages. All facilities are helpful for the student with short term memory problems. Words, phrases, definitions and notes can be saved which reduces the amount of time that would otherwise be spent on reading. The material can be transferred to an electronic notebook for revision purposes. Lecturers can enter whatever documents or information they wish to give to their students. It uses a large clear typeface. There is an option for the text to be read aloud.

Choosing a computer for a dyslexic pupil

The computer is to the present day child what the ballpoint pen was to the writer in the 1950s or the calculator to the mathematician in the 1970s. The trend is for the pupil to have his own computer. Increasing numbers of students are being enabled to buy their own computer with the help of the Disabled Students Allowance. Prices of computers are falling sharply relative to their power and performance, and it is not unrealistic to predict that the personal computer will be as universally accessible to the learning disabled population as the pen and calculator.

When buying a computer the major decisions relate to the choice of:

• computer hardware (the machine itself)
• computer software (the programs to be used).

Computer hardware

There are several categories of computer. All have advantages and disadvantages. When buying a machine, it is important to check what software, for example a word-processing package, is included in the package that comes with the machine.

Desktop machines

These are robust and usually general purpose – they can be used for a variety of tasks including word processing, spreadsheets and games. They tend to be large and heavy and therefore can only be moved with some difficulty. If a desktop machine with word-processing software is available to the dyslexic pupil, even if it has to be shared, it is well worth the effort of learning to use it – and of perhaps waiting for one's turn to use it.

Portables

These tend to be more expensive than desktop machines because their components need to be more resilient to cope with being carried around. Their primary advantage over desktop machines is their flexibility. Their instant availability and facility to be truly 'personal' usually outweighs the question of cost. Power can be supplied from the mains or from batteries. They are very suitable for the dyslexic pupil, who requires a good set of word-processing tools that are portable and personal. They make it possible for the pupil to work in his own time and anywhere he chooses, which may mean that he has additional time to catch up on work at home, for example. He does not have to wait his turn to use the classroom desktop and he does not monopolize it to the frustration of classmates. It can even be taken on fieldtrips to write notes. **Notebooks** are small portables which have the same functionality as the desktop and can fit into a briefcase for portability.

Organizers

These have many enthusiastic users, not least because of their size. They are pocket sized and weigh only about 250 g. They include a diary, spreadsheet, spellchecker, database and a word-processing facility. Work can be transferred to a desktop machine. An example is Psion Series 3a.

Palmtops

Palmtops are pocket-sized and are admirable for spelling aids and other word manipulation tasks. Their small size means that their keyboards require greater dexterity and are difficult for touch typing. An example is a Franklin Wordmaster.

Dedicated word processors

These machines have been designed just for the purpose of word processing. They are not general purpose computers. They can be desktop or laptop. The word-processing software provided may be the same as that in a general purpose computer. The files that are created may perhaps be transferred to other computers via disk, though this is not necessarily the case.

The Tandy Dreamwriter is popular and can hold 40 text pages but only ten lines of script can be viewed at any one time.

A machine such as the Canon StarWriter 30 comes with an internal disk driver and includes an integral printer. It also has the advantage of a flick-up screen.

A Sharp Fontwriter 710 has a 35 line back-lit screen, an internal disk drive and its own integral printer, as well as a clamshell case.

Guidelines

for choosing a portable computer

- Price is important, so shop around. Big discounts are available for the discerning shopper. Buying in 'bulk' often warrants a discount. Some outlets, such as Tandy Education Supplies and Services, have an 'education price'. They run a parent/teacher/student purchase scheme, giving a discount of between 20 to 33 per cent of the retail price in their Tandy stores.

- Consider the size and weight of the machine. It is better if it comes with its own case as dust, dirt and liquids are major enemies.

- Durability is important. Will it withstand the wear and tear of being carried backwards and forwards to school or college on the coach or train? Many suppliers sell 'carry cases'. These help to minimize breakages but make the computer distinguishable and attractive to the thief.

- Security is of prime importance as portable machines attract thieves. The machine will be safer if it can be carried discreetly and can be locked into a cupboard or a desk during breaks. Engraving the owner's name on the machine can help identify it. It is important that some form of insurance is arranged and that this covers the machine when it is taken away from the household. LEAs pay the insurance on the machines they lend to pupils with special needs or who are Statemented. It is an advantage if it can only be used by someone who knows the password. This is known as 'logical' security. It may reassure the pupil to know that his work can only be 'accessed' by somebody else at a time of the pupil's choice.

- It is important, when buying a computer for personal use, that the machine is one that is compatible with the existing technology in the educational institution being attended. If it is not, life can be very complicated.

  a) The school's printer should be able to print from the pupil's diskettes.

  b) Files and programs should be capable of being interchanged. According to Singleton (1994), 'in general, an IBM-compatible system (generally known as a 'PC') is recommended as this is the most widely-used system in education and business (*though not in school*)'. It is important to discuss the purchase of equipment with whichever school or institution the pupil attends to ensure that it is compatible with their own technology.

- The manual and instructions should be user-friendly. Is the layout clear?

- Routine maintenance should be easy for the user to perform himself, such as changing the cartridges, charging the batteries, cleaning or changing the printer.

- It is best if there are servicing facilities available locally. Does the manufacturer run a helpline?

- Is it easy to 'reboot' after it crashes?

- It should have a warning system when batteries are running low. Battery-operated computers should have sufficient power to last for two to four hours in use. It is important to have a battery adapter which can be plugged in to the mains overnight. This means that the machine is ready for use in the morning, it can be used anywhere, and it cuts down the cost of the batteries.

- Does the machine have the facility to switch itself off automatically if not being used, thus saving power?

- The screen size is important. A large, back-lit screen is desirable. A screen that is not flat is easier to use.

- Can the colour of the screen be modified? Some find it easier to read on a different coloured background, for example black printing on a lighter background.

- The keyboard is an important feature of any computer. For a dyslexic user it is vital that it is well laid out and clear.

- It should have enough memory to run the programs required. Many programs need 12 or 16 megabytes (Mb) of RAM (Random Access Memory) and games in particular need a lot of memory, as do talking wordprocessors. It is very irritating if a machine takes a long time to do its job.

- If it has been bought via mail order the cost of returning it to the supplier by post (for repair) can be very expensive and there may be an additional charge to cover for insurance costs.

Guidelines

for buying a second-hand computer

- According to Birkle (1994), 'the most important "don't" is don't look at second-hand machines until you have decided on the exact make and model that meets your size, durability, compatibility and operability criteria'. Then investigate the thriving market in second-hand machines that has grown as users trade up, lose interest or outgrow their machines.

- Auctions, often of bankrupt stock for example, can be a good source of machines which may sell at a fraction of their retail price. The disadvantage is that the purchase is entirely at the buyer's risk.

- Local newspapers, 'free' newspapers and the many personal computer magazines are also good places to look. Some magazines have a Buyer's Guide.

- Some retailers specialize in second-hand machines.

- Check with local retailers and find out the retail price of the machine when new. It is not unknown for advertisers to ask as much for their three-year-old machine as the brand new model costs in the shops.

- Don't be afraid to haggle.

- Check the condition of the machine and the manual. If it is in pristine condition and its box is still in good order, it can be taken as a good indication that the machine has been well looked after (or the owner did not know how to use it) or that it has had little use.

- Try and establish its life history. How old is it? Who used it? How much use has it had – every day in a classroom, or just occasionally to write reports?

- Has it got enough memory? It can be expensive to upgrade a two-year-old machine if it has only four Mb. Many programs, and voice-activated packages, now require at least 12 or 16 Mb of RAM.

- 'Test drive' it. Try before you buy with a number and variety of software programs. See it switched on. Type 'A B C' and ask to see it printed.

- Use a credit card to pay. Payment by credit cards may give some protection under current Consumer Protection Legislation.

Word processing

The ability to word process is a basic requirement when using computers to maximize benefits and, according to Hutchins (1994a), 'typing skills, whether touch typing or keyboarding familiarity, are vital for effective use of word processing'. A word-processing package is software. It provides a set of tools to enable the user, whether dyslexic or not, to express himself on paper or electronically. Word-processing packages contain a variety of functions, such as a spell checker, grammar checker or a thesaurus. Some of these functions are available as separate software packages.

Why is the word processor such a powerful ally?

The dyslexic teenager Paris Innes (1990) commented that 'writing takes all my concentration, especially if I want to write neatly'. Word processing on a computer frees the creative process for dyslexic learners. Adult dyslexics say that word processing and a spell checker have transformed their lives and made the mechanical writing operation effortless and efficient.

Word processors help in many ways:

- The pupil with fine motor, including handwriting, difficulties can be saved the manipulative task of writing because the machine creates letters and text from simple finger movements. The voice recognition systems are even more helpful because the pupil can talk to the computer and does not have to type.
- The machine can identify spelling mistakes and grammatical errors and suggest corrections. A thesaurus can find suitable alternative words.
- The machine can take the slog out of drafting, redrafting and editing material. It can file, edit and search for a word. It can help with the lay-out of material.
- It can help with proof reading.
- It can reduce the load with which the pupil must juggle:
  '. . . because word processing enables the separation of highly complex activities in writing which are normally carried out simultaneously. It reduces the information load on the brain and facilitates a systematic approach to detection and correction of errors, and editing and improvement of text' (Singleton, 1994).
- It has the ability to store work for reference or revision.

The arguments for teaching word-processing skills to all pupils with special educational needs

The Times (Brown, 1996) issued a challenge and asked 'in an era when so much adult work is done on keyboards, why is touch typing not generally taught in primary schools?' particularly as '90 per cent of school leavers are going to need touch typing skills'.

- Word processing improves motivation. Pupils who have good spoken language skills often fail to use their vocabulary and their ideas because they are overwhelmed by the effort writing manually requires. The quantity increases and the quality of the pupil's work improves.
- Pupils can often pick up more of their own errors on the screen because the print looks more like what they see in books. Word processing is a multi-sensory use of technology which we know enhances learning for the pupil with special educational needs.
- Pupils develop pride and confidence in their work when they can produce neat and error free work.
- It is faster. It can be easier and quicker to press a key than to write a letter, providing the pupil has good keyboard skills. The pupil therefore has more time to prepare, draft and redraft. This is particularly important for pupils doing coursework. However, if the pupil cannot type as quickly (or as accurately) as he can write, it is less satisfactory.
- Essays need no longer be rewritten by hand, risking the introduction of further errors, especially as the pupil becomes tired or stressed.
- The pupil with illegible handwriting can 'write' neatly. The machine turns his creativity into communication.
- Adult learners find it less demeaning to learn or practice basic skills on a computer because it is 'different' from what they have learned at school. Technology is regarded as innovative and more advanced.
- Motor memory is enhanced and users say that their spelling improves because they are also using kinesthetic memory.

How do computers help the classroom teacher?

- The same criteria can be used to evaluate the work of all the pupils, whether dyslexic or not. Marks are not lost for untidy presentation or poor spelling.
- Examples of the pupil's work can be mounted on the wall for display, kept in folders for reference, or included in the school magazine or class newspaper.

- Worksheets can be produced that are custom made for the individual pupil – spelling or punctuation exercises for example.

- Computers can be used when teaching essay writing. Pupils can be encouraged to 'brain storm', to trigger ideas and information. There are programs, for example *StoryBook Weaver*, with story beginnings and ways that incorporate pictures in stories that can encourage the most timid writers.

- Model answers and standard letters can be stored on diskette for the pupil as reference.

- The pupil can be taught how to make revision notes which are instantly accessible and quickly retrievable. This saves having to search through files which may easily be lost or misplaced.

- It helps with time management. The dyslexic pupil can be set a separate task if other pupils are working on something he finds too difficult.

- It helps with record-keeping for reviews and meetings with parents.

- The pupil can work at his level and he is not made to feel aware that he is struggling behind his peers.

- The pupil can reinforce whatever the specialist teacher may be doing with him, either with games or parallel exercises.

- It helps to boost the pupil's confidence because he is enabled to produce neat, legible work with few spelling mistakes.

Guidelines
for choosing a word-processing program

- Does it have a variety of different typefaces (fonts) for different purposes?

- Can it handle pictures/graphics?

- How effective and efficient is the spell checker?

- Is there an in-built safety device? This should ensure that the pupil's work cannot be wiped out by a clumsy touch on one key.

Keyboard skills

The word processor is a tool and the text it produces is only as good as the operator. It confers no unfair creative advantage upon the dyslexic writer over his peers who write in long hand. Some observers say it levels the playing field for the dyslexic learner. The

National Curriculum (1995) concurs with the view that 'pupils should be given opportunities, where appropriate, to develop and apply their IT capacity in their study of National Curriculum subjects'.

Why is it necessary to learn to touch type?

Keyboard skills have to be taught and practised. Like all motor skills, they improve and get better with practice.

Experts have different views on whether the pupil should be taught touch typing (using all his fingers and not looking at the keys) or whether the 'pick and peck' method will suffice. The advocates of the two finger approach say that children's enthusiasm can be dampened if they have to go through the monotonous, dreary routine of learning to touch type. The advocates of touch typing argue that word-processing skills are life skills, and the additional effort required to learn to type 'properly' is worthwhile. Stoecker (1985) found that the average student, without training and practice, can produce 6.5 words per minute. This can gradually increase to 18 words per minute after 20 minutes daily practice for four weeks. Thirty minutes practice per day for five weeks can produce a speed of 28/30 words per minute for the average pupil. There are no set rules. The aptitudes and weaknesses of the individual learner must dictate the chosen approach.

In the UK many of the specialist schools for dyslexics teach all their pupils touch typing from an early age. There is no conclusive research regarding the age at which children are able to touch type. Anecdotal evidence suggests that the pupil needs to be 10–11 years to have the manual dexterity to touch type. Some dyslexics take to it quickly and easily, particularly if they already have experience of a keyboard. Others find it slow and difficult to master.

Teaching keyboard skills

Specialist schools have developed a multi-sensory approach to teaching keyboard skills and teach the pupil to say the letter name as he types it. Some pupils find this beneficial, others find it distracting. Skills should be taught in a structured and systematic way.

Software packages that might be helpful

The following software should provide the pupil with a comprehensive basis for most of his homework requirements:

- A word-processing package which includes a spell checker, thesaurus and a grammar checker.

- A reference source, such as CD-Rom with an encyclopaedia, (for example Microsoft's Encarta, or items from the Dorling Kindersley set of educational titles).

Recommended programs
Micro Type: Fairley House Touch Typing Program
Fingers for Windows: Type to Learn

Spelling and spell checkers

'Whatever their individual pattern of difficulties, all dyslexics have persisting problems with spelling.' (Hutchins, 1992)

Modern technology can free the dyslexic from the mechanics of writing, leaving him to write down what he knows and wants to say. Higgins and Zvi (1995) reported that 'the use of the computer as an assistive device appeared to have a liberating effect on students, generally increasing productivity and in many cases releasing them from long-standing difficulties such as severe spelling disabilities...' and 'the use of speech recognition technology directly encouraged the expansion of more mature and complex vocabulary'. 'Godsend' is a frequently mentioned epithet by the dyslexic user – perhaps 'revolutionary' would be a more appropriate word.

Spell checkers can be an integral part of the word-processing package purchased, or they can be purchased separately.

Choosing a spell checker
There are several options available when choosing a spell checker:

1 The spell checker that makes a 'bleep' to warn the writer of a possible mistake. Not many professional word processors have this facility but some portables do. Paris Innes (1990) commented 'when I am on my word processor and it "bleeps" to say that I have spelt a word wrong, I feel livid, but when the spelling comes up and it's corrected, I feel better again'. Some pupils find the 'bleep' distracting and intrusive. Others report that the 'bleep' acts as a trigger and this in itself can often make them focus on the correct spelling of the word.

2 The spell checker that corrects the document when it has been completed.

3 There are now spell checkers that include a phonetic spelling option. They can predict words after the first two letters have been typed in.

4 There are also talking spell checkers.

Guidelines
for choosing a spell checking program

- Does it use English rather than American spelling?
- Can the pupil add his own list of words that he frequently misspells?
- Can the pupil read the choices of spelling offered to him? If the list is too long or too difficult then it will defeat the objective.
- Does the package have a word prediction facility? This can be useful for the slow typist or very poor speller. It cuts down on the amount that needs to be typed by presenting the user with a choice of words.
- How does it identify errors? Does it use a bleep, which can be distracting or irritating to other pupils in the classroom? Does a mark appear on the screen when a word is wrong?
- Can the whole document be checked for errors once the work has been 'finished'?
- Can the program be reconciled with the spelling pattern being taught or programme being followed? The following teaching programmes are compatible with the following programs:
  Alpha-to-Omega – Word Shark 2
  Spelling Made Easy – Starspell Plus
  The Bangor Dyslexia Teaching System – Xavier Software

The advantages of spell checkers

- More sophisticated programs are better at handling the 'phonetic approximations' that many severely dyslexic pupils use: 'kof' for cough
- A spell checker aids visual memory and consequently can improve the pupil's automatic response to the spelling of a word. Just seeing the word correctly printed on the screen is a powerful reinforcer.
- For the very seriously dyslexic writer who has become paranoid about attempting to write because of his almost total inability to spell, the predictive word processor can be very helpful, providing the pupil has good reading skills. On being presented with two or three letters, it will offer a range of words from which to choose:
  'The weary soldier sat down in the tr ...' train/tree/tram/traffic
- It is a boon for proof reading and corrections. The advent of the

talking spell checker is a huge breakthrough. Examples are the Longman Logotron *Pendown* with the Superior Software speech program called *Talking Pendown* or iAnsyst Ltd's *TextHelp*.

- Many specialist teachers of dyslexic pupils encourage their pupils to develop proof reading skills, particularly for spelling errors. David Moseley (1991) commented that 'many teachers report that most children detect only a small proportion, 25–30 per cent of their own spelling mistakes'. The spell checker can improve on this.

- It is possible to program the spell checker with a list of the individual pupil's most frequently misspelt words and with specialist subject words.

- It can help to develop the vocabulary and the language skills of the user. It can also have a stimulating effect by giving a sense of the choice and options of words available, without the constant worry of trying to remember how to spell the word.

- It is faster than using a dictionary.

The limitations of spell checkers

- They were not designed specially to meet the needs of the dyslexic speller. They are better at coping with typing errors, such as using a wrong letter or an incorrect vowel, than the idiosyncratic spellings of a dyslexic pupil. The more elementary spell checkers assume that the first two letters of the word are correct.

- The spell checker cannot cope with 'homophones' (words which are pronounced the same but spelt differently and which are one of the greatest problems for the dyslexic speller). Grammar checkers can correct this type of error and are consequently very useful.

- The spell checker does not pick up a word used inappropriately: are/our or were/where.

- Spell checkers are not appropriate for the very young pupil. Some teachers argue that the pupil will not bother to learn to spell the word if all he needs to do is type a few letters. They liken it to attempting to teach mathematics to a child by just using a calculator. It can dissuade the young pupil from understanding the necessity of learning spelling rules and patterns. This can be a serious handicap in his understanding and use of expressive language skills in later life.

- Examination boards forbid the use of a spell checker when knowledge and use of language is being tested expressly. It is important that the dyslexic pupil is encouraged to try to learn to spell and does not become reliant on mechanical aids.

- The biggest drawback for many dyslexics is that the whole computerized spell checking process is dependent on good reading skills. Scheib and Lillywhite (1994) said that 'spell checkers are suitable for children with a reading age above ten years'. The pupil with poor literacy skills may not know the meanings of the words he is offered when given a choice. This can make selection of the appropriate word problematic.

- The biggest criticism made of spelling programs for dyslexic pupils is that there is not enough multi-sensory input, which is regarded by many experts as essential.

Handheld spell checkers

The handheld spell checkers have been available for some time and their performance has been improved and modified by the advances in technology. The choice should depend on the pupil's needs, priorities, expectation and budget. The *Franklin Elementary Spellmaster*, suitable for primary school pupils, secondary school pupils and dyslexic adults with primary levels of literacy is typical of handheld spell checkers on the market.

Facilities offered by the Franklin Elementary Spellmaster

- It works on a long life battery which cannot be recharged, but it does last a very long time.

- It has a small screen which can be made darker or lighter to suit the light conditions, or the dyslexic pupil's preference or toleration of light or colour.

- The pupil types in a word and if it is correctly spelt, it says 'correct'. If it is wrong, it gives a list of options to choose from. It has a list of over 30,000 words.

- It has been designed to be linked to the pages of the *Oxford Children's Dictionary* (2nd edition, 1985). It gives the dictionary page number and therefore instant access to word meanings. This saves the dyslexic, particularly one with sequencing difficulties, the work of having to hunt for the word. This facility can also be used to help build vocabulary skills. This is useful for checking the meanings of the homophones.

- It has an option called a 'User List' which can be personalized by the owner. He can add a list of his own frequently misspelt words, as well as a specialist vocabulary list. Up to fifty words can be stored.

- It can be used to play a number of spelling 'games'.

- The 'Wildcard' option can be used in a variety of ways, for example to examine letter patterns and make lists of words with prefixes and suffixes.

- It is often easier for the weak reader to type in the word he wants and then check the meaning on the named page of the dictionary, than to grapple with a list of words that the spell checker has given.

- Its relatively cheap cost makes it affordable for many pupils. It is also an easy way to introduce the pupil to simple technology, and can stimulate experimentation with more advanced machines.

Guidelines

when choosing spelling software programs

- Look at the catalogues of the specialists in the field. A handful of names appear constantly in the recommended 'best buys' of experienced practitioners in the field.

- Try before you buy. Many suppliers are happy to do this and a few companies will send their programs on approval.

- The programs produced by established teaching centres and university departments who are working in the field of special needs are usually worth investigating.

- The BDA Computer Committee reviews and updates information on what is currently available. Its members are drawn from different disciplines and have differing views on and experience of the methodology being used in the independent and maintained sectors of education. The committee publishes lists and descriptions of its recommended 'best buys'. The Dyslexia Computer Resource Centre at the University of Hull has copies of most of their recommended programs.

- Buy from specialist publishers, usually by mail order. High Street outlets' materials are usually not appropriate for the special educational needs of dyslexics.

- Gauntlett (1991) produced a list of words which he recommended to test whether the spell checker could cope with the idiosyncrasies of a dyslexic's spelling:

Gauntlett's list of spelling gaffes

altruistic	*ultrustic*
dyslexia	*dislexer*
written	*wrten*
writing	*writting*
exacerbate	*exaserpate*

exasperate	*exasperat*
received	*recieved*
necessary	*neccessary*
learnt	*lernt*
aquatic	*equaitic*

Source: Gauntlett D. (1991) *A Review of Spelling Aids for the Dyslexic*. BDA, Reading.

Voice recognition technology

Voice recognition technology is a blessing to many dyslexic pupils, and is particularly useful for those with very severe spelling problems, or those who who are unable to master keyboard skills. Higgins and Zvi (1995) found that 'significantly more students obtained a better score when writing essays using speech recognition technology' and 'subjects found significantly more of their own errors overall using speech synthesis/screen review than when proof reading without assistance or when having the essay read aloud to them.' They also found that 'the use of speech recognition technology directly encouraged the expansion of more mature and complex vocabulary after suitable training and practice'.

Speech and talking computers

There are two speech options available with talking computers:

- 'digitized' or 'sampled' speech, which uses real, live reconstructed speech. It can only use words that have been recorded in its memory.
- 'synthesized' speech, which is robotic-like.

Speech is used in educational and specialist teaching programs such as *Word Shark 2* (compatible with *Alpha-to-Omega*). Talking books, such as *Oxford Reading Tree*, are available which display the page on the screen and provide a recording of the text for the pupil to listen to at the same time. Talking word-processing packages such as *Talking Pendown* or *Write: Outloud* are available. Word prediction software which is useful includes *Penfriend and Co: Writer.*

Guidelines

on using talking word processors

- Some dyslexics have word retrieval problems, so they may find voice recognition technology challenging to use initially.

- It imposes additional strain on the user who has a poor short term memory because he is required to think and speak simultaneously.

- An interruption may mean losing the train of thought or the flow of ideas.

- Reviewing what has been said will require a replay.

- The system has to be trained to recognize the pupil's voice and may not handle fast speech.

- The pupil needs to leave gaps between the words as he says them.

- Most spellings are handled well, although some homophones can cause problems, for example in a sentence like 'the two cars were going too fast to stop in time'.

Many of the difficulties can be overcome with effective training. Any irritations are far outweighed by the joy of being able to see the text on the screen of what has been said, even at speeds of up to 60 words per minute.

Talking software is an eminently suitable way of incorporating multi-sensory methods in teaching literacy skills such as touch typing, numeracy and writing.

DRAGONDICTATE and KURZWEIL VOICE, available from iAnsyst Ltd, are two of the most poplar systems available for PCs.

Computers and mathematics

Many dyslexics have difficulty with mathematics, particularly with arithmetic (see Chapter 7). Some have visual perceptual problems, for example they may not remember what a figure '5' looks like, and others may have difficulty in writing the number. Many have poor auditory short term memory, making them unable to recall a string of numbers. Their auditory sequential memory is weak, making it difficult to learn the times tables or to use mathematical processes such as formulae. Their directionality difficulties lead them to confuse left and right and up and down. Not many computer programs can teach these skills but they can provide the drill and practice to reinforce them.

A computer is excellent for the rote activities, such as teaching number bonds and times tables. The pupil can sit quietly and practise his times tables using one of the many programs that are available.

- The pupil with poor motor skills can be encouraged when he discovers that he does not have to remember how to form a number, and only has to press the correct key.
- The pupil who has difficulty setting out his work can be helped with the clearer presentation he sees on the screen.
- The pupil can practise the same skill repeatedly. The computer can keep a record of his score and the learner can aim to beat his own score. This improves motivation if his performance is progressing, but can lead to frustration if he is not.
- The pictorial representations, such as pie charts or fractions, are often clearer than in a textbook. The program can often be adapted to the pupil's environment.
- The computer is endlessly patient and never criticizes.
- The scientific calculator is useful for checking calculation errors because it lists what has just been entered.
- The spreadsheet facility is very helpful when doing graph work.

How to evaluate
a maths computer program

Read the BDA Computer Committee's recommendations and obtain updates of their literature. Then consider the following:

- Is it appropriate and will it reinforce what has been taught in the lesson?
- How often can the program be used?
- Are there varying levels of difficulty suitable for pupils with different skills and aptitudes?
- Can the pupils cope with the reading content of the program?
- How long does the program take to use? Can the speed of presentation be varied to suit the individual learner?
- Cost – is it reasonably priced?
- How useful/helpful are the maths games?

- Does it test understanding of concepts and principles as well as memory?
- Does it encourage and promote problem-solving skills?
- Is there a facility to reinforce basic maths vocabulary?
- Are the graphics age appropriate? The adolescent can be alienated if asked about counting teddy bears.

Information access via the computer

Many books, journals and newspapers are now available in computer readable form on disk or CD-ROM. Computers can access multimedia materials involving audio and visual presentations. The Internet has made available vast channels of information and interpersonal communication. The versatility and flexibility of the computer enables it to present material in a form which is helpful to the dyslexic pupil: sound and moving images reinforce written text. Schools, universities, colleges and libraries increasingly have access to computers and to the sources of information that can be accessed by computer.

Computers and examinations

Dyslexic pupils who use a word processor as their 'normal means of communication' can apply to use it in the National Curriculum tests at Key Stages 2, 3 and 4, as well as in GCSE and 'A' Level examinations, and also at colleges and universities. In Scotland any candidate can use a word processor for examinations providing the spell checker facility cannot be operated, and other candidates are not disrupted.

Preparation for the examination

The following remarks can apply to GCSE and GCE pupils:

- Using a word processor is a mechanical skill that needs practice. The pupil should be encouraged to start using his word processor the year before he begins his course. Ideally he should already have learned to touch type.
- The pupil should use the word processor as 'his usual method of working in the classroom'. This will strengthen his case when applying to the examining board for special consideration. The GCE Examining Boards ask for historical evidence of the candidate's needs and expect to see that the candidate's needs

have been recognized over a period of time. It is also important to develop the skills of 'thinking' at a keyboard rather than drafting in longhand on paper and then typing it in.

- The word processor and laptop computer are ideal to use for taking notes and for making revision notes.

- All candidates are allowed to do coursework on a word processor. This is even more important for the candidate with a specific learning difficulty because the mechanical skills are taken care of by the machine. The pupil is then able to concentrate on content and comprehension. The Joint Forum for the GCSE and GCE (1996) states that 'candidates may, without the need to request permission from the examining group, use spelling aids, for example dictionaries and word processors with spell check facility, in coursework unless a set task to be undertaken under controlled conditions specifically forbids their use'.

- Candidates who have a 'Statement' of special educational needs should ensure that access to information technology is specifically mentioned in the Statement, and that it continues to be included at each annual review if necessary. 'All provisions, including those for candidates with Statements of Special Educational Needs, are subject to application for permission from the examining groups.' (Joint Forum for the GCSE and GCE, 1996)

- Records of all coursework done on disk should be kept so that when the time comes to submit the best examples, clean copies are readily available.

Guidelines

for applying for concession to use word processors in examinations

Some candidates may be allowed to take their examinations using a word processor. The timing of a request to use such equipment is important. The Examining Groups have produced *Regulations and Guidelines* (Joint Forum for the GCSE and GCE, 1996) to help when making requests of special assessment needs in the GCSE, GCE and National Curriculum examinations. These are common to all GCSE and GCE examination groups. The reason for these arrangements is to enable the candidate 'to demonstrate their attainment in relation to the assessment objective of the syllabus' but 'it must not give the candidate an unfair advantage over other candidates'.

- A request for special examination arrangements must always be supported and arranged by the Head of Centre.

- The school should write to the examination board when the pupil starts the course (two years before he is due to sit a GCSE examination), to inform it of the pupil's difficulties, enclosing an educational psychologist's report, prepared within the two years prior to the examination, as evidence in support.

- Early in the Autumn term prior to the examinations, the Statement, or the educational psychologist's report, should be checked to see that it is up-to-date for the examination board. The report must not be more than two years old.

- In December or January, the internal school 'mock' examinations should be taken using a word processor. It is not worth pursuing the request for this in the final examination if this is not the case. The examining boards will require evidence that a word processor is the candidate's usual method of working in the classroom.

- The Head of Centre must submit a formal application to the appropriate examining group using the official form JEB/SA. By the 28 February in the year of examinations to be taken in the Summer term (30 September for examinations to be taken in the Autumn/Winter term) the school makes a final statement of entry and tells the Board what subjects and modes of examination are being taken and the special considerations being requested.

- The examination boards reply to requests for concessions between January and March.

- If the examination board refuses a request, the school's director of studies/examinations secretary should appeal.

- By April, a copy of the concessions and provision being made should have been received.

- The pupil should be given a copy of these to take in to the examination on the day, in case of any lack of communication, or misunderstanding by the invigilator.

Conditions made by GCSE and GCE Examining Groups for the use of a word processor in the examination

- Any provisions and concessions have to be made by prior arrangement, as stated above.

- The word processor must not have any access to files or material stored on it. Electronic calculators and spell checkers are not allowed in certain examinations, such as English language.

- The examination should be conducted away from other candidates.

- The printing of answers may take place after the time allowed for the examination has expired and the candidate should be present to verify that the printing is complete.

- No considerations will be given if there are technical problems with the machine. The centre/candidate must ensure that the computer is working properly and should have a supply of reliable batteries.

- The operating manual is not permitted.

- The candidate must operate the word processor himself.

- The examination centre is responsible for ensuring that all these conditions are fulfilled.

Source: Joint Forum for the GCSE and GCE (1996) *Candidates with Special Assessment Needs: Special Arrangements and Special Consideration*. Manchester.

Summary and conclusions

1   There are many exciting technological breakthroughs which will enhance and empower the dyslexic learner. Computer literacy 'including the confidence to solve problems and communicate will be a fundamental facet of literacy in the 21st century' (Heppell, 1995).

2   Computer Assisted Learning is one of the most significant breakthroughs in the lives of dyslexic people. The National Curriculum puts computer literacy on all school timetables as a statutory requirement and states that by Key Stage 4 all pupils should be able to 'use IT to handle and communicate information in a variety of contexts'.

3   Computer literacy and word processing build confidence, improve motivation and enhance skills as well as removing much of the stress and strain in studying. Employees now

require multi-disciplinary skills and information technology at work. Information technology literacy is as important as manual skills or intellectual training.

4 Teachers who have responsibilities for SEN can be helped by using the computer. According to the *Code of Practice 1994*, 'to assist in the early identification of children with special educational needs, the school will wish to make use of any appropriate screening or assessment tools'. The computer is designed to do this easily, effectively and efficiently.

5 Computer Assisted Learning requires certain basic literacy skills, such as reading, but it cannot readily substitute the traditional methods of teaching literacy skills.

6 Laptops are a great asset to the dyslexic person. It is advisable to shop around before buying a machine, either new or second-hand, and to ensure that the machine is capable of doing all that the pupil may need it for.

7 There are many sources of advice and information on computers, both nationally and locally.

8 All dyslexics should be given the opportunity to learn word processing and keyboard skills. They should ultimately learn touch typing, but, according to Hanbury King (1985), the conventional methods of teaching typing do not work well for the dyslexic. They must be taught as a motor process not as a visual process.

9 Spell checkers make the life of the poor speller easier and more productive.

10 There are many maths programs available which are excellent for reinforcing and revising processes and skills.

11 Computers are part of modern life and are now commonplace in the classroom, lecture hall, office, factory and home. CD-Roms, which include encyclopaedias, books, journals and newspapers, provide sophisticated and often user-friendly facilities to gain access to information. Modems enable computers to communicate with other computers, such as on-line reference libraries, and information can be obtained from institutions all over the world. The Internet provides access to global sources of information and knowledge.

12 Some pupils with severe special educational needs may be allowed to use a word processor when sitting examinations. There are strict criteria laid down for the use of this concession.

Chapter 11

Music

- the implications of dyslexia for the musician
- how to help the dyslexic musician

Introduction

The problems of the dyslexic musician have not been recognized until recently, and talent has languished because of a lack of understanding of his specific difficulties. There has been little research into or information produced about, the problems faced by dyslexic musicians.

Critchley, in the early 1970s, reported cases of professional musicians who were members of London symphony orchestras who had difficulties, because of their dyslexia, with certain aspects of their work. Greater awareness of their problems is due mainly to the disclosures of talented, but often frustrated, musicians who have gone 'public' about their struggles. The experiences of the dyslexic Delos Smith (Pollack and Branden, 1982) gave a fascinating insight into his difficulties, which include not being able to carry a tune and no sense of pitch or rhythm. He was unable to read music or tell whether a scale was being played in ascending or descending order. In the UK professional musicians, such as the singer Annemarie Sand and the composer Nigel Clark, have allowed knowledge of their dyslexia to be made public in order that other dyslexics can benefit from their experiences.

The Disabled Living Foundation and Violet Brand helped increase public awareness of the dyslexic musician's problems. In l983, a working party was set up to examine the problem which drew attention to the difficulties of the many musical, dyslexic people. This later evolved into a sub-committee of the BDA. The BDA itself made a further contribution by including music in its definition of dyslexia:

*A specific difficulty in learning, in one or more of reading, spelling and written language which may be accompanied by difficulty in number work, short-term memory, sequencing, auditory and/or visual perception and motor skills. It is particularly related to mastering and using written language – alphabetic, numeric and **musical notation**. In addition oral language is often affected to some degree.*

Source: 'What is dyslexia?'. In Crisfield J. and Smythe I. (1993) *The Dyslexia Handbook 1993/4.* BDA, Reading: 8.

Margaret Hubicki, who was a professor at the Royal Academy of Music in London, has also played an important role in making her colleagues aware of the implications of being dyslexic for the musician and has contributed much to practical ways of helping these aspiring musicians.

What specific problems do dyslexic musicians have?

Time and again there have been reports of dyslexic pupils who showed a talent and interest in music but who gave up, because they encountered problems with the written forms of music and with certain aspects of theory or performance. Their teacher may have influenced this decision by becoming exasperated or perplexed by these pupils' peculiar errors and their lack of progress, perhaps attributing their problems to lack of effort or concentration, or to carelessness.

Notation

'Notation' relates to the symbols written down to represent the notes and directions for pieces of music. It is a code, just as the alphabet is used to make words which convey meaning.

The notes on a stave are symbols used to represent the sounds which make music. It should not, therefore, be surprising that processing these symbols can cause confusion and difficulties for the dyslexic musician since there is much evidence to show that dyslexics have difficulty decoding (reading) and encoding (writing) letters. Atkinson (1991) confirmed that 'many dyslexic children were significantly worse on both the sight reading and sight singing than non dyslexics'.

Reading and writing music

'These children may be as "musical" as anybody else but their achievements as musicians are hindered by the problems of having to read notation' (Beaumont, 1994). Visual perceptual difficulties and weaknesses in dyslexic pupils can cause nightmares when reading and writing music. Florence, ten years old, who won a music bursary at her school, said, 'I look at a note, then I play the wrong one.'

- The symbols used to represent the notes are very small and very similar in shape and configuration thus causing confusion for the dyslexic:

𝅝	= semibreve	= (4 beats)	= whole note
𝅗𝅥	= minim	= (2 beats)	= half note
𝅘𝅥	= crotchet	= (1 beat)	= quarter note
𝅘𝅥𝅮	= quaver	= (1/2 beat)	= eight note
𝅘𝅥𝅯	= semiquaver	= (1/4 beat)	= sixteenth note
𝅘𝅥𝅰	= demisemiquaver	= (1/8 beat)	= eighteenth note

- Remembering the names of these notes, and the names of the lines and spaces on a stave, can present great difficulties to the pupil who may have both a word retrieval problem and problems learning to read. The pronunciation of the polysyllabic names such as 'semidemisemiquaver' or 'hemidemisemiquaver' can be impossible stumbling blocks for the pupil with a phonological deficit. Atkinson et al (1992), while researching the musical ability of children with dyslexia at King's College Choir School, Cambridge found that pupils had significant problems in 'remembering names of lines and spaces on the stave'. These same pupils may also reverse letters, such as 'b' for 'd', when reading; lose their place on the line; or omit parts of a letter, for example confusing 'u' and 'y'. When reading music they may have difficulty because the horizontal lines are so close together.

- The use of alphabetical names for notes which do not correspond to the alphabetic sequence can cause problems: H does not come after G.

- The sharp sign is easily confused with a natural sign:

A sharp sign.   A natural sign.

- 'Rests are as difficult as commas, they don't register', an adult dyslexic musician commented. This is not surprising if a pupil has a visual memory problem.

The semibreve rest hangs below a line (on the fourth line if there is only one melody on the stave).

The minim rest sits on top of a line (normally the third line).

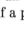

- The dyslexic with poor visual perceptual skills may confuse the sign for a tie, the slur and the phrase.

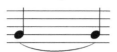

The tie is a small curved line joining two of the same notes. The second note is not played separately, but is held for its value.

The slur is a curved line covering two notes. These notes are to be played in succession smoothly.

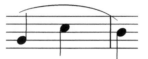

A phrase mark is similar to the slur and tie. It joins several notes together to form a segment of melody.

Time signature and key signature

Reading the time signature, which is represented like a fraction, can present problems for the dyslexic pupil experiencing difficulties with mathematics. He may have problems remembering which number goes at the top (which tells how many beats there are in a bar) and which number goes at the bottom (which tells what kind of beat it is):

$\dfrac{3}{4}$ = 3 beats in a bar
= 4 denotes crotchets

Before he plays a note the pupil also has to read the key signature and identify what key the piece is in. If it is in G major he must remember that every 'F' note he meets in the piece will be an F sharp not an F natural.

Clefs

Reading music of different clefs presents problems. Most music is notated using one of two clefs, the treble clef and the bass clef. These are both notated on the five lines of a stave (which look similar), but the notes on each line and space have different letter names. Many pupils, not just dyslexics, who sing or learn an instrument which uses the treble clef only, such as the descant recorder, have great difficulties when they begin to learn an instrument which uses the bass clef, such as the cello or trombone. According to Jason Hazeley (1994), 'its equivalent in verbal terms would be learning the alphabet again and assigning entirely different sounds to the letters'.

The bass clef problem is probably the single, most common preliminary stumbling block that piano pupils face. Many find this to be the last straw and it prompts their decision to abandon learning the piano.

Losing his place on the page

The pupil may lose his place when he has to follow the notes on the page, especially if he has simultaneously to keep his eye on the conductor. The notes for the soprano and alto voice are often on the same stave, differentiated only by the direction in which the note stems go (soprano notes are indicated by the stems of the notes going upwards and alto notes by the stems going downwards). Add to this the difficulty of reading the words of the song and life becomes very difficult, especially if compounded by the need to sight read.

Sight reading

Reading music can be very hard for the dyslexic pupil, and 'sight reading music is the most difficult thing a musician can undertake' (Brand, 1995). Singers and all professional musicians, such as members of the Chorus at the Royal Opera House in Covent Garden, London have to re-audition from time to time. Part of the audition involves sight reading. According to Brand (1995), 'it is an ongoing problem throughout their careers'. The percussion player in the orchestra, with several instruments to play, may have difficulty finding his place in the music score. An orchestral musician will often be required to 'rest' for some time (when not required to play) and so will need to count how many bars rest before he plays again. For those with sequencing difficulties this can be a nightmare if he forgets where he is or loses count.

Even the size of the music and the words can cause problems: 'I have problems with reading the words in the hymnal when I sing in the church choir, because the words are too small. It helped when my mother got one with large print for me.' (Stuart, 12 years old)

Backhouse (1994) when writing an account of a dyslexic international concert pianist and Professor of Piano at one of the London colleges of music, confirmed the tremendous strain that reading music can put on the dyslexic musician. The descriptions of the way this musician learns a new piece give great insight into the dyslexic musician's strengths and weaknesses. She learns new pieces partly by ear, listening to a recording of the piece, and partly by remembering the fingering patterns on the score. She uses motor, auditory and musical memory, as do the many musicians who have never learned to read music or who are unable to do so. She stated that the music score interferes greatly with her learning process, because then all her efforts have to go into decoding the notes. For this woman 'the score is an active distracter, taking away her attention from the music' (Backhouse, 1994).

Writing notation

When writing notes on the stave, dyslexics may reverse or invert the stems of the notes. For somebody who has directionality confusion when reading, such as 'b'/'d', 'p'/'q', how difficult it must be for him to remember that:

- the stem may go either up or down from the notehead:

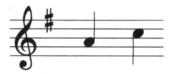

- if the stem goes up the stave, the notehead is placed on the left of the stem, not on the right and that the 'tail' is always on the right for a single quaver/semiquaver or demisemiquaver.

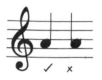

These rules are broken in music made up of many lines or 'parts'. If two parts are written on the same stave, the higher normally takes the stems upwards and the lower, the stem downwards.

The language of music

The dyslexic pupil may encounter difficulties with both the written and the spoken aspects of the language used in music.

According to Jason Hazeley (1994), 'there are two schools of thought on note names. One advocates using the terms semibreve, breve, minim, crotchet, etc., the other, whole note, half-note, quarter-note etc.'. This is an added confusion to the pupil who may be struggling with residual language difficulties as well as coping with the visual representations of the notes.

The vocabulary

Music has its own language and musical scores use words from a variety of languages.

The hybrid origins of the language of music are revealed in the use of Italian, Latin, German and French words to give directions for performance. We know from the work of Done and Miles (1978) that 'many new names have to be learned' and in 'name-learning tasks (paired associate learning), dyslexics are likely to have considerable difficulty' and 'regularly remain slow at reproducing them'. Cantwell (1992) found 'that adults with written language difficulties have object-naming problems'.

Memorizing words of songs

Some pupils, such as solo and choral singers, are expected to memorize the words of songs, especially for performances. For the pupil with poor auditory sequential memory, this can prove very difficult, to the extent that in some cases they may not be permitted to participate in performance.

Words and music

Added to the difficulty of remembering the meaning of the word is the difficulty caused by similar-looking words:

affettuoso (tenderly) with *affrettando* (hurrying)

The terms for dynamics (how loud or soft music is to be played) can also create problems, particularly for someone who has sequencing and directionality difficulties.

Musicians regularly meet marks such as *f*, *p*, *mf*, *mp*, *ff*, *pp*, *sfz* and *sfp*. These all have subtly different meanings musically, but are visually difficult to discriminate between, particularly when they have to be read from a score and acted upon very quickly.

Words used in a musical context do not necessarily mean the same as words used in other contexts:
'mezzo' means 'half' as loud and relates to the mood or the pace of the piece (it does not mean 'half' as used mathematically).

Simple words such as up/down can cause confusion. You can go up and down the piano keyboard in the horizontal position. But up/down on a string instrument is often in the vertical position.

High/low have special connotations for the musician. They can refer to pitch, such as high C, and also to notation on the page.

For the pupil with severe language difficulties or for literal thinkers, familiar words such as note, key, bar, sharp, flat, left and right, can cause problems. Hubicki (1994) pointed out that 'it isn't the differences of sound which are the problem; the problem lies in these words "high" and "low" familiar enough in daily life, being used in relationship to music':

'Give me a note' refers to the sound made by a singer or an instrument

'What note is that on the page?' refers to the written symbol for the sound

'Make a note of that' means write it down

'Note carefully' means pay careful attention to what is being done

'Note' may also refer to a finger-key of the piano, organ or accordion

Directionality confusions

Left and right
Many dyslexics have difficulty distinguishing between left and right.

The guitar
The guitar can be easier to learn to play at a basic level because one hand does the strumming (a simple movement of the wrist) while the other hand does the more complicated action of fretting the chords on the finger board (requiring the fingers to be moved and stretched into various positions).

The piano
The piano, on the other hand, involves an almost identical technique in both hands. There is often a near equal level of difficulty in each hand, making it more difficult for the dyslexic pupil to master. Music for the piano has two staves, each consisting of five lines on which the notes are written. Each line and each space can represent a note which can cause problems for the pupil who has poor visual perception and has a tendency when reading to omit words. The pupil has to remember that the top stave is for the right hand and the bottom stave is for the left hand and that the higher notes are situated towards the right-hand end of the keyboard and the lower notes to the left. He has to use the little finger of the right hand to play the highest notes on the treble clef, but the thumb of the left hand to play the highest notes on the bass clef. This can be a great problem for the pupil who cannot remember which is his right hand or which is his left hand! 'I am slower at finding notes with my left hand. I sometimes play a line of music for the right hand with my left hand.' (Edward, 10 years old) It may take some time and a lot of practice for such a pupil to respond automatically when he is asked to play the treble clef with his right hand and the bass clef with his left hand.

The pedal
To compound the problem, some dyslexics may have even greater difficulty remembering the left and right foot when using a foot pedal. When it comes to remembering hands, the fact that their

watch is usually on their left wrist may give them a quick point of reference. An instruction such as 'use the right pedal for this chord' or 'use the left pedal here' may cause panic.

Beating time

Pupils are taught to beat time to music to help establish a sense of rhythm and an appreciation of time signatures. Directional difficulties and a tendency to confuse left and right may cause the dyslexic pupil problems.

Beating four four (or common) time requires the pupil to:

- hold his hand out in front of himself and to move it in a definite action downwards
- move it horizontally to the left across his body
- retrace the movement horizontally across to the right side of the body
- to swing his arm diagonally anti-clockwise in an upward direction back to the starting point.

The left-handed pupil will have to mirror all the actions. When the majority of the pupils are right handed, and particularly if the teacher is right handed, this can be very hard.

Fingering patterns

Fingering patterns for string, brass and woodwind instruments require the use of both hands but the music is written on only one stave. An illustration of the implications of this may be given when a pupil picks up, for example his recorder. He has to remember that his left hand should go at the top of the instrument and his right hand at the bottom. The dyslexic left hander may automatically put his right hand at the top. Oldfield (1987), a flautist, said she has difficulty because the finger chart is written vertically whereas the flute is played horizontally.

Performance directions

Performance directions can be another source of confusion.

- Some reverse the 'hairpin' signs for crescendo and diminuendo:

Crescendo (cres).   Diminuendo (dim).

- 'Da capo' is often abbreviated to DC, meaning 'from the beginning'. This can be confused with 'Dal segno' abbreviated to DS, which means 'from the sign'.
- The names of the notes (letter names) can be sequenced in a different order to the alphabet – a descending scale is C B A G F E D C.

- Directional confusion can arise when dealing with the signs for an octave.

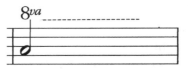

This tells you to play the notes an octave higher than written on the stave.

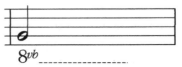

This tells you to play the notes an octave lower than written on the stave.

Laterality

Delos Smith reported that his breakthrough came when he was introduced to retrograde (the backwards) playing of music as used by Bach. 'I realized there was true laterality in music, just as there is in language' (Pollack and Branden, 1982). He was particularly inspired by a piano concerto written by Ravel for the one-armed pianist Paul Wittgenstein. There is right-handed music as well as left-handed music (with the melody and power in the left hand). Prokofiev and Scriabin, for example, also wrote music for one hand only. Almost every composer who has written for keyboard instruments has allowed the left hand to dominate the right at times.

Rhythm

Bradley and Bryant (1983) showed that many dyslexic children have difficulty with rhyme and this can have many effects on their musical skills. Ganschow, Miles and Lloyd-Jones (1994) defined 'rhythm [as] a recurrent pattern formed by notes of differing stress and duration'.

- They find it difficult to sing some of the easy and familiar 'rounds' such as 'London's Burning'.

- They cannot remember the words of popular songs or hymns or Christmas carols.

- In choral singing, dyslexic singers may 'come in' at the wrong place.

- Psalms are particularly difficult to sing since there is often little tune and the words have odd stresses and unusual syllable divisions.

- The orchestral player may miss his cue or may not play in time.

- Dancing with a partner may be difficult, resulting for example in constantly treading on his partner's toes and causing social embarrassment. Formal ballroom dancing is difficult and the intricacies of Scottish dancing, which involves remembering the steps and at the same time remembering the sequence of movements, can be beyond many dyslexic people's abilities. Most complaints are about male dancers. It is highly speculative to compare this with the known ratio of approximately 4:1 males to females in the dyslexic population. Geschwind (1984) confirmed this, saying that a dyslexic reported that 'in spite of efforts of friends, relatives and even dancing teachers, he found that this skill, attained without effort by the overwhelming bulk of his contemporaries, was beyond his ability to perform except at the most mediocre level as a result of his insensitivity to rhythm'. The pupil may be sent to sit on the side because he is unable to follow the sequence of movements of the other children and 'spoils' their performance.

- Young recruits to the armed services have often been penalized on the parade ground by their inability to master drill. A young Officer Cadet at Sandhurst was most disconcerted when his childhood dyslexia difficulties came back to haunt him and gave him difficulties when marching on the parade ground.

Theory

To the music student, 'theory' means the written aspects of his studies. Time and again one hears evidence from dyslexic pupils who struggle desperately with this aspect of their work. Music teachers should be aware of the particular difficulties experienced by dyslexic pupils and adopt a flexible approach to their teaching and the demands they make on their dyslexic pupils. The mastery of theory should not be allowed to quench the fire of musicality in the dyslexic pupil. It is of paramount importance that the music theory does not overshadow the importance of the music and performance. There is much anecdotal evidence of talented musicians and of composers, such as Irving Berlin, who were unable to read or write music.

Musicians themselves have different opinions about the role and importance of teaching and mastering the theory of music. Some point out that performance by others of the works of the greatest composers depends on an ability to read and play their music. Others comment that in certain cultures music was not written down at all and was often played by 'ear', for example jazz or traditional Irish music, and in the Orient there are many different examples of folk music that are not written down. The composer needs to write down his music so that others can play it and record it. There are many highly successful pop stars and musicians who cannot read or write a note of music. Many modern composers also use tape before notating their ideas – John Adams and Steve Reich are two examples. The essence of the matter is that if the music is to be performed by someone other than the composer, it probably needs to be written down. If the original musician cannot write down the music, record companies are often prepared to have it transcribed by someone else so that it can be reinterpreted into other media.

Melodic dictation

Melodic dictation is part of many music examinations. It has two purposes. The first is to establish whether the pupil can identify notes and intervals. The second is to prove that the pupil has a comprehensive understanding of musical notation. The pupil has to listen to a tune and then write down the notes. This presents the dyslexic musician with a host of difficulties (just as taking notes at a lecture may).

Practical suggestions
to help with teaching music to dyslexics

- Remember that often it is musical notation, and not music making, that lies at the root of the problem for many dyslexic pupils.

- Use multi-sensory teaching methods:
  – play the piece while the pupil listens
  – encourage the pupil to rehearse his fingering while listening, to develop motor memory
  – allow the pupil to sing or hum the tune where appropriate. Brand (1993) said that 'singing the tunes as well as playing them, can ensure that the musical ear and memory continue to support the eyes that are dealing with those written notes'
  – it may be useful if he beats time
  – record the demonstration on tape. This can be played back later and used for rehearsal and practice. 'RS' agreed and said 'listening to recordings of the music and pounding the melody out on the piano until she remembered it' helped her to learn a piece (Ganschow, Miles and Lloyd-Jones, 1994).

- Many pupils find scales and arpeggios difficult. This is not necessarily laziness, it is often related to their sequencing problems. Encourage them to sing along while practising.

- Be consistent with the language being used when referring to music and notation:
  - always give the symbols the same name, don't mix 'crotchet' with 'quarter note'
  - use 'treble clef' consistently, don't refer to it occasionally as G clef

- Use a structured, systematic and where possible multi-sensory approach. Introduce one concept at a time. It is helpful if the teacher puts each concept on a card index for revision and reinforcement.

- The pupil learning the piano should begin by learning the right hand of the piece.

- Be aware of the possible language confusions of the pupil, such as up/down, left/right. It can be helpful to put a mark on the right hand to help pupils quickly to identify their right hand.

- Some pupils find it helpful if certain notes or performance directions are highlighted. For example, repeat signs can be difficult:

Repeat signs.

Pupils cannot find the place where the repeat starts. This may be dealt with by cutting out and inserting the notes to be repeated in position on the music score. Another way of dealing with this problem is to use a coloured arrow.

One dyslexic pianist said that 'she finds that writing her fingering on the score is absolutely vital as it links the distances and patterns on the keyboard with her own image on the music' (Backhouse, 1994).

- Introduce musical notation from the earliest opportunity. Demonstrate its importance by asking a pupil to compose a tune. Then explain why it is necessary to be able to write this down – so that he can play it another time or that someone else may.

- Large print music is readily available and can help many musicians.

- Allow the pupil to have a sheet of music in front of him and allow him to play from this when he is performing. The additional burden of having to remember the words and the music may result in a poorer performance from a singer.
- For those who have difficulty in remembering the clef lines and spaces and what notes they represent, the following mnemonics may help:

Treble clef lines
'Every Good Boy Deserves Fruit'

Spaces
'F A C E'

Bass clef lines
'Great Britain Designs Faster Aircraft'

Spaces
'All Cows Eat Grass'

Music teachers

There is little formal training for teachers of music in the special needs and difficulties of dyslexic pupils, despite the fact that 'for many years professionals who work with dyslexic people have reported on how creative many of them are in music' (Pollack and Branden, 1982).

The BDA (1992) noted that 'it is vital that any teacher working with a dyslexic musician should have some understanding of the nature of their student's difficulties'.

Music examinations

The Associated Board of the Royal Schools of Music has recognized the particular difficulties experienced by dyslexic candidates, and published guidelines for the examination of such candidates.

Associated Board of the Royal Schools of Music

Guidelines for the Examining of Dyslexic Candidates

Wherever possible the Board makes provision for any candidate facing particular challenges, but without granting concessions in terms of the standards expected at each grade.

Dyslexic candidates may take advantage of these provisions by attaching a letter to the entry form and supporting their request with a certificate from an Educational Psychologist or teacher with RSA (SpLD) Diploma or AMBDA.

The nervousness which anyone may have at an examination is likely to be intensified for a dyslexic candidate because of the fear that he/she may 'make a fool of themselves' – caused by (apparently) 'stupid mistakes'. Awareness of and allowance for a dyslexic candidate's possible point of view can avoid an examination being remembered as 'just one more dreadful experience'.

Examiners will aim to convey the impression:

(i) that there is *plenty of time and space*: no one is being rushed;

(ii) that they will not be surprised by anything that happens – they are prepared for it.

Examiners will be aware that any kind of misplaced sympathy such as 'talking down' to a candidate or a 'poor old chap' attitude is neither appropriate or appreciated.

The following specific arrangements have been made:

1. Practical examinations

(a) An additional five minutes will be allowed for each examination;

(b) Examiners will not offer the usual choice of beginning with scales or pieces but will expect the pieces to be played first;

(c) Examiners have been asked:
  (i)   to speak *clearly* and not too fast;
  (ii) to repeat an instruction if asked or if a candidate is slow in responding;
  (iii) to understand that a candidate can become muddled with his/her own words when asked to name what has been heard;
  (iv) to be aware that *memory lapses* can occur in:

    (a) *Scales* – a candidate can forget what scale they were playing. A replay will be allowed;

    (b) *Sight Reading* – having lost the place in the music a candidate may have particular difficulty in re-finding it;

(d) Examiners will not refer to 'right' or 'left' but to 'this hand' or 'the other hand', demonstrating if necessary;

(e) Candidates will be allowed up to two minutes to study the Sight Reading test rather than the usual 30 seconds;

(f) Examiners will be prepared to give an additional attempt at the Aural Tests;

(g) Candidates experiencing particular difficulties with reading from white paper may bring with them to the examination a tinted overlay sheet.

Written comments

Marks, naturally, must always reflect the standard of the candidate's performance. However, examiners will aim to avoid comments which directly relate to the above mentioned points and would seem to emphasize them.

2. Written examinations

(a) Additional time will be allowed for the completion of each examination as follows:

Grades 1, 2 and 3	an extra 30 minutes
Grades 4 and 5	an extra 40 minutes
Grades 6, 7 and 8	an extra hour

(b) Markers are aware that copying out poses special difficulties. However at the lower grades, where the skill itself is assessed, all candidates are required to do the best they can. At the upper grades, where the skill being assessed is primarily that of continuing a melody based on an opening fragment, the instruction to copy out the fragment may be ignored without penalty.

(c) The Board will endeavour to simplify rubrics in all written papers.

(d) Candidates who may benefit from working theory papers printed on non-white paper may request a paper printed on blue, green, pink or yellow paper, and should do so when making entry.

(e) In cases of exceptional difficulty an amanuensis is allowed, provided the examination takes place at a private centre, without additional cost to the Board. The Board must be satisfied that the examination will be conducted in all respects strictly by the Regulations. The theory papers would be sent direct to the invigilator named by the applicant on the entry form.

Source: Associated Board of the Royal Schools of Music (1995) *Guidelines for the Examining of Dyslexic Candidates. London.*

Application to music colleges

Different colleges have different arrangements regarding provision for and their attitude to the admission of dyslexic pupils. Currently many colleges are not particularly sympathetic towards dyslexic pupils but there are notable exceptions. It is best to check carefully on all the details relating to their entrance requirements and their admission procedures.

Royal Academy of Music

If a dyslexic candidate hopes to study at the Royal Academy of Music, it goes without saying that it would be to everyone's advantage if his problem is known in advance so that the maximum help can be given to that student. The Academy's current entry form contains the following paragraph under 'Health':

> *'Have you any medical history (disability, learning difficulty) that might affect your musical studies or you feel might influence your audition? In the little box provided tick 'yes' or 'no'. If 'yes' give details on a separate sheet.*
>
> *Source:* Royal Academy of Music (1996) 'Entry form'.

The Academy has felt it vital to keep this query muted so that if a student is unwilling for information to be given nothing needs to be said. But the college in question can do little to help that dyslexic student if it has not been told. Help is needed on both sides. If a student is wise enough to take advantage of this part of the entry form, then he should be met by sympathetic understanding, awareness and help.

The Guildhall

The Guildhall has a section on its entry form which has to be completed by the academic referee. It states that comments will be treated in the strictest confidence and adds that it would be very much appreciated if the statement could include information on a number of points including:
a) the applicant's physical ability to stand up to long hours of rehearsal and his/her general state of health
b) the applicant's ability to organize work without supervision
c) the applicant's ability to mix with other students
d) any direction in which the applicant might need guidance other than in his/her studies.

Summary and conclusions

1   There is evidence that some dyslexic people are gifted musicians. Some of these may have difficulties with certain aspects of music. Oglethorpe (1996) summed these up: 'The common denominator for music is sound – that which our ears hear and translate into something meaningful. Second to that is the score – that which our eyes perceive. Pictures are sent to the brain which in turn send messages to the muscles telling them how to act. These two aspects, sound and sight, are two of the primary areas in which dyslexics have difficulty'.

2   Reading and writing music present great challenges to many budding musicians who are dyslexic.

3   Many dyslexic pupils have difficulties with language, both the spoken and written forms. The idiosyncratic language of music may cause horrendous problems for such a pupil.

4   Dyslexic pupils often have additional problems because of their confusions with laterality, sequencing and orientation, especially when they are playing an instrument.

5   Many dyslexic musicians report that rhythm causes problems. Bradley and Bryant (1983) have shown that dyslexic children have difficulty with the spoken aspects of rhythm, and lack of phonological awareness is now regarded as a cardinal feature in the long list of symptoms. It is not too difficult to hypothesize that words and sounds when translated into music will also cause difficulties.

6   Much can be done to help these talented musicians if their teachers are aware of possible problems and if they deal with them in a positive and sympathetic fashion. According to the BDA (1992) 'many dyslexic musicians have found the piano to be difficult, demanding tremendous co-ordination skills and an ability to scan a number of lines of music simultaneously. If this is the case, it might be worth trying an instrument which reads only from a single line of music'.

7   There is little formal training and no qualification for music teachers who may have to teach dyslexic musicians. The BDA Music Committee has been holding discussion with one of the music colleges about setting up such a course and hopes to report a satisfactory outcome (Hubicki, 1996). The BDA (1992) noted that 'it is vital that any teacher working with a dyslexic

musician should have some understanding of the nature of their student's difficulties'.

8   The examining boards are sympathetic and have an exemplary policy towards dyslexic candidates. Such provision is aimed at ensuring that dyslexic musicians when they take examinations, are not penalized for lack of skills which are irrelevant to the examination's purpose' (Miles and Augur, 1992). The teachers of candidates should be familiar with the policy and should apply for these concessions for their dyslexic pupils.

9   Some colleges of music are highly sympathetic, if approached, about the needs of dyslexic students, but not all are.

10 There are many highly successful (and dyslexic) professional musicians who have succeeded despite their difficulties. Hazeley commented that, 'The ability to be a musician does not rely on the ability to read music. There are scores of talented musicians – many in the rock/pop world – who have never been able to read music and never need do so.'

11 Technology has made music more accessible and penetrable. As music comes in increasing numbers of digital formats, devices such as MIDI disc recordings and C-D Roms (which allow access to all the different musical lines individually) make music more attainable. Hazeley noted that, 'The advent of sampling (recording and reproducing music digitally) allows entire songs to be written without a note ever being played, enabling the most severely dyslexic musician to make music'.

12 Music is aural, emotional, physical, intellectual and artistic and dyslexic musicians should be enabled to share in this heritage.

Recommended text
Instrumental Music for Dyslexics. A Teaching Handbook.
Oglethorpe (1996)

Chapter 12

The adult dyslexic

- guidelines on identifying dyslexia in an adult
- guidelines for adult literacy and learning support tutors
- the implications of dyslexia for employer and employee

Introduction

Dyslexia is a lifelong condition and cannot be 'cured'. The BDA give the number of dyslexics in the UK as two million, but this figure is not broken down to give the prevalence for adults and children. Dyslexic children grow up to be dyslexic adults. During the BDA's awareness campaign in 1990 the helplines in its head office alone received over 8,000 calls.

If the difficulties experienced by dyslexic children are not identified, they will persist, and even if they are addressed, many dyslexics continue to experience the symptoms in adulthood because of the congenital nature of the difficulties. Literacy is one of the greatest challenges faced by a dyslexic. It is not a problem faced solely by dyslexics, but the adult dyslexic will need to address it slightly differently from the average adult or the dyslexic child. McLoughlin, Fitzgibbon and Young (1994) reminded us that adult dyslexics are not simply children with a learning disability 'grown up'.

Emotional and social implications

Dyslexia may be less of a handicap for some than others. For many the handicap can remain hidden. The less fortunate may suffer from the frustrations, anger and despair that dyslexia brings to many aspects of their lives, both in the home and at work. Some adults suffer from low self-esteem because of their feeling of failure. Others are continuously under pressure because they are afraid of constantly making mistakes and of being humiliated by employers and colleagues. This can lead to anxiety and stress which may require counselling and support from family and friends.

Lifelong implications

There is an increasing awareness of literacy problems which persist into adult life. These problems may lead to and 'take the form of limited academic achievement, economic hardship, restricted vocational choice, emotional stress and loss of self-esteem' (Beare, 1975).

How to recognize dyslexia in an adult

McLoughlin, Fitzgibbon and Young (1994) suggested that 'an inefficiency in working memory' is 'the key to understanding developmental dyslexia'. Vellutino (1987) described this difficulty as a 'problem of short term memory storage'.

An adult dyslexic may show indications of some, or many, of the following difficulties:

Reading
- Misreads words:
  computers for commuters
  revolutions for resolutions.
- Omits or confuses small words.
- Struggles to remember the content of what he has read and finds it hard to follow instructions in manuals or guidelines.
- Finds it difficult to read aloud.
- Reads very slowly.
- Loses his place on the line of words, or at the end of a sentence.
- Frequently has to re-read a text to make sense of it and to understand it.
- Dislikes reading long or detailed reports or books.

Spelling (see Chapter 6)
- Misspells familiar words, such as forty, or names of relatives.
- Has difficulty remembering when and how to use homophones:
  their/there/they're
  of/off
- Sometimes gets letters in the wrong order in words:
  flied/feild for field
  thier/thrie for their
- Has good days and bad days with spelling.
- Finds remembering punctuation a problem:
  the boys hats' for the boy's hats
- Uses capital letters in the wrong places.

- Has a tendency to use phonetic spelling.
- Finds it difficult to fill in forms, such as job application forms, particularly where dates have to be included.

Mathematics (see Chapter 7)

- Forgets telephone numbers and sometimes dials the incorrect numbers.
- Has difficulty remembering car registration numbers.
- Always uses pen and paper or fingers when doing arithmetic.
- Difficulty with the times tables.
- Has difficulty working out foreign currency when abroad.
- Frequently makes mistakes when using a calculator. Pushes the wrong button.
- Has difficulty remembering mathematical formulae.
- Loses his place when doing a mathematical operation, such as long division, or miscopies numbers from a computer screen.
- Has difficulty remembering dates.
- Finds filling in cheques difficult, particularly getting the numbers and words to tally.
- Has difficulty with time. Forgets the time of appointments, is often late for meetings or may go to the wrong venue. Forgets to pay credit card bills by the date stipulated.

Sequencing difficulties

- Has to keep saying the alphabet when trying to use a dictionary, for example to remember what letter comes after 'g' or before 'n', or when using a filing system.
- Finds it difficult to use a dictionary, telephone directory, filing system or reference system in a library.
- Has difficulty remembering a telephone message accurately.
- Loses track of the content of a meeting or a lecture.
- Has left/right confusion, for example giving directions to other people or following instructions given.
- Finds map reading difficult.
- Has difficulty finding the car in a carpark.
- Loses the shopping trolley in a supermarket.
- Has difficulty in remembering right/left, for example needs to look at a wrist watch to remember which way is left. Peer (1994) recounted that when she was testing a fourteen-year-old boy she told his father that his son did not know left or right. 'Neither do I' retorted the father, who was an airline pilot. 'No problem!

I put a tiny yellow sticker on the left side of the panel in front of me and that way I don't forget.'

Language/speech

- Has difficulty in remembering the names of familiar people, places, objects.
- Mispronounces words, especially multisyllabic words: pacific/spercific for specific
- Has difficulty learning new words and needs to see them written down first before being able to remember them
- Has difficulty remembering the words of familiar hymns, songs and carols.
- Finds it difficult to speak in public and may lose the train of thought and dry up.

Diagnosing dyslexia in an adult

There is much debate and difference of opinion on how to deal with dyslexia in adults. The protagonists are separated by their background, training and occupation. Those who work in the field of adult literacy are aware of the need for quick responses, available resources and financial restraints. Klein (1994) argued that 'if an educational psychologist's assessment continues to be required, the high costs and lack of agreement as to who should pay mean that many students could be denied access to special exam provision'. Time is short so adults demand answers and solutions for their immediate problems. But as so often in life the quick and easy answer is not necessarily the best or cheapest way of dealing with the problem.

An adult dyslexic is often diagnosed as a result of investigations of the problems experienced by their child. During the course of the child's assessment the diagnostician usually takes a detailed case history and attempts to establish whether others in the family have had similar difficulties with reading and spelling (frequently there is a link of dyslexia between members of a family). On one such an occasion a successful chartered accountant, on being asked if he had had any difficulties with spelling, sat bolt upright in his chair and replied, 'Yes, and I now know as a result of this conversation why I failed my English Language 'O' Level exam thirteen times.'

The Dyslexia Institute (CBI, 1995) carried out a survey of its adult students in 1995. The key findings from the responses to the questionnaires were:

- 70 per cent were not diagnosed dyslexic until after the age of 21 years

- 73.3 per cent were male
- 49.4 per cent were unemployed
- Eighty were diagnosed by the Dyslexia Institute, 69 by the Placing, Assessment and Counselling Team (PACT)
- Funding for tuition came from family or self in 70 cases and in 76 cases from PACT
- Fifty-six had no qualifications, either academic or vocational
- 67 per cent of their employers were aware of their problems.

Is formal testing necessary?

There is a very strong case for formal assessment. West (1991) stated that 'they [dyslexics] need to know that the problems that they experience are real and not imagined. The relief and sense of personal vindication that comes from a positive diagnosis based on a professional evaluation should not be underestimated'. Experts who come from a teaching background often dismiss the need for formal testing, making the valid criticism that there are few suitable standardized tests available to use with adults, and those that do exist are mostly 'closed' tests that can only be administered by psychologists. Klein (1994) argued against adults and students being subjected to 'intelligence tests or tests which determine reading and spelling ages. Such tests are unnecessary and may distress students and undermine their confidence as learners'. McLoughlin, Fitzgibbon and Young, psychologists themselves, made cogent arguments for the central role of psychologists in any investigative and diagnostic procedures involving adults. But a growing number of psychologists and teachers agree that all evaluations should include a case history, a cognitive ability test and tests to ascertain attainment levels in reading, spelling and writing and should be followed by counselling and career guidance.

Criteria for and content of adult assessments

Case history
A careful and detailed case history should give information gathered during an interview and from previous reports on age, education, school reports (if available), examinations, qualifications, work experience, occupation, family circumstances (including marital status) and an examination of family history (to establish whether there are any other members of the family who have similar difficulties). The reason for requesting an assessment should be ascertained. This helps to establish the person's goals and expectations. The diagnostician should question the person

informally and should ask many questions relating to the points indicating dyslexia listed on pages 277–9. Responses must be carefully, but discreetly, recorded and the good clinician should observe the reactions and processes by which answers were given.

Arguments in favour of the use of psychometric tests

The underlying cognitive (intelligence) ability of the individual needs to be established. Thomson (1990) stated that 'the appropriate assessment of intelligence is one of the most crucial factors in the diagnosis of dyslexia'. There are some very sound arguments for this opinion:

- It can help to eliminate a fundamental lack of ability as a cause of difficulties and banish the misconception of being 'stupid', 'thick' or 'dumb'.

- It can restore the battered ego of the severely dyslexic, and give him a sense of purpose and the motivation to prove to himself and to the world that he is not dullwitted.

- It is important for all concerned to be able to establish the person's potential and 'to close the gap between potential and achievement' (Johnson, 1980).

- The tests used in the hands of an experienced and qualified diagnostician can identify and clarify the underlying areas of difficulty.

- It can help with setting realistic goals for further study or in the choice of career. Many occupations require basic aptitudes or talents. Job satisfaction is important; the converse can lead to stress and unhappiness.

- It can pinpoint aptitudes, such as good visual and spatial skills, which may have important ramifications for future education and employment.

The most reliable and respected way of establishing cognitive abilities is to administer an IQ test. The Wechsler Adult Intelligence Scale (WAIS–R^{UK}) is the most widely used test and is suitable for adults over the age of sixteen. The whole subject of IQ testing is emotive and confrontational to some people. Some commentators decry the whole notion of measuring intelligence and the notion that it is inborn, general or fixed, saying that the nature of the tests produces bias against some individuals and some groups in society. Others say it does provide a measure of the individual's strengths and weaknesses and academic potential.

If it is not possible to give an IQ test, measures of cognitive attainment skills can be used.

Attainment tests

To establish the attainment levels of the person in reading, spelling and writing is not quite as straightforward or as simple as it might seem. Some practitioners liken the results of such tests to the rubbing of salt in the wound of the person because they draw attention to and reveal weaknesses in the basic skills, which so many other people find simple and automatic. The testing in itself can be stressful, but the indignity of being told that one has a reading age equivalent to that of a seven-year-old child can be soul-destroying. McLoughlin, Fitzgibbon and Young (1994) pointed out that 'adult dyslexics are frequently reluctant to admit to their illiteracy because of its association with stupidity'. However, in order to be able to offer the appropriate kind of help, problems that have dogged the client for many years must be identified.

Reading

Not all adults will have obvious difficulties with reading. Simpson (1979) confirmed this when she remarked 'dyslexics do learn to read, but much later, with much more effort, and more slowly than others'. It is therefore important to administer a battery of reading tests to look at different aspects of reading and to remember that 'while valuable, assessment based on reading age [alone] says little about how well or poorly someone can perform everyday tasks' (ALBSU, 1994).

- Word recognition tests are useful because there are no contextual cues to help. It also helps to observe the tactics used by the individual to decode a word, for example a visual approach, a phonic approach or a semantic approach.

- A prose reading test is invaluable because it provides the equivalent to reading in the 'real' world.

- A reading comprehension test is essential because it helps to establish how much of what has been read has been remembered.

A running record of the reading errors should be made. These miscues should be analysed when making the diagnosis and should appear in the report. They will help the tutor plan how to teach the student. (See also Chapter 4.)

Spelling

'Spelling has been considered the most "tell-tale" symptom of dyslexia' (Saunders, 1990). It is important to keep giving the words to spell even though the person has apparently reached his ceiling, because the patterns of errors made is helpful when the analysis of errors is made. Some authorities advocate the inclusion of a passage of dictation because of its approximation to using spelling in context. Adolescent and adult dyslexics sometimes spell words correctly in isolation, such as when taking the spelling test, but may be unable to spell the same word when writing essays or reports. Critchley (1966) said: 'In the case of the "cured" dyslexic, defective writing and spelling may continue long into adult life. The mistakes are of such a nature as to make it often possible to diagnose the reading defect from a mere perusal of the script.'

Written expression

It is crucial to see a sample of the person's creative writing, for example a short narrative about a favourite hobby. The diagnostician can make observations on the collection or organization of ideas, structure, syntax, punctuation, speed of writing and quality of written work. The spelling test and the dictation will indicate what, if any, handwriting difficulties there may be.

Other diagnostic tests

These might include tests of:

- laterality
- sequencing
- arithmetic.

The assessment report

The format, content and tone of the written assessment is important. The person may have great difficulty, because of his language problems, in remembering most of what has been said. But he will want to be able to read the report, consider the implications and act upon the advice given. He must feel relaxed about showing this to a tutor, employer or personnel manager. In view of this, the person should feel reassured and encouraged by what is being said and written about him. It may be helpful to offer to let him see a draft of the report which he can study in his own time. If he is unhappy about a phrase or comment it can be open to amendment in the final copy. The person must give permission to allow others to see the report.

Test results

Should the report include the test results? This question generates widely differing opinions. On one hand, some question the point of administering tests of reading and spelling if they are not to be used in planning the future remedial programme. McLoughlin, Fitzgibbon and Young (1994) supported this view and advised putting the test results on a separate sheet. The person can then choose whether or not to include the results when using the report. Some feel that it is crucial to have this information and necessary to use it in order to plan appropriate intervention, and to set realistic goals and targets for the person. On the other hand, others feel that it is demeaning and destructive for the person if information provided by the test results is revealed to him or to others.

Plan of action

The assessment report should end with recommendations and a 'plan of action' to help the person. These will be often be broad guidelines. The details and the priorities which have been established should be discussed and advice on the action to be taken should be given. It is important that the language in the report is free of jargon and 'psychobabble'. The report should include the following:

- Names and addresses of adult literacy tutors/agencies, and support groups.
- Suggestions to help with reading, for example where to obtain books on cassette.
- Spelling recommendations, for example useful dictionaries or spell checkers.
- Recommendation to learn typing or word-processing skills or to practice dictation skills, or for study skills to be learnt.
- Recommendation about concessions to be given to the candidate in examinations.
- It is important to be specific because the person may wish to apply for the Disabled Students Allowance or for other provisions.

What can be done to help the adult learner?

It is essential that all those who teach adult dyslexics are fully aware of their specific needs. These are different from those of the dyslexic child, both emotionally, psychologically and socially. They have to be treated as mature people, and ideally as partners, in any discussion of the outcome and results of the testing. They already know this because of their relentless daily battle to overcome their learning difficulties. They also know the emotional stress and strain if they choose to try to conceal their difficulties from family, friends and colleagues.

Counselling is essential and should involve a detailed and extensive explanation of the adult's difficulties and weaknesses, for example of short term memory. Even more important is to discuss with the adult what help is available, where to seek it and what to tell their partner and employer. The assessor must be positive and supportive. It is often constructive to cite examples of individuals who have had similar difficulties and to describe their responses to the help available and the successes they have had in overcoming or coming to terms with their dyslexic difficulties. It can be enormously reassuring if the person can be encouraged to 'compare notes' and discuss difficulties with others who have (had) similar experiences. The value of group therapy is well-documented and help and support organizations, such as the Adult Dyslexia Organization and the BDA's local association's adult groups can be invaluable.

Admission or denial?

Many adults expend enormous energies hiding their disabilities, either for fear of ridicule or discrimination. West (1991) opined that 'there are no rewards for revelation, and the penalties can take the most humiliating forms'. People have different reactions to being told they are dyslexic, ranging from relief, through anger and disbelief to denial. In the medical world it is considered important to name the disease in any situation where doctor and patient are in consultation with each other. When an appropriate disease label has been reached, the management of the condition is, on most occasions, correspondingly easy. Recognition of the condition can reduce confusion and misunderstanding for all concerned.

Individual strategies for coping

Many adults have grown to live with and come to terms with their difficulties. 'By the time they reach adulthood, most dyslexics (whether they realize they are dyslexic or not) have learned to avoid situations which might expose their disabilites to others' (Singleton, 1992). They devise means of coping and compensating for their difficulties, such as the infant school teacher who knew she had a spelling problem and used to keep a little black book of her problem words on her desk which she would check when in doubt.

Emotional scars caused by lack of awareness

Some adults, unaware of the cause of their struggles, grow up with poor expectations of themselves. In this group are often to be found people who have low self-esteem and who suffer from depression as a result. Bryant (1978) commented that 'the feeling of failure breeds many other feelings – feelings of self-doubt and uncertainty, of guilt and shame, of resentment and the wish to blame, of rage and despair, of deep inadequacy and worthlessness... the progression is from mild to clinically significant depression, with severe emotional problems, some are suicidal, a few do take their own lives'. Lord Renwick (1990), when speaking on illiteracy in the House of Lords during the 'International Literacy Year' Debate, reported on the contents of a letter received by the BDA from a mother whose son was diagnosed as dyslexic late in his school career. He eventually achieved an engineering degree but 'sadly' she wrote 'the damage to his self-esteem was such that at the age of 22 he committed suicide'. Peter Bradford (1993), a successful film maker, confessed in a television documentary that 'at 19 I really was suicidal'.

Identification and recognition brings rewards

Some seek help and persist with their quest for the standards and the education they feel they are capable of. One of the first documented case histories in this country was that of David Gauntlett (1978), who said 'for the early part of my life I lacked an explanation of my language disability and was simply advised not to continue further studies. This was after 'O' Levels but for me at least, the knowledge that there was a recognized problem provided much needed motivation'. He detailed his struggles and told of how he finally, at the age of 40, obtained a degree in Psychology, going on to obtain a doctorate from the Open University.

The climate of understanding is improving and there is great tolerance for dyslexic people who may work differently but who can produce good results.

Where and how do adults find help?

The adult dyslexic's first priority should be to obtain an assessment. This can be arranged with the help of a number of agencies. There may be a waiting list and a delay in obtaining an appointment. Some of these assessments are free, others involve fees.

- The Specialist Careers Officer can help (16–19-year-old) school leavers seeking employment or waiting to enter further or higher education. She can make a referral to the Schools Careers Service or to the Department of Employment's Occupational Psychologist (who will be part of PACT). If the student is already in further education the same arrangements for assessment apply.

- The Placement Assessment and Counselling Team (PACT) can also be contacted direct by an adult seeking help. The local County Hall should direct the caller to the appropriate department in his area. There are 80 of these nationally. The BDA has a list of their locations.

- The Job Centre will have a Disability Employment Adviser who can refer to PACT, which is part of the Employment

Rehabilitation Service, to arrange an appointment. The Parliamentary Under-Secretary of State at the Employment Department said, at a conference organized by the CBI in London on the 28 February 1995, that 'disabled people also have a priority for a place on the main schemes and programmes for which they are eligible and suitable. These include Job Clubs, Restart Courses, Training for Work, the Job Interview Guarantee Scheme and Work Placement Schemes'.

- Help may be obtained through the NHS. This requires a referral by the general practioner (GP) to a clinical psychologist who works for the NHS. It can be difficult to obtain help through this channel.
- A number of private teaching centres also offer assessments.
- There are a number of support agencies for adult dyslexics:
  The Adult Literacy and Basic Skills Unit (ALBSU)
  Adult Dyslexia and Skills Developmental Centre
  Adult Dyslexia Organization
  Local Associations of the BDA
  Dyslexia Adult Support Group
  The Prince's Youth Business Trust

Recommended text
Adult Dyslexia Assessment, Counselling and Training
(McLoughlin, Fitzgibbon and Young, 1994)

Dyslexia as a recognized disability

Severe dyslexia is recognized as a disability. There are some advantages for a dyslexic adult being on the Disabled Person's Register:

- Funds are sometimes available for training people between the age of sixteen and eighteen years and in some cases, up to 21 years old.
- Help and advice with finding a job is provided.
- Help with approaching an employer and with disclosing the extent of the disability is given.
- Equipment to help with a job, such as a personal computer, can be loaned.
- The green card provided can be produced as evidence of a disability.

Help can be arranged for paying for an assessment which is necessary to be included on the Register.

The Disability Discrimination Act 1995

The Disability Discrimination Act aims to tackle discrimination against disabled people in a number of areas, including the workplace. It defines disability as a 'physical or mental impairment which has a substantial and adverse long-term effect on a person's ability to carry out normal day-to-day activities. People who have a disability and those who have had a disability and no longer have are covered by the Act'.

Philip Oppenheim (1995) said that 'people substantially affected by dyslexia will be covered by the Act on this basis' and that they will have access to ACAS conciliation and the right to complain to an Industrial Tribunal.

According to the BDA, the Act will be responsible for monumental changes in the way disabled people are treated. It gives disabled people new rights and will have implications for employers, schools, colleges and retailers. It will be against the law for an employer to treat a disabled person less favourably than someone else because of their disability' (Department of Social Security, 1995).

Some suggestions for adult literacy and learning support tutors

We believe that teachers can present every subject in a multisensory way and thus reach every kind of learner in the classroom ... Never just show students what they need to learn ... they will forget 90 per cent. Never just tell them. They may remember 20 per cent, but briefly. Instead both show and tell them (they will remember 50 per cent). Let them also talk through, walk through, draw through or in some way rehearse an example activity. If they understand, they will both remember and retain up to 90 per cent.

Source: Cox A. (1983) 'Programming for teachers of dyslexics'. *Annals of Dyslexia*, 33:223

There are as many opinions and theories as there are methods on how to tackle the problem of teaching adults to read and write, both in the UK and abroad. There is a growing consensus, based on the results of scientists and practitioners, that the essential ingredient for success is multi-sensory teaching. This was given official recognition in 1989 when the United States' Senate passed the National Literacy Act (to which an amendment was added in 1990) which stated that 'tried and proven methods such as Orton/Gillingham, Spalding, Carden and many other programs where intensive phonics is used' were to be incorporated into adult literacy education.

Qualities and skills required by adult literacy and learning support tutors

- Need to understand the nature of the difficulties.
- Must discuss and involve the adult in his programme, for example by asking him to bring along spellings that he wants to learn to do his job more efficiently.
- Must be available for out-of-hours counselling and support.
- Must be able to react sensitively to indications that the adult is under pressure or stressed because of work. The adult may need to talk about this before he is ready to learn.
- There should be critical appraisal of work being covered as progress is made.
- Must be conversant with different teaching methods. Must use the many technological aids currently available and must tailor these to the adult's needs.
- Must tap into the adult's strengths, for example the person with good visual skills can be encouraged to use these when note-taking or making essay plans.
- It is always productive to take the time to discover the adult's interests, hobbies and talents. Reference can then be made to these in the lessons to help spark interest, sustain motivation and foster pride and a sense of achievement or personal worth.
- Exchanging roles can encourage the adult to teach his tutor something about which he has perhaps superior knowledge, such as using the computer. It develops a 'feel good' factor.
- A sense of humour and great flexibility are vital!

Establishing the adult dyslexic's strengths and weaknesses

McLoughlin, Fitzgibbon and Young (1994) and Klein (1993) recommended that advantage should be taken of the dyslexic's skills and weaknesses.

What type of learner is he? It is important to establish this at the outset.

Good visualizers

Some dyslexic people are strong visualizers. Evidence of this is found in West (1991) when he pointed out that 'one of the common indicators of bright dyslexics and others like them is a distinctive peak-and-valley pattern in intelligence tests and other measures of ability. They have good spatial ability and are good at pattern recognition and visual thinking. Therefore, they should capitalize on this by using charts, maps, posters and pictures to help with spelling and reading'. The notebook and the filofax will play an important role in their daily lives.

Strong auditory skills

The person with strong auditory skills will find listening to cassettes and reading aloud helpful.

Kinesthetic learners

Some students are kinesthetic learners which means they need to see, read and write what ever it is that they seek to memorize.

Multi-sensory learning techniques

Multi-sensory learning techniques provide the key to teaching all dyslexic people. Guyer and Sabatino (1989) confirmed this and said that 'because all the pathways to the brain are being used, the strong senses help the weak ones'. Ideally it is useful if some lessons are on a one-to-one basis so that the teaching programme can be tailored to the specific needs of the individual, and so that the recommendations made by the assessor can be implemented. It helps to establish a rapport and mutual trust.

Reading

Reading skills have to be acquired. The multi-sensory training programmes help with these. Research suggests that it is crucial for the novice reader to build an 'internal lexicon', that is a bank of readily recognized sight words. This needs to be reinforced on a daily basis.

One of the greatest challenges facing the tutor of an adult dyslexic is finding suitable reading materials. It is pointless, frustrating and counter-productive to ask a weak reader to attempt to read something he has to struggle through and consequently not understand or remember the content of what he has read, yet 'simpler' material often means material designed for younger readers. West (1991) said that 'it is so important to use adult materials in adult literacy programs. Even if the vocabulary is considered difficult, the serious interest and sense of genuine accomplishment may easily outweigh the additional difficulties'.

Suitable reading material can be obtained from specialist suppliers (see Appendix III). Abridged versions of classic novels (for example the Oxford Abridged Classics) may be helpful.

Another excellent source of readable material is provided by books produced for Teaching English as a Foreign Language (TEFL).

Special interest hobby magazines and newspapers are also a useful resource. Anecdotal evidence suggests articles, for example the Sports Page for the football fanatic, as suitable and stimulating for the adult reader with problems.

Reading research has consistently shown that a *code emphasis program* in which the reader uses his intelligence and previous experience to make sense of what he reads (*'Wash your hands after you go to the ... lavatory?*) produces superior results with school aged children' (Anderson et al, 1985). 'Some adult educators argue that a *meaning emphasis approach* [semantic cues] works best with adults because of their cognitive maturity and extensive vocabularies' (Chall, 1986).

Reading is crucial for improving comprehension skills and it is vital to practice if reading ability is to improve. We read to learn and until we can do that, much of the printed word is inaccessible.

Spelling

Spelling is the most persistent and greatest stumbling block for many adult dyslexics. Many become obsessed by their inability to spell. Anecdotal evidence comes from a parent of a woman who gave up her job in a shoe shop after she was asked to write a list and keep a record of the various names of the shoes they stocked in the store. She was unable to spell the names and, being too embarrassed to disclose her dyslexia, resigned instead.

Spelling needs to be taught using a formal approach in tandem with the person's own immediate problem words and irregular spellings. The adult dyslexic needs to follow a structured spelling programme and to be taught spelling rules. The English language orthography does have some structure. This can be taught. For the dyslexic, it is not which spellings they are taught, but how they are taught and how relevant they are that is of lasting importance. The person can be taught the major spelling rules, and work on them using multi-sensory learning techniques and dictation to help establish the rule in long term memory. They may not remember the working of the rule but as they study the word family, they will have visual and semantic cues to help them.

It is often useful to begin with words that are causing immediate concern, such as the specialist vocabulary necessary for a course currently being taken. Put these words alphabetically in a small notebook and highlight the tricky or problem letters with a felt tip pen, for example, <u>ca</u>len<u>da</u>r. Some people find it easier if the word is broken up into syllables which they can tap out as they spell them. This 'chunking' of the letters is a visual stimulus. Specialist vocabulary can be built gradually and reinforced using multi-sensory learning techniques, such as the SOS method (see Chapter 6).

Dyslexics should be taught how to use a dictionary quickly and easily. The four quartiles of the alphabet are important concepts to teach as they will help to find the right section in the book: A–E, F–M, N–S and T–Z. A mnemonic such as 'Edward May Stink' may help remind the dyslexic which letter each quartile ends with.

In reality the electronic device has become the favoured method of spell checking for most adults because of its speed, ease of use and efficiency.

A variety of spell checkers are available, including hand-held spell checkers, spell checkers with a thesaurus feature and voice-activated spell checkers. Some hand-held spell checkers are designed to be compatible with a particular dictionary, giving the word, followed by the page number where it can be found in the dictionary. This saves wasted time and energy for the poor speller.

There are many people who are successful and who are doing important jobs who cannot spell very well. A. A. Gill has triumphed over dyslexia to become one of Britain's most prolific, entertaining and controversial journalists. He said 'the message is more important than the medium. I have a marketable skill: I can write. I just can't spell' (Margolis, 1995).

Writing

Handwriting may be a problem for some. It is worth taking a careful look at a specimen of writing, as often a few cosmetic touches can make it more legible. Help may be needed to improve a few problem letters, such as an 'a' which fails to close at the top, so it is easily confused with 'u'.

Learning typing and word-processing skills may be the answer for the person with illegible handwriting.

Grammar

Basic grammar might need to be taught. Klein (1993) suggested using the acronym WEE to teach the concept that a paragraph is a group of sentences about one subject:

W   What is the point?
E   Explain what you mean
E   Example of what you mean.

Planning

Strategies to plan written work can improve the dyslexic's writing hugely. A good plan will reduce the effort involved and help to eliminate the rambling, confused and irrelevant material that often characterizes the writing of the dyslexic.

Letter writing

The protocols for letter writing need to be taught, as well as the difference between the formal and the informal letter.

Proof reading and editing skills

One of the most important skills any dyslexic has to learn is the ability to proof read. Training is necessary to heighten the awareness and practise the skill. McLoughlin, Fitzgibbon and Young (1994) said 'proof reading one's own work is difficult because one anticipates what should be, rather than what actually is, written'. It is possible to train the dyslexic to recognize and correct many of the more obvious basic errors by following this procedure:

1   Leave the draft and re-read it the next day.
2   Read the passage aloud and check that it makes sense.
3   The acronym COPS is useful to remember what to look for when proof reading:
    C   Capitalization
    O   Omissions of words
    P   Punctuation
    S   Spelling.

Theory test for drivers

Problems with practical skills can occur where it is necessary to have a theoretical backup. One such example is driving.

The driving test in the UK used to consist of a practical test with oral questions. Now candidates must take a written test which examines their knowledge and comprehension of the Highway Code. The 40-minute test comprises 35 multiple choice questions and covers up to twelve subjects, including law, first aid and road etiquette. It must be taken and passed before the practical test is attempted.

Types of problem likely to be encountered by dyslexic candidates

*   Reading and assimilating the 600 questions and answers in the *Complete Theory Test for Cars and Motorcycles* (HMSO, 1996).

*   Directionality problems may make it difficult to answer theoretical questions about positioning of a car, for example on a roundabout.

- Sequencing difficulties make, for example, stopping distances hard to remember.
- Visual perceptual difficulties could cause confusion regarding road signs.
- Word retrieval problems make it hard to remember specific details. Mnemonics may help.
- Questions can be misread easily.
- Stress and pressure in the test could lead to a higher number of errors.
- If the test is to be taken orally because of dyslexic difficulties then auditory imperceptions could cause problems. The person with a word retrieval problem could find it difficult to 'find' the word for the answer.
- Poor visual sequential memory could mean that the dyslexic may have forgotten the question by the time he has finished reading it.

Concessions for dyslexic candidates

Enquiries with Drivesafe Services (who handle the arrangements for the Ministry of Transport and the Automobile Association as to the provision of concessions for candidates with learning difficulties) elicited the following information:

- Candidates will be asked if they have any form of reading/writing difficulties.
- If they are dyslexic they will need to notify the test centre in advance so that any special arrangements necessary can be made. 'Dyslexic candidates will be allowed one-to-one help with both reading and scribing their test. Requests to repeat any section, sentence, line or word will be complied with in full'.
- An extra time allowance of up to 80 minutes might be given to enable the candidate to complete the paper.
- Evidence of the candidate's genuine need must be provided.

The motoring organizations and a number of pressure groups say that a computerized examination in which learners watch simulated traffic situations on a screen and are then tested on their perceptions and reactions would be a better test and one that would demonstrate skills rather than theoretical knowledge. 'It is hoped that there will be an opportunity for some dyslexic candidates to take the test on a scroll CD-Rom computerized version of the test.' (Lilleyman, 1996)

Practical suggestions
for management of day-to-day activities

- Keep a list of words needed for filling in cheques in the same place as the cheque card. Keep a duplicate of this in a convenient place.

- When planning a car journey, write the directions on a sticker and put this on the dashboard of the car. When giving directions to other people, use landmarks rather than road numbers.

- Telephone numbers can often be remembered more easily if they are broken into pairs – 78, 84, 92. Some find it helpful to say 'seventy eight, eight four, ninety two'. Others report that it helps if they rehearse dialling the numbers on a phone. Many telephones can be programmed to hold a bank of frequently-used numbers. Some display the number dialled on a screen. Some watches can be programmed to store telephone numbers, as can personal organizers.

- British Telecom has a free Directory Enquiry Service for people with learning disabilities. An application form for this service is available from BT, Freepost, Sheffield S6 2NT FreePhone 0800 919195. Dyslexia is one of the conditions mentioned.

- The switch card helps those who find it difficult to fill in the figures and words on cheques, particularly when in a rush at the checkout in the supermarket or department store.

- Mnemonics and rhymes help to remember the spelling of tricky words.

- Obtain professional help with preparing a CV and have it typed. Keep one to hand and file one in the home computer. It can be very helpful when filling in forms, such as when applying for a driving licence or a job.

- When applying for a job, telephone beforehand and enquire whether they are willing to send application forms in advance. It may also be possible to take the form home and return it completed the next day, or to photocopy it and fill in a draft as preparation. Keep copies of completed forms for reference.

- Keep to hand a supply of BDA leaflets which give a simple description of and information about dyslexia. This reduces the burden of trying to give an explanation to employers, friends or colleagues.

- Keep a selection of standard letters on the personal computer. These often will just need 'topping and tailing' and will save a great deal of time and energy.

- Many adults report that they have found it helpful for their own reading if they practise their newly acquired skills by reading aloud to their own children.

- Keep a personal list of spellings which frequently cause problems.

- Use a book-mark or a ruler to help keep the place on the line when reading and copying from a text. It speeds up the process and lessens both the strain on the eyes and the concentration required.

- Ask the manager or supervisor to tell colleagues about their dyslexic co-worker. It can save embarrassment and confrontation in the long term.

- To help with time keeping it is useful to have a watch with an alarm which can be programmed to help with times of appointments. A stop watch facility is also useful to work out times of journeys or how long a particular task takes when being undertaken for the first time.

- Electronic diaries and personal organizers are very helpful to those dyslexics with poor memories and lack of organizational skills. The press of a button can recall the date of a special birthday or anniversary.

- Use a laptop to take notes at meetings.

Dyslexia and its implications for an employee and employer

Scarborough (1984) said 'judging by our research, most dyslexics remain diagnosably dyslexic throughout their lives'. Many overcome some of their difficulties or develop strategies to cope. Others do not develop strategies and their dyslexia can affect the way they do their jobs. In the Kershaw Report (1974) there is a poignant quotation which puts into words the fate of a sizeable number of the adult population: 'I have to take jobs which I can do with my hands, instead of my head'.

Some dyslexics don't want anybody to be aware of their dyslexia and develop many ingenious strategies to cover up, from claiming to have left their glasses at home to asking someone to quickly check some written material. Some are simply afraid that they will lose their job if they admit to dyslexia. Indeed, a Manpower Services Commission survey in 1987 estimated that 20 per cent of the long term unemployed had literacy problems.

Dyslexia: The hidden resource

The tide is turning and dyslexic employees are being treated more sympathetically when they admit that they are dyslexic. The CBI held a conference in 1995 to alert companies to the hidden resources that they have in their dyslexic employees. 'Companies cannot afford to stay ignorant of employees' potential and need to develop all their employees to stay competitive' (CBI, 1995). Many people are underemployed because they do not seek promotion or responsibility because of their dyslexic difficulties. 'There is no doubt that adult dyslexics are employed in jobs that underuse their capacity or subject them to potentially damaging stress and strain.' (Kershaw, 1974)

Problems typically experienced by dyslexic employees

Employers are often baffled by a dyslexic employee. What is so difficult to understand is that performance is inconsistent and variable. Many of the following difficulties will be experienced on an individual basis from time to time by a large number of the population, but the dyslexic will do so more frequently and with greater regularity.

- He may take a long time to read straightforward standard English, such as a letter or report.
- He may misread and fail to follow the instructions given.
- He may forget colleagues' names or job titles.
- He may be hesitant, and find it difficult to explain processes or give instructions or directions to others.
- He may forget to give telephone messages, not remember the details correctly or give the incorrect telephone number.
- He may not be punctual for work or for meetings because he loses track of the time, or is unable to estimate how much time he needs to allow for a specific activity.
- Written work often has many spelling errors and may be inferior to oral work. This can lead to verbal abuse. An industrial tribunal recently awarded £9000 in damages to a green keeper at a Yorkshire golf course who claimed he had tried to take an overdose after being bullied and embarrassed by his supervisor about his poor spelling (*Daily Mail*, 1996).

- He may always want to give oral reports and try to avoid writing.

- Mathematical difficulties might cause problems. It can have devastating effects if a digit is omitted. An accountant working for an airline used to omit digits and it resulted in a shortfall in the accounts. He put £200,000 where it should have been £2,000,000.

- The employee can create additional work for colleagues who may have to check his figures, or search for misfiled work.

Summary and conclusions

1   Dyslexia is a lifelong condition. It can be remedied but some of the residual difficulties remain. West (1991) pointed out that 'since there is no "cure" for dyslexia, its symptoms may be diminished over the years but never disappear'. Dyslexic adults fall into two categories: those who have had their dyslexia identified when they were children and who may have had help, and those who are identified only after they have left school.

2   There is a need for short, easily administered screening tests, such as a computerized test, to identify the adult dyslexic.

3   Basic literacy is a major problem facing many of the population but dyslexia can affect people's lives in many other ways too, including finding and remaining in employment.

4   The adult dyslexic needs to master the fundamental skills of reading, spelling and writing. There are a number of organizations that can help him with this.

5   Dyslexia can cause low self-esteem, depression and even in some cases suicidal tendencies.

6   Employers should be aware that 'difficulties with literacy do not necessarily mean lack of intelligence or education' (McLoughlin, Fitzgibbon and Young, 1994). Many dyslexics are highly talented and good at creative, artistic design, science and engineering activities. The Disability Discrimination Act 1995 should ensure that dyslexics will not be discriminated against in the workplace.

7   The 'dramatic changes during the past few years with respect to dyslexia have not been restricted to changes in attitudes. There has also be an explosion of alternative channels of learning ... inexpensive, varied, and easily accessible forms ideally suited to dyslexics' (West, 1991). Educators, employers and dyslexics must capitalize on these.

Chapter 13

Education legislation

- Special Educational Needs Code of Practice
- The role of SENCOs and School Governors
- Statementing and Tribunal appeals

Key legislation

Chronically Sick and Disabled Persons Act 1970
Required LEAs to provide 'special educational facilities for children who suffer from acute dyslexia'.

Education Act 1981
'A child has **special educational** needs if he has a "learning difficulty" which calls for **special educational provision** to be made for him'.

Education (Special Educational Needs) Regulations 1983

Circular 1/83: Assessments and Statements of Special Educational Needs within Education, Health and Social Services

Education Reform Act 1988
Resulted in The National Curriculum. Several government circulars ensued.

Education Act 1993
'A child has "**special educational needs**" if he has a learning difficulty which calls for special educational provision to be made for him.' The latest legislation for children with SEN is contained in Part III of the Education Act 1993 and is called 'Children with Special Educational Needs'. It is accompanied by a *Code of Practice* designed to give guidance to schools and LEAs on how to make effective decisions about provisions for the identification and assessment of children with SEN. **The Education Act 1996** incorporated unchanged the provisions of the 1993 Education Act.

The Education (Special Educational Needs) Regulations 1994

The *Code of Practice for the Identification and Assessment of Special Educational Needs (1994)* brought into effect by the Regulations spells out the fundamental principles concerning the identification, assessment and education of children with SEN as directed by the Education Act.

Events leading up to the issuing of the Code of Practice

The Committee of Enquiry into the Education of Handicapped Children and Young People

In 1978 the Committee of Enquiry into the Education of Handicapped Children and Young People was entrusted with examining children with SEN. The chairman was Mary Warnock and the report became known as the Warnock Report. It considered that 'twenty per cent of children might be expected to have special educational needs' (Warnock, 1978). This was at a time when two per cent of children with special needs were being taught in special schools and were described as handicapped under the Education Act 1944 criteria. The Education Act 1944 focused on the individual child and on categories of handicap. Warnock turned on its head this policy of separating pupils with learning difficulties out of mainstream schooling and spearheaded an integration policy, saying that 'special educational needs should be met in the ordinary classroom of the ordinary school' (Warnock, 1978). There was great debate on whether or not to 'label' children in an attempt to describe their difficulties. The report recommended that the term used should be 'children with learning difficulties'. Speaking many years later, Warnock (1994) said, 'We were expressly forbidden to use the word "dyslexia" in the report'. The issue of the terminology to be used remains contentious, particularly when a psychologist's report is written. Many educational psychologists were reluctant to use the term dyslexia, preferring to use the term 'specific learning difficulties' (SpLD). This was confirmed in the results of a national inquiry coordinated and written by Pumfrey and Reason and a working group of educational psychologists.

Education Act 1981 for England and Wales

Many of the recommendations made by the Warnock Report were enshrined in the Education Act 1981. This Act made many major changes to the education of children with SEN, their identification and the arrangements to be provided for them. It stated that a child who has a learning difficulty has:

- *a significantly greater difficulty in learning than the majority of children of his age.*
- *a disability which either prevents or hinders him from making use of educational facilities of a kind generally*

> *provided in schools within the area of the local authority concerned, for children of his area.*

Source: Education Act 1981. HMSO, London.

LEAs were instructed that they had to establish whether the child had a learning difficulty by using formal assessment, and if so they had to issue a statement of his needs. They had to make a Statement if they were 'of the opinion that they should determine the special educational provision that should be made'. The wording of the Education Act 1981 meant that there were wide discrepancies over decisions on whether or not to Statement a child. This failure to identify or help children with SEN was one of the root causes of litigation under the Education Act 1981, as parents sought Statements for their children to try and ensure that they received the help their condition required.

Further legislation and changes in the law

Since the Education Act 1981 there have been many changes in the recognition of, acceptance of and provision for children with SEN. It was widely recognized that legislative changes needed to be made. The government and educationalists wanted reforms but pressure for change came as a result of issues being tested in the courts. There were a number of high profile court cases which were widely reported in the media. Parents and members of the BDA, its Local Dyslexia Associations, Dyslexia Institute and the other dyslexia organizations actively campaigned for change.

Education Act 1993

With the implementation of the Education Act 1993 the government hoped to 'eradicate some of the worst difficulties – delay over issuing Statements, inconsistency between LEAs in their policies and practice on Statementing and the lack of parental involvement in some cases' which can, according to the Department for Education and Employment's (DfEE) own research, 'cause undue anxiety to parents and, in the worst cases, damage to a child's education at a critical stage of development' (DfEE, 1992).

The Education Act 1993 gave the LEA the responsibility to determine the special educational provision 'for any learning difficulty [the child] may have'. The Education Act 1993 states that 'for the purposes of the Education Acts, a child has "special educational needs" if he has a learning difficulty which calls for special educational provision to be made for him'.

The **Education Act 1996** incorporated unchanged the provisions of the 1993 Education Act.

Code of Practice

One of the most important provisions of the Education Act 1993 was the directive to publish a *Code of Practice*. This is aimed at making wider, fairer and more open accountability by schools to pupils in need of special education and to their parents. The Education (SEN) Regulations 1994, made under the Education Act 1993, came into effect and the *Code of Practice* was issued. This has been instrumental in raising the profile of SEN in mainstream education.

Objectives of the Code of Practice

1   It gives practical guidance 'to LEAs and the governing bodies of all maintained schools' about the needs of children with SEN and the help available and states how and by whom and to whom it should be provided. Friel (1995) had reservations about this claim and said that 'the Code contains a great deal of statements of good intention rather than guidance, or firm practice'.

2   It is designed to 'ensure greater consistency in the making of Statements'.

3   There are strict time limits for the various procedures to be followed.

4   There should be 'greater precision in the contents of Statements' (Minister of State, 1993).

The *Code of Practice* places duties and responsibilities on LEAs and schools, the health services and social services. The BDA responded enthusiastically to the *Code of Practice*, but despite this reported that 'callers to the BDA National Helpline and our local Dyslexia Associations continually report concerns about the Code of Practice' (BDA, 1996a). The Code is designed to help schools make effective decisions. It gives guidance, but it does not or could not tell schools what to do. Friel (1995) stated that 'the Code was intended and is intended to promote a consistent approach to SEN across England and Wales'. Greater accountability on the part of the educational institutions involved is demanded, and parental involvement and co-operation is actively sought in the new legislation. The *Code of Practice* has been generally welcomed by parents, teachers, voluntary organizations and LEAs, according to the enquiry and report of the House of Commons Education Committee (Healey, 1996). But 'all those to whom the Code applies have a statutory duty to have regard to it; they must not ignore it'. Professor Davie of the National Association for SEN (NASEN) said 'it put special needs at the top of the educational agenda for the first time in most people's lifetime' (*The Sunday Observer*, 1994).

The principles underlying the Code of Practice

1 The needs of all children who have special educational needs throughout, or at any time during, their school careers must be addressed.

2 Children with special educational needs should be given the greatest possible access to a broad and balanced education, including the National Curriculum.

3 Provision for most children should be met 'in the mainstream, and without a statutory assessment or Statement of SEN'.

4 Some children may have special educational needs before they reach compulsory school age.

5 Partnership between parents and their children and schools, LEAs and other agencies involved is vital.

Education Act 1993/1996
Glossary of terms

Annual review
This is the review of a Statement of SEN which a LEA must make within twelve months of issuing a Statement, or of the previous review.

Code of Practice
This contains fundamental principles concerning the education of children with SEN.

Independent School
It is a private school which can be privately owned or have charitable trust status, but it is neither maintained by a LEA nor is it a grant-maintained school. Much of the legislation which applies to mainstream schools does not apply to independent schools.

Individual Education Plan (IEP)
It is a detailed personal plan for the child concerned. It should detail the following:

• A description of the child's learning difficulties.

• Action to be taken, staff involved, external specialists involved, frequency and timing of help provided.

• What parental help can/should be given.

• Targets and deadlines.

• Recommendations for help for medical, emotional or social problems.

- Arrangements for monitoring progress and for assessment.
- Date of review and with whom it is to be discussed.

Learning difficulties

A pupil has SEN if:

- He has a 'significantly greater difficulty in learning than the majority of children of his age'. This could include problems with literacy, behavioural problems, or physical disabilities.
- 'He has a disability which either prevents or hinders him from making use of educational facilities of a kind generally provided for children of his age in schools within the area of the LEA'.

Mainstream School

An ordinary school funded by the government and subject to government legislation.

Maintained Sector of Education

This is made up of schools which are funded by the government. The following types of school are included in the maintained sector of education:

Nursery schools: for children under five years old

County schools: owned by the LEA and run by staff appointed by the LEA

Special schools: to educate children with SEN

Grant-maintained: schools that have 'opted out' of LEA control and are funded by the DfEE

Voluntary: usually founded by voluntary organizations such as a Church, these have greater independence from LEAs than other schools have

City Technology Colleges: funded partly by private donations and partly by the government.

Named Officer

An officer of the LEA who will deal with the child's statutory assessment and the making of a Statement.

Named Person (more often called a 'Befriender')

A person chosen by the LEA and the parents. She should normally be independent of the LEA and can be a friend or relative of the parents, or a member of a voluntary organization. She should be able to give the parents accurate information and advice about the child's SEN and the assessment process, and help with the negotiations with the LEA. It is useful if this person is willing to attend meetings and has experience of advocacy, for example the appeal procedures at an SEN Tribunal. There are a number of voluntary organizations who provide this help. The BDA also has trained volunteer Befrienders and says that they can support parents through the administrative and legal processes of special education but that they do not have legal training.

Note in Lieu of a Statement
This is a note in which the LEA will set out its reasons for not issuing a Statement when a statutory assessment has been made. It should describe the child's SEN, explain why the LEA is not making a Statement and make recommendations about what help, if any, the child should receive. It has no legal status and is not binding on the school concerned.

OFSTED (Office for Standards in Education)
OFSTED is responsible for the inspection of all schools in England and Wales. It carries out inspections and makes reports on its findings and has the power to close down schools which are not meeting required standards.

Proposed Statement (formerly called Draft Statement)
It is the first Statement of SEN made by the LEA. It may be changed after consultation with the child's parents.

Responsible Person
This refers to the head teacher or chairman of the school governors (unless the governing body has designated another governor) who must ensure that all those who will teach the child know about his SEN. The LEA must inform this person when a child has been given a Statement.

Special Educational Needs (SEN)
For the purposes of the Education Acts, a child has special educational needs 'if he has a learning difficulty which calls for special educational provision to be made for him' and should have extra help at school. Most of the help should be given in mainstream education. Up to 20 per cent of children will have SEN at some time in school.

Special Educational Needs Co-ordinator (SENCO)
Each school must have a member of staff who is responsible for:

- managing and planning all aspects of the school's SEN support
- ensuring that the child is included on the school's SEN register
- helping the child's teacher or tutor to gather information to access the child's needs, and to update and keep records of children with SEN

- informing, advising and supporting those who teach the child
- liaising with parents and other support agencies, including voluntary organizations
- contributing to the in-service training of staff
- drawing up the Individual Education Plan (IEP) for children with SEN.

SEN Tribunal

The SEN Tribunal was set up under the Education Act 1993 to give parents a forum in which to appeal against the LEA's decisions regarding their child's SEN. It is an independent body appointed by the Lord Chancellor and the Secretary of State. The decision of the Tribunal is binding on both parties in the appeal. It consists of three people appointed by the DfEE: a legally qualified chairman and two 'lay persons'.

Special Educational Provision

For a child who is over two years old this is defined as follows:

Educational provision which is additional to, or otherwise different from, the educational provision made generally for children of his age in schools maintained by the LEA other than special schools in the area.

Source: Code of Practice for the Identification and Assessment of Special Educational Needs (1994). Department for Education and Employment, London.

Staged Assessment

This is a five stage model of principles, practices and procedures to be followed by the school and LEA when dealing with a child with SEN. Stages 1–3 of the assessment are carried out in school. At stages 4 and 5 the LEA shares the responsibility with the school.

Statement

A Statement of SEN is a document that sets out a child's needs and all the extra help he should get. Friel (1995) pointed out that 'essentially, therefore, a statement is intended to protect in practice children with the more severe or complex type of problem'. The Code states that 'only in a small minority of cases – nationally, around two per cent of children – will a child have SEN of a severity or complexity which requires the LEA to determine and arrange the special educational provision for the child by means of a statutory Statement of SEN'. It must set out the SEN in terms of the child's learning difficulties, and must enumerate the special education provision, including equipment, staffing arrangements and curriculum. The *Code of Practice* says of the Statement that 'the provision should normally be specific, detailed and quantified (in terms, for example, of hours of ancillary or specialist teaching support)'. It should also specify arrangements for monitoring and reviewing the Statement. It should name the school for which the parent has expressed a preference. It may also specify non-educational needs or non-educational provision. Statements should be reviewed every twelve months.

Statutory Assessment

The Statutory Assessment 'is a comprehensive study of the abilities and learning difficulties of a child who has or may have special educational needs'. 'It should be undertaken only if the authorities believe that they need or probably need to determine the child's special educational provision themselves by making a Statement'. Its job is to determine and identify a child's needs and to establish what provision is required. It is undertaken by a number of different professionals. The LEA calls it a multi-professional statutory assessment.

The LEA must give parents:

* written notice of its intention to make a Statement
* a Named Person who is preferably independent of the LEA who can help with advice
* information about voluntary organizations who may be able to help
* the opportunity to submit private advice or opinion, such as advice from a qualified educational or clinical psychologist, or specialist teacher's assessment
* information about provision in mainstream schools.

The child's feelings and perceptions should be taken into account during the assessment, and older children and young adults should be treated as partners in the assessment along with their parents.

A Statutory Assessment is a necessary part of the formal procedure required in order to get a child Statemented.

Transition Plan

This should form part of the review after the child's fourteenth birthday. It sets out steps to plan the young person's transition to adult life.

School Special Educational Needs (SEN) Policy

The Education (SEN) Regulations 1994 state that governing bodies of schools must draw up a policy document for children with SEN and that they must report annually to parents on its implementation.

A SEN policy should set out the following:

1   Basic information about school policy.

- State objectives of the policy and give details of the provisions to be used to overcome specific areas of difficulty.
- Name the school's SENCO or teacher responsible for the day-to-day operation of the SEN policy.
- State arrangements for coordinating educational provision.
- State admission arrangements.
- State any SEN specialism and any special units.
- Describe any special facilities which increase or assist access to the school by children with SEN.

2   Policy on identification and assessment.

- Allocate resources to and among children with SEN.
- Set out procedures for identifying, assessing, monitoring and reviewing.
- Make arrangements for providing access to a balanced and broadly based curriculum, including the National Curriculum for children with SEN.
- Show how children with SEN are integrated into the school as a whole.
- Set out the criteria for evaluating the success of the SEN policy.
- Make available any arrangements for considering complaints about the SEN provision within the school.

3   Staff arrangements and liaison with outside bodies.

- Give information on SEN in-service training.
- Give details of the use of specialist teachers outside the school, including support services.
- Describe links with parent helpers and voluntary organizations.
- Describe links with other mainstream schools and special schools.

- Describe links with social services, educational welfare services and dyslexia organizations.

Source: Office for Standards in Education (1996) *The Implemation of the Code of Practice for Pupils with Special Educational Needs*. HMSO, London:15

It is very important that every need has been identified and that provision made for each need is itemized. The Statement should say which provision is to come from the LEA and which is to come from the resources of the child's school. It should describe 'all of the SEN, and provision must be specific for each and every one'.

Model for identifying and assessing children with SEN in England and Wales

The *Code of Practice* states that 'all children with special educational needs should be identified and assessed as early as possible and as quickly as is consistent with thoroughness'.

Five stage model

There is a five stage model for this help, but it does not have to be followed rigorously or sequentially by the LEA or school. The first three stages are school based. The school governors are responsible for implementing stages 1 to 4. The LEA is legally responsible for Stage 5.

Stage 1
Involves the initial identification and registration of a child's SEN. The class teacher should identify the child's SEN and record these and speak to the child's parents. The **trigger** is an 'expression of concern' by anybody involved with the child.

Stage 2
The school's SENCO 'takes the lead in assessing the child's learning difficulties and planning, monitoring and reviewing the special educational provision'. The **trigger** follows when there has been further discussion after the initial concern and when the SENCO considers that 'early intensive action' is necessary.

Stage 3
Specialist help from outside the school is sought from an educational psychologist or a specialist teacher who may need to test the child. The **trigger** comes after discussion with those involved with the child when the SENCO 'having consulted the head teacher, considers that early intensive action' is necessary from 'other agencies'. The SENCO will then draw up an Individual

Education Plan (IEP) which describes the education action and 'new strategies for supporting the child's progress'.

Stage 4

The need for a Statutory Assessment must be considered by the LEA after consultation with the child's parents. 'Where a school refers a child for a statutory assessment the head teacher may' according to the Education Reform Act 1988 'give a special direction either modifying or disapplying the National Curriculum for the child for a period of up to six months'.

'An assessment under Section 107 of the Education Act 1993 should be undertaken only if the authorities believe they need or probably need to determine the child's special educational provision themselves by making a Statement'. This will involve other professionals and a multi-disciplinary assessment may be made.

Stage 5

The LEA should consider the need for a Statement of SEN. It should then issue a Proposed Statement or Notice in Lieu including provisions for any special arrangements including the choice of school. If appropriate, the LEA must then issue a Final Statement and monitor and review the Statement thereafter.

Timetable

The time limits for the completion of stages 4 and 5 are set at no more than 26 weeks in total. These limits may only be extended in exceptional circumstances. There is a strict timetable for the procedures leading to a Statement:
Six weeks: for the LEA to decide whether to make an assessment
Ten weeks: to make the assessment
Two weeks: to draft a Proposed Statement or to issue a Note in Lieu
Eight weeks: to finalize the Statement.

Parents as partners

At each stage the parents must be consulted and informed of the steps that are being taken. 'The relationship between parents of children with special educational needs and the school which their child is attending has a crucial bearing on the child's educational progress and the effectiveness of any school-based action'. Furthermore, the *Code of Practice* says that 'the school-based stages should therefore utilize parents' own distinctive knowledge and skills and contribute to parents' own understanding of how best to help their child'.

How do parents obtain a Statutory Assessment of their child?

Normally the school should instigate and request the Statutory Assessment. But under Section 172 or 173 of the Education Act 1993 parents may ask the LEA to conduct a Statutory Assessment and 'whatever the background it [the LEA] must take all parental requests seriously and take action immediately'.

Under the Education Act 1993 the LEA can agree to the parental request for a Statutory Assessment at its own discretion. This discretion is based on whether the LEA feels 'it is necessary' for it 'to determine the education provision' or whether the child's needs can be met from 'resources generally available to the school.' Parents of a child at an independent school also have the right to apply to a LEA to have their child assessed and the same provisions apply.

Schools are required to send evidence of a learning difficulty to the LEA. If the LEA decides that it may be necessary for it to determine the provision, then the LEA must arrange an assessment, and must notify in writing the social services department, the district health authority and the head teacher that a request has been made for an assessment.

The LEA must contact the school to ask for more detailed evidence of the child's learning difficulty. The LEA must look at the child's Individual Education Plan (IEP) and the steps taken to identify and assess the child's SEN, as well as the records of the child's attainments, including the results of tests in the core subjects of the National Curriculum. *The Code of Practice 1994* states that they should look for evidence of the child working at a level significantly below that of his or her contemporaries in any of the core subjects of the National Curriculum. *Of particular interest* are some children [who] may have significant difficulties in reading, writing, spelling or manipulating numbers, which are not typical of their general level of performance. There should also be reports about the child's behaviour and details of health, general development and information from parents, the GP or social services department. The child's views should be sought and recorded.

The Statutory Assessment process

The Education (SEN) Regulations for the Education Act 1993 state that an assessment must include:

- parental advice
- educational advice
- medical advice

- psychological advice
- social services advice
- any other advice deemed necessary, for example speech therapy
- child's views.

The contents of an educational psychologist's report

The advice of the educational psychologist will be the linchpin in the assessment proceedings. The report is the core document. It should outline the nature and extent of the child's problems and should enumerate the help and the provisions that need to be made for the child. The Statutory Assessment is concluded when the LEA decides whether or not it will make a Statement.

The educational psychologist's assessment report should include the following information:

1 Name and address of the child and the school attended. Date of birth and chronological age when assessed as well as the date of the assessment.

2 The reason for referral, for example at the request of the parents to establish the child's current attainments and to establish whether he has a specific learning difficulty. It should also chronicle the delay or difficulties in speech or physical skills he has experienced. His acquisition of basic literacy skills in comparison with that of his peers, including how he is coping with the demands of the National Curriculum, should be examined.

3 A note of the specific tests used and the results obtained, for example an intelligence test such as WISC–III^{UK} with figures obtained for the Verbal IQ, Performance IQ and Full Scale IQ (very occasionally the Full Scale IQ is not quoted if there is a huge discrepancy between the verbal and performance scores as this can undermine the reliability and accuracy of the Full Scale IQ score). The report should say how the child responded and reacted in the testing situation.

4 The main body of the report should explain in some detail the child's abilities and difficulties and include the results of the educational attainment tests – reading including single word recognition and continuous prose, spelling and arithmetic age as measured by standardized tests. There will probably be comments on the child's strategies when reading. Handwriting skills, such as pencil grip, fluency, speed and style of writing will be considered. A 'free writing' test is important because it reveals the full extent of the child's problems, including the

child's spelling, punctuation, sentence structure, expressive language skills and use of vocabulary. It may also highlight his spelling difficulties.

5   Other diagnostic tests may be administered depending on the child's performance. They could include tests of laterality and tests of visual and auditory memory, such as digit span, immediate visual recall, recall of designs and fine motor and ocular motor control.

6   Background information should include a précis of the child's schooling, developmental history, a case history and a brief medical history. It should also include a family history which should help to establish whether there are other members of the family who have similar difficulties in reading and spelling. Details of behavioural or emotional problems may be included.

7   Conclusions usually comment on the level at which the child should be achieving and provide a description of the specific learning difficulties.

8   Recommendations on the nature and type of specialist help for the child's SEN should give the following information.
   • How many sessions per week should be given.
   • How long the sessions should be.
   • Details of non-educational provision, including extra physical education or physiotherapy required if the child has gross motor problems.
   • Say whether provision is to be mainstream or otherwise.
   • Say whether a support teacher is to be provided for general curriculum work (and indicate provisions for emotional support).
   • Specify appropriate aids, for example word processor, laptop or computer or electric typewriter.
   • Say, if appropriate, that the child should be offered an opportunity to enhance self-esteem through Art, Drama or Sport (these subjects are often the first to be lost when time tabling for specialist lessons is being considered, whereas these very activities may be crucial for the child's emotional or physical well being).
   • Say if speech therapy would be appropriate.
   • State if there are to be 'disapplications' (exemptions) or modifications to the National Curriculum and for how long.

9   It should recommend a placement which gives the name and type of school where the special educational provision specified can be carried out.

The above information is used to prepare the Proposed Statement of SEN. The advice from the other agencies who were consulted must also be included in the appendices.

When is a Statement necessary?

A Statement is necessary when a child:

- has a severe or complex learning difficulty
- needs to be exempt from some part of the National Curriculum, or
- when the normal school is unable or unwilling to make the appropriate help available for the child.

The Proposed Statement

Once the LEA has decided to make a Statement it must give written notice of this to the parents within two weeks of the date of the Statutory Assessment. The LEA must then send the parent a copy of the Proposed Statement, and a notice setting out the arrangements for parental preference of schools, both maintained and non-maintained, which cater for children with SEN. Parents are allowed fifteen days to make comments on the Proposed Statement and/or ask for a meeting with an LEA official to discuss the contents. At this stage, it is often very helpful to have an objective third party on hand – a Befriender to put the parents' point of view in an unemotional and cogent manner.

Parents can request a further meeting with the professionals who gave the advice. The LEA must consider any oral or written representations from the parents, and it has a duty to name the parents' preferred school in the Statement, providing it is appropriate to the child's needs and concerns. The *Code of Practice* says that 'taking parents' concerns seriously may ensure that there is mutual understanding and respect and may help to avoid conflict'.

The Final Statement

The LEA must issue to the parents a copy of the Final Statement which should state in detail:

- the child's SEN
- the special provision to be made to meet these needs
- placement, giving name and type of school
- objectives and targets for the child's progress, including details of how these are to be monitored
- non-educational needs, such as specialist equipment, speech therapy or occupational therapy

- non-educational provision to meet these needs
- appendices, including evidence from parents, the child's views, medical specialist, teacher or anybody from whom the LEA sought advice.

If all the parties involved are happy the Statement can be finalized. The Final Statement, which should be signed and dated, is a legally binding document, and the LEA must deliver whatever has been stated.

The Final Statement must also include information on how to lodge an appeal to the SEN Tribunal and it must name an individual for further contact. The school must ensure that the child's SEN are made known to all those who teach him.

Monitoring and annual review

It is important that the child's progress is reviewed at least once a year. The LEA can amend or cease to maintain a Statement, but if so it must serve notice of this. Parents then have fifteen days to respond. The first annual review that follows the child's fourteenth birthday is very important because it should set out the details in a Transition Plan for the child's transfer to further education. A Statement will remain in force until the LEA ceases to maintain it or until the child is no longer the responsibility of the LEA.

The hypothesis and the reality

Obtaining help for a dyslexic child

The *Code of Practice* makes it abundantly clear that the government expects that only a small number of cases – nationally, around two per cent of children – will have SEN which require the full blown treatment of a Statement. Orton (1996) highlighted the huge gap between the number of children who actually receive Statements and the number of children who are put forward for a Statement.

It is widely regarded in many parts of the UK that the only guarantee of receiving teaching appropriate to the child's needs is to obtain a Statement, hence the stampede down this road and the rush to the door of the SEN Tribunal. The BDA has been attempting to monitor LEAs nationally and to establish the quality and quantity of help available. It is widely recognized 'that the process was often taking far too long with dismal statistics about the average time taken and many horror stories of children not getting their Statements until they were about to leave school'

(BDA, 1996b). The time limits set by the *Code of Practice* should help alleviate this. The Audit Commission publishes information about Statements which on close scrutiny provides evidence of the wide discrepancies in the provisions made nationally. St Helens in Lancashire, for example, issues Statements to the highest proportion of children of any LEA, begging the question why other LEAs have much lower records.

Many issues remain to be resolved, not least that there is a wide gap between the figure of two per cent of children considered by the government to require special help and the numbers quoted by the BDA regarding the prevalence of severe dyslexia, which it says exceeds four per cent of the population. Pumfrey (1994) demonstrated the problem facing schools, educationalists and LEAs:

> *Pupils with SEN and dyslexic-type difficulties*
> *IQ 120 Reading Ability 6.0 years*
> *IQ 100 Reading Ability 6.0 years*
> *IQ 80 Reading Ability 6.0 years*
> *Which pupil should be Statemented?*

> *Source:* Pumfrey P. (1994) 'The management of specific learning disabilities (dyslexia): Challenges and responses'. Unpublished paper. *Towards a wider understanding. Third International Conference of the British Dyslexia Association, Manchester.*

There has been great emphasis placed on the children with severe and profound learning difficulties. With the more enlightened approach of the *Code of Practice* a large number of these are being helped through Statementing. But it is clear that significantly more children will ultimately need to be formally assessed and provided with Statements if they are to receive teaching appropriate to their needs. Problems remain for the thousands of children who do not fall into the Statemented category. The BDA (1996b) stated that the child's SEN have 'to be more severe before he is regarded as having learning difficulties'; furthermore 'parents are being told "we cannot help him until he is three (or more) years behind" in reading in comparison with his chronological age'. The BDA goes on to say that 'LEA criteria for Statutory Assessments and Statements are becoming more simplistic and severe'.

Resources

Children with SEN are to receive help according to the Stage models specified in the *Code of Practice*. The *Code of Practice* assumes that the expertise is already in place in all schools and it has put enormous pressure on SENCOs and the teachers who have responsibility for special needs of the children in their classrooms.

There are not enough specialist teachers trained to assess or to give the specialist teaching that most experts in the field of dyslexia deem to be necessary to comply with 'the teaching appropriate to the child's needs'. Healey (1996) argued that 'there needs to be agreement on the qualifications for a specialist teacher for specific learning difficulties'. The BDA has criteria for accepting and approving courses for the training of such teachers, but according to Professor Davie (*The Sunday Observer*, 1994), 'the amount of money Ministers have allocated to train teachers is too little'.

The word 'dyslexia' is only once mentioned in the 134 pages that constitute the *Code of Practice*. Yet some observers, such as Brereton (1995), commented that 'we are delighted with the comprehensive description of dyslexic difficulties. The real problem is that schools are assumed to have the expertise to deal with the difficulties, using their own resources without the pupil having a Statement'.

Pupils aged between 16 and 19

The LEA must inform the social services about a young person aged between sixteen and nineteen years who has been Statemented. The LEA has a duty to young people over sixteen years who have a Statement whilst that young person is still at school and must provide for him in accordance with his Statement. When the young person leaves school and enters further education responsibility for the provision of appropriate help is the duty of the Further Education Funding Council (while the young person is in full-time education).

School governors' role

The school governors have a duty to:
- make the necessary provision for any child who has SEN, including children without a Statement
- designate a 'responsible person', either the head teacher, an appropriate governor or the chairman of the governors. This person is responsible for making the child's learning difficulties known to all who teach him
- ensure that all the teachers in the school are aware of the importance of identifying and providing for children with SEN
- report annually on the school's policy for children with SEN and on the effectiveness of their SEN policy

- ensure that the child joins in school activities and mixes with other children in the school
- liaise with the LEA or other bodies involved.

Governors have a duty to 'use their best endeavours' to see that there are provisions in their school for children with special needs. They should establish whether individuals are receiving the education they require. There should be a nominated governor who is responsible for informing other staff and liaising with parents and other professionals concerned with the child with SEN. They must publish a SEN policy for their school. They must report annually to the parents on how effective their SEN policy has been and on how resources have been allocated. There have been reports that primary school governors have used the SEN budget to create an extra class (thus reducing class sizes) benefiting all the children in the school, rather than targeting just the SEN children. The justification for this is arguable.

Parents' rights

The *Code of Practice* encourages co-operation between parents, schools and LEAs. It requires schools and LEAs to pay particular attention to the role of parents and includes precise guidelines for the involvement and contribution of parents to the Statutory Assessment. This should include provision of information on the child's early years, current skills, health and behaviour. It also gives parents the opportunity to express their opinions and concerns.

Guidelines
for parents on how and where to obtain help

- Obtain copies (free) of the following literature from the Department for Education and Employment (DfEE):

  Code of Practice for the Identification and Assessment of Special Educational Needs (DfEE, 1994)

  Special Educational Needs: A Guide for Parents (DfEE, 1994)

  Special Education Handbook: The Law on Children with Special Needs (The Advisory Centre for Education (ACE), 1996)

  Children and Young Persons with Special Educational Needs Assessment and Recording Circular 4/96 (1996) (Circular No 4/96, Scottish Office Education and Industry Department, 1996)

A Parent's Guide to Special Educational Needs
(Scottish Office Education and Industry Department, 1996)

- Contact the LEA and ask for a copy of their policy on educating children with SEN.

- Ask the school for information on its SEN provisions and obtain a copy of their SEN policy. Try to find out how many children are in their special needs department, how many teachers there are and what the teacher/pupil ratio is. Find out how many children in the school have a Statement, and how many are on the Special Needs Register or Staged Assessment.

- Obtain the name and address of the governor or 'responsible person' who is in charge of SEN at the school and establish what they have done for children with special needs.

- Contact the BDA Local Association nearest to the LEA catchment area. It may have a parent volunteer who has had training as a Befriender. It may have had experience of dealing with schools and LEA officials, and with the LEA psychologists. Its knowledge and experience can be invaluable, and its relationship with the personalities involved may be helpful and save effort. The *Code of Practice* states that 'assessment can be stressful for parents. The value of early information and support to parents cannot be over-emphasized'.

- Keep written records of all meetings and telephone conversations, including the dates. Make copies of and file all correspondence. Try to obtain written replies from officials. Ask for written confirmation of important points discussed on the telephone.

- Talk to the child's class teacher. Some issues to discuss are 'Does the teacher think the child is underachieving?', 'Is he having difficulties coping with classwork?' or 'Does he have a learning difficulty?'

- Talk to the head teacher. It is helpful if both parents/partners attend the meeting to discuss their views and concerns for the child's needs. Try to establish whether the head teacher is sympathetic to the needs of dyslexic children. It is a great help if the head teacher is supportive. At this meeting try to find out about the help being offered, if any, to other children with SEN in the school. Request that the child is put on the school's SEN register.

Enquire whether the school will put the child on a Staged Assessment.

- Arrange to meet the SENCO and enquire about the following:
  - the ratio of dyslexic children to others
  - whether the SEN children are taught with, and in the same way as, the slow learners, the emotionally disturbed or the children with behavioural problems
  - what training the teachers working with the SEN children have, for example RSA Diploma in Specific Learning Difficulties or AMBDA Diploma
  - whether they use a multi-sensory structured teaching programme such as *Alpha-to-Omega* (Hornsby and Shear, 1994), *The Hickey Multi-Sensory Language Course* (Augur and Briggs (eds), 1992) or *The Bangor Dyslexia Teaching System* (Miles, 1993)
  - the amount of time children spend in the unit if there is one
  - help available with the National Curriculum
  - whether typewriters, computers, word processors or tape recorders are readily available and whether they are used by the SEN children
  - arrangements to inform and enlist the assistance of other members of staff to help dyslexic children.

- Visit the SEN unit on a working day. This is a very useful way of establishing the nature of help being given.

- A very good indicator of the type of provision being given can be gained from looking at the books, materials and resources in use. If the parent is unsure about this, it is still important to ask and note the response which can be discussed later with someone who can advise on the appropriateness of the materials being used.

- Find out about the examination results of the SEN children. Information on the number of GCSEs sat by the dyslexic children, which examining boards were used and the grades obtained, particularly in English Language, gives an indication of the standards and success rate of the children. Bear in mind that it is not fair to use the same criteria to judge the dyslexic child as other children in the school and that it is difficult to judge what individual children should achieve without knowing their ability levels, IQ, the severity of the dyslexia, at what age their problems were identified and the quality and quantity of specialist teaching they have received.

- Find out how many of these dyslexic children stay on for 'A' Levels (if the school has a sixth form) and how many 'A' Levels they usually sit.
- Find out if the school curriculum includes the option to study GNVQs.

Do parents have a right to choose their child's school?

Parents have a right to express a preference for a school in the maintained sector or outside it under the Education Act 1993 . 'The LEA must comply with a parental preference for a maintained special school so long as the three following conditions – appropriateness for the child and compatibility with the interests of other children and the efficient use of resources – are met'. If parents name an independent school as their preferred choice, the LEA must discuss with the parent why that provision is deemed necessary. Some independent boarding schools are well-known and established as centres of excellence for teaching dyslexic pupils and give intensive, highly skilled tuition.

Parents often turn to the law in their attempts to get the LEA to pay the fees for their child to attend the school which they feel is best placed to give the child the help required to overcome his learning difficulties. Devon County Council (1996) pointed out 'when nationally more than half (22/39 – SEN Tribunal Annual Report 1994–95) of appeals naming independent schools are being upheld, the Tribunal's decisions have the effect of placing a mandate upon LEAs to make provision that is more costly than would normally be allowed for in LEA budgetary. This does not sit easily with the cost-neutrality of the Education Act 1993 and the Code of Practice'. But the 'decisions of the courts suggest that LEAs do not have to place children with SEN in independent schools even where it offers better provision than in maintained schools, provided that the education available is suitable (R v Surrey Health County Council Education Committee, 1984; and R v Mid-Glamorgan County Council, 1988).

Parents may decide to educate their Statemented child at a fee-paying school at their expense. In those circumstances the LEA still has a duty to maintain the child's Statement and to review it annually.

What if parents fail to get the help they believe to be their child's right?

After a Statutory Assessment has been carried out the LEA may decide not to make a Statement. The LEA must give its reasons in writing and it must produce the evidence for its decision. Sometimes a Note in Lieu of a Statement is issued. This may contain helpful advice and suggestions for the child's future education but it has no legal status and is not binding or enforceable on the school or LEA.

Parents may appeal to the SEN Tribunal. This is an independent body.

Appealing to a SEN Tribunal

What are the grounds for appealing to the Tribunal?

Parents may appeal if the LEA has:

1 refused to make a formal assessment

2 refused to issue a Statement

If they are unhappy with:

3 the description of the child's special needs as described in the Statement

4 the description of the type of special educational help

5 the school named

6 not having a school named

7 the fact that the Statement is not maintained

8 a refusal to re-assess the child if the LEA has not made a new assessment for at least six months.

The Tribunal may not deal with:
- the provision made by the school to meet the child's needs
- the school's failure to meet the child's needs
- delay in assessing or making a Statement
- the descriptions of non-educational needs
- the way the assessment was carried out.

Appeal process

There has been much disquiet about the appeals procedure. Many parents are frightened by it, particularly if the LEA involves its legal department. Despite the reassurance of the SEN Tribunal, appeals are often conducted in a legalistic manner, and the LEA is often legally represented. The BDA (1996a) suggested a compromise to redress this unfairness and said 'there should be a "concordat" that LEAs should not take a lawyer when the parents do not. Some parents employ a lawyer, but the expense involved can be prohibitive for many for SEN Tribunal appeals'.

Legal Aid

Legal Aid is not available to the child's parents for a tribunal appeal but:

Children may be entitled to Legal Aid in their own name and since very few have income or capital most comply with the financial criteria. Legal Aid is available for court proceedings only (ie judicial review or an action in negligence.) It is not available for any part of the statementing process, including appeals. In appeals from the SEN Tribunal it has been found that the parent, not the child, is the party to the appeal. This means Legal Aid is only available if the parents qualify, usually only if they are on Income Support.

Source: Educational Law Association (1995).

Using the SEN Tribunal

Devon County Council (1996) pointed out that 'the large overall number of cases being heard suggest that the Tribunal is being used by parents not as a last resort as intended but as a first resort to be exploited at the earliest signs of a difference arising between the parents and the LEA'. Children with SEN were the largest group making use of the SEN Tribunal.

- There are strict time limits on SEN Tribunals. Parents must appeal within two months of the LEA's decision not to Statement, that is within two months of the date of the finalized Statement letter from the LEA.

- The final Statement letter contains a form (on the back inside cover) entitled 'Notice of Appeal to the SEN Tribunal'. This should be filled in and sent off with a copy of the final Statement.

- The SEN Tribunal will then ask the LEA for the documents relating to the case. The Tribunal has to consider all the evidence and the LEA must submit all the documentation it has.

- Parents should attend the hearing if possible. Parents may have two witnesses.

- The decision will often be made at the SEN Tribunal. If not, parents will be informed in writing of the decision within ten working days of the hearing.

- Both parties, if dissatisfied, have a right to appeal to the High Court on a point of law within 28 days of the decision.

How to prepare for an appeal to the SEN Tribunal

Sources of help

- Volunteers belonging to support organizations offer help.
- The BDA runs 'Befriender' training courses to help members of BDA Local Associations to guide and advise parents through the legal processes.
- The Befriender can assist in the preparation of the case, and may also appear with parents before the SEN Tribunal.
- It may be necessary or wise to have legal representation but parents will have to pay for this since there is no Legal Aid for representation at a Tribunal.
- The Citizens Advice Bureau has information on the 'Green Form' scheme which entitles a parent to up to £80 worth of legal advice prior to the appeal. The ceilings on income are very low and this amount is but a drop in the ocean if further legal advice is necessary.

  More difficult or complex cases, and certainly those parents who go to the High Court, would be well-advised to have legal representation if possible.
- The Education Law Association (ELAS) members, including solicitors and barristers, have specialist knowledge of the workings of the Education Acts.
- Obtain a free copy of *Special Educational Needs Tribunal: How to Appeal* (DfEE Publications, PO Box 2193, London, E15 2UE. Telephone 0181 533 2000).

Children and young persons with SEN in Scotland

Scotland has its own legal system and it has a body of education legislation for special educational needs which is as follows:

The Education (Scotland) Act 1980

There were a number of amendments and Regulations made to this Act. The most important are as follows:

The Education (Scotland) Act 1981

The Education (Record of Needs) (Scotland) Regulations 1982

Disabled Persons (Services, Consultation and Representation) Act 1986
Self-Governing Schools, etc. (Scotland) Act 1989
Children and Young Persons with Special Education Needs
Assessment and Recording *Circular No 4/96 (1996)*.

Key definitions of the Education (Scotland) Act 1980

'Children and young persons have **special educational needs** if they have a learning difficulty which calls for provision for special educational needs to be made for them.'

They are said to have a **learning difficulty** if they:

(a) 'have significantly greater difficulty in learning than the majority of those of their age; or

(b) suffer from a disability which either prevents or hinders them from making use of educational facilities of a kind generally provided for those of their age in schools managed by their education authority.'

According to Circular No 4/96 (1996), 'In the [Scottish Office] Department's [of Education and Industry] view, as a rule of thumb, it should be assumed that children or young persons have a "learning difficulty" if additional arrangements need to be made to enable them properly to access the curriculum'.

Glossary of Terms

Assessment
A formal procedure which assesses the child's educational needs and seeks to establish the nature and extent of these. This is carried out by an educational psychologist, a medical officer, school staff and other professioals whose opinion is sought.

Case Conference
A meeting and discussion of the findings by all the professionals involved in the assessment. It should include the child's parents.

Discontinuance of a Record of Needs
This takes place when the education authority decides that a Record of Needs is no longer necessary and ceases to have effect.

Education Authority Appeal Committee
This committee hears appeals arising from decisions made about the assessment and recording of special needs procedures.

Future Needs Assessment
An assessment carried out to determine the future educational needs of a child nearing school leaving age.

Individualized Educational Programme (IEP)
Plans written for an individual child. They list the aims and objectives for the child's education, goals to be achieved, timescales, arrangements for assessment, resources, the staff involved and the involvement of the parents.

Named Person
A person who should be able to provide help and support for parents, including help with understanding what is contained in the Record of Needs.

Record of Needs
A confidential folder opened by the education authority. It contains a description of the child's special educational needs, including information on how these are to be met and giving details of where and how the child is to be educated.

Review of the Record of Needs
A formal review of the child's or the young person's progress. For the purpose of the Act a 'child' is one who attends school and is between the age of five and sixteen years. A 'young person' is over sixteen years and is not yet eighteen years.

Special School
A school or special class which forms part of a primary or secondary school. It makes provision wholly or mainly for children with a Record of Needs.

The Statutory Assessment Process
Schools may request that a child is formally assessed. Parents have to be informed and consulted about this and a named member of staff must be available to give information about the process. Parents also have a right to ask the education authority, with a view to opening a Record of Needs, to assess their child and this request cannot be refused unless the request is deemed unreasonable.

The assessment will involve the school staff, educational and health professionals employed by the education authority and administrative staff. Parents have a right to be present throughout although the educational psychologist may wish to test the child without the parent being present. In this case the educational psychologist should report and discuss her findings with them.

The Disabled Persons (Services, Consultation and Representation) Act 1986 made changes to the process of assessment. '. . . the change substituted a process of observation and assessment, which must include educational, psychological and medical assessment.' But in certain circumstances, formal assessment is not necessary, and 'assessment may often be best carried out by careful and discreet professional observation in the home or in the school'. Circular No 4/96 (1996) states that 'all contacts with parents, particularly when giving information, should use straightforward, plain language'.

The Record of Needs

There are two stages involved in issuing Record of Needs:

1 Sending a draft of the proposed Record of Needs to the parents. They may respond or comment in writing within fourteen days of the issue.

2 The finalized record which is then signed and which becomes legally binding.

According to Circular No 4/96 (1996), 'the education authority needs to give very careful attention to the wording of the Record of Needs and to any preparatory drafts so as to ensure that their meaning is precise and clear and "the language used in the Record needs to be clear, concise and jargon free"'.

Contents of the Record of Needs

The Record of Needs should include the following ten specific parts:

Part I – details of the child or young person, information about the transfer, discontinuance or preservation of the Record

Part II – details of the parents and Named Person

Part IIIA – a general description of the child's strengths and weaknesses; an assessment profile

Part IIIB – a statement of the causes of the child's special education needs

Part IV – a description of the child's special education needs

Part V – a statement of how the education authority proposes to meet the child's needs

Part VI – details of the school nominated for the child to attend

Part VII – a summary of the parents' views or child's views

Part VIII – a summary of reviews of the Record

Part IX – information about disclosure, that is, who has been allowed to see it.

Formal appeals process

If, after an assessment, parents are unhappy with the provisions made in the Record of Needs, they may appeal to the local Appeals Committee on the following grounds:

- the statement describing the child's learning difficulties
- the description of the child's special education needs
- the school named.

The Appeals Committee can make decisions about the school. If parents are dissatisfied with this they can appeal to the Sheriff nominated against the Appeals Committee's decision. Other questions or disagreements must be referred to the Secretary of State. His decision is final and is based on the advice of his medical and educational advisers.

Appealing against the Local Authority's choice of school

According to Circular No 4/96 (1996), 'recent legislation has changed the law where educational authorities reject a placing request on the grounds that they could make provision at a lower cost at one of their own schools. Now authorities must give the appeal committee a satisfactory reason if they refuse to place your child in an independent or grant-aided special school. Moreover, they must accept your request unless it can be shown that it is not reasonable to grant it, having regard to the extra benefit which is likely to result from the school placement proposed by you compared with the extra cost'. It also notes that 'the Self-Governing Schools, etc. (Scotland) Act 1989 made it possible for parents in Scotland of children with Record of Needs to make placing requests for their child to attend a special school suited to their particular special education needs anywhere in the United Kingdom.'

Provision for children with SEN in Northern Ireland

The provisions contained in the Education and Libraries (Northern Ireland) Order 1986 mirror the arrangements in the Education Act 1981 for England and Wales.

The Education (Northern Ireland) Order 1996, with effect from September 1997, makes provisions similar to those in the Education Act 1993/1996 and likewise includes a Code of Practice on the Identification and Assessment of Special Educational Needs. It also establishes a Special Education Tribunal to determine appeals by parents and Education and Library Boards.

Summary and conclusions

1   There is now official acceptance that there are children who have special educational needs, many of whom are dyslexic. There is a large volume of legislation to cater for children with these needs.

2   Great improvements have been made in the early indentification and assessment by schools of children with SEN as a result of the *Code of Practice*. Many SENCOs, however, feel that they have not been given sufficient training or resources to carry out their task effectively.

3   The *Code of Practice* is a huge step forward. It presents an ideal and an example of best practice. It is a valuable source of information and advice for all who are involved with identifying, assessing and making provision for children with SEN. However, some critics claim that it is unrealistic and that it does not address fully all the main issues.

4   There is a myopic approach by the government as to the size, extent and variation in the needs of children with SEN. 2.6 per cent of pupils are Statemented. The rump of the 4–10 per cent with dyslexia are not always recognized nor are their special educational needs fully provided for.

5   Much remains to be done to ensure that *all* dyslexic children receive teaching appropriate to their needs and ability, not just the children with severe learning difficulties whose problems are obvious to the majority of parents and educationalists.

6   The *Code of Practice* encourages a partnership between parents, schools and LEAs and urges that the school-based stages should therefore utilize parents' own distinctive knowledge and skills and contribute to parents' own understanding of how best to help their child. It encourages parents to become involved and better informed about their child's education. Parents still have to battle with teachers, schools and LEAs to obtain the help they know their child needs. Friel (1995) said that 'even after the long period of time since the implementation of the Education Act 1981, through a form of omission, many children with severe special educational needs have not been the subject of a Statement'.

7   The *Code of Practice* puts huge demands on individual classroom teachers, tutors and the SENCO. The *Code of Practice* makes little mention of how they are to be trained. It presumes that SENCOs are specialists in diagnosing a multiplicity of learning difficulties which can range across the whole spectrum of special needs, from the deaf child, to the partially sighted child, to the dyslexic child. The report of the SEN Tribunal Select Committee on Education in 1996 highlighted this and said of SENCOs: 'Many of them do not have sufficient time to undertake their duties effectively ... and there is evidence that they receive inadequate support from school management ... and there is evidence that LEA learning support services have been reduced in recent years and that SENCOs are now receiving less support from them.'

8 More parents are appealing to the SEN Tribunal if they are not happy with the treatment that their child is receiving. Surrey County Council in 1996 said that there should be an 'enquiry into the issue, to help remove the principal cause of rancour between parents and LEAs'. The BDA (1996a) said that '40 per cent of all appeals heard by the Tribunal concern dyslexic children. This reflects both the high prevalence of dyslexia (at least 10 per cent of the population) and parents' concern that their children's needs are not being met'.

9 The question of finance and funding has not been fully addressed. LEAs are under pressure from the Audit Commission to keep within a tight budget and limit the number of Statements issued. A central issue in the services provided is the question of who is to pay.

10 The BDA has launched a campaign to try to instigate changes in initial teacher training courses so that in future teachers will be taught how to identify and teach dyslexic children. It is also seeking to improve inservice training for existing teachers because 'parents want their dyslexic child to be taught by a teacher who has gained additional qualifications to teach dyslexic children' (BDA, 1996a).

11 Scotland has legislation which caters for the needs of children and young persons with special educational needs. These are identified by way of assessment, after which the education authority may decide to issue a Record of Needs which 'facilitates the identification of the learning difficulties of a child or young person, so that long term educational strategies can be developed especially for him or her. It also enables progress and requirements to be monitored and reviewed in a structured way throughout the entirety of a pupil's school career' (Circular 4/96, 1996).

12 Provision in Northern Ireland for children with SEN, provided for under the Education and Libraries (Northern Ireland) Order 1986 and the Education (Northern Ireland) Order 1996 is similar to that in England and Wales.

Chapter 14

The eyes

- their significance and importance in the dyslexia debate
- visual factors: eye movements, reference eye, coloured lenses

Introduction

It is not surprising, when a child is having difficulty with reading, that his parents' or teachers' first response is often to question whether he might have something wrong with his eyes. For many children this is a sensible supposition and the prudent parent should always have the child's eyes tested by an optometrist. In cases where there is a positive family history of learning difficulties it is important that the eye care professional has some knowledge of dyslexia. 'Unfortunately there are no specific qualifications that eye care practitioners can take to indicate specialist expertise in the assessment of people with specific learning difficulties' (Evans, 1996a) but the College of Optometrists has introduced a module on dyslexia as part of the training and education of their students. For a long time researchers have been studying the possibility that visual factors might be a cause of reading difficulties and they have remained a leading suspect as a cause of delay or retardation in learning to read.

Are the eyes themselves responsible for reading difficulties?

In 1887 Adolf Kussmaul coined the term 'word-blindness' which he used to describe a stroke patient who had normal sight but could not recognize written words. Other physicians, the most notable of these being James Hinshelwood, a Glasgow University surgeon and ophthalmologist, began to investigate the working of the eyes in his quest for solutions to the baffling problems of the intelligent children who failed to learn to read. He concluded that 'the study of the cases of acquired word-blindness is necessary to the proper understanding of congenital word-blindness' (1912). Orton and his researchers contributed to the debate with their neurological and psychiatric investigations from the late 1920s onwards.

Orton had studied the work of Hinshelwood and, as a result, recognized his first case of congenital word-blindness in 1925, reporting that the patient's 'visual perception was normal'. Geschwind (1982) observed that 'it is intriguing to consider how often this important observation, which we now all know to be true in the majority of cases of dyslexia, has been forgotten and then rediscovered'. By 1937 Orton had concluded that 'there is nothing wrong with the vision of these children but we feel the demonstrable fact that their difficulty lies in recalling previous exposures of the word rather than seeing it' (Orton, 1937).

Orton (1946) found that many of the children he saw were cross-lateralized, for example they had a dominant right hand but a dominant left eye. He coined the word 'strephosymbolia' (which literally means crossed symbols) to describe these people and to explain their difficulties with reading. He noted, among other things, the frequency with which they tended to reverse letters in words. Ocular dominance relates to what is generally regarded as necessary for good vision: the brain receives signals from one, dominant eye rather than confused information from two eyes.

It is not uncommon to hear a diagnostician say 'this child is cross-lateralized' and offer this as an explanation for the child's difficulties. However, Newman (1989) studied 323 children and found that 'those children who failed to show a dominant eye when assessed by the Dunlop test (see page 336) were just as likely to be good readers as poor ones'.

Are there sub-types of dyslexia?

Scientists realized that dyslexia seemed to take different forms. Johnson and Myklebust (1967) described 'visual' dyslexia and 'auditory' dyslexia. Boder (1971) argued that there were three different types of dyslexia:

1 dysphonetic dyslexia – which she used to describe the reader who could recognize whole words and who consequently had a small sight vocabulary

2 dyseidectic dyslexia – which she used to describe the reader who had to decode words letter by letter each time he sees them

3 dysphonetic-dyseidectic dyslexia – which she used to describe the reader who had difficulties with both whole words and letter-by-letter decoding.

Dysphonetic dyslexia became known colloquially as 'visual dyslexia' and dyseidectic dyslexia as 'auditory dyslexia'. It was acknowledged that some readers had a combination of both.

Determining the cause of the reading disability is vital. According to Aaron (1993), 'the issue whether developmental dyslexia is a homogenous entity or consists of two major sub-types is not a trivial one because the two sub-types may call for drastically different remedial approaches'.

Why visual defects were often considered a cause of reading disability

Stanovich (1985) said that 'the hypothesis that a deficit in a basic visual process is a critical cause of reading failure has garnered enormous attention in the learning disabilities and dyslexia literatures'. One of the reasons for this is that the symptoms described by or observed in dyslexic children and adults often suggest visual defects, such as 'blurred print, moving print, diplopia (double vision), losing place [on the line], omitting words and a resultant fatigue and aversion to reading' (Stanley, 1994). This list has a familiar ring to it for many practitioners and diagnosticians in the dyslexia field. Not surprisingly, these observations have sparked further investigations in the past twenty years, but, according to Stanovich (1985) 'this attention has not, however, been accompanied by a commensurate amount of solid empirical evidence'.

An examination of the evidence for a visual dyslexia

Aaron (1993) pointed out that there are two major issues to be considered when examining the evidence for a visual dyslexia:

1 definitions of dyslexia

2 the methodology for identifying dyslexia.

He argued that sensory deficits such as 'myopia' or 'scotopic sensitivity' are not usually given as causes of dyslexia, and he concluded that 'by definition, therefore, reading problems caused by sensory defects cannot be included in the category of dyslexia'. Furthermore he asserted that it is a well-established fact that dyslexics are 'slow and erratic readers' but that they also have problems with 'output' of words, that is, spelling. He said that 'sensory processes cannot satisfactorily account for [this]'.

Aaron (1993) examined the type of spelling errors made by older dyslexic pupils and 'found that younger poor readers produced phonologically unacceptable spelling errors, whereas older poor readers produced more phonologically acceptable errors than unacceptable ones'. He concluded that spelling involves more than just remembering visual patterns of letters because the pupil will also use his knowledge of sounds and meanings of the word to help him spell.

The search for a quick and easy solution

The media is always ready to look for ready-made answers and to champion anyone who offers these. Reports on eye research findings have made the main news on radio and television in the UK on a number of occasions and have had sensational coverage at times, such as 'Experts hail cure for child dyslexia' (Brace, 1993). Finding a physical (visual) cause for dyslexia is an attractive proposition since the implication is that a remedy can then be designed to 'cure' it easily.

Research into visual causes of dyslexia

There have been three main areas of research involving visual factors: eye movements, the reference eye, and coloured lenses.

Eye movements

Work has gone on for many years into the way in which skilled and disabled readers move their eyes across the page when they read. 'There have been a number of reports that the little jumps, or saccades, that the eyes make as they scan a line of text are more erratic in reading disabled individuals than in normal readers' (Newman, 1989). These movements are mostly in a left-to-right direction, moving from right to left at the end of a line. Zangwill and Blakemore (1972) found that disabled readers moved their eyes more slowly across the page as they scanned lines of print and that they were more prone to making regressions. They called this 'an irresponsible tendency to move the eyes in a right-to-left direction'. Generally speaking, with more difficult reading material or with less expert readers, the number and duration of fixations (stops to inspect the word) is increased, resulting in slower reading and an increased number of regressions. Evans (1993) concluded that 'treatment regimens based on training eye movements [tracking exercises] are generally unlikely to be effective' because people think that eyes move slowly across the page when reading, and do exercises to improve this. Poor tracking could also be explained by lack of concentration (Evans, 1996b). A key issue is whether these atypical eye movements are, as has been suggested, the result of the poor reading skills or whether they are underlying causes of poor reading.

Observation of a dyslexic's reading suggest that speed and accuracy in reading a text is dependent on the reading ability of the person, the difficulty of the text and the size of the print.

Pavlidis (1981) continued to research this area. He claimed that dyslexic readers showed abnormal eye movements and that the presence of these could be used to diagnose dyslexia in young children.

The hypothesis that dyslexics have atypical eye movements was promulgated in some circles as a cause of the reading difficulties of dyslexics, and it was suggested that if it could be treated it would be a remedy for dyslexia. This research was not successfully replicated, despite many attempts to do so both in the UK and the USA, and has now been discredited. If dyslexia were caused by defective eye movements, which could probably be treated, then how does one account for the continuing spelling and writing problems experienced by dyslexics? Miles and Miles (1990) made an interesting observation and said that the 'consequence of treating erratic eye movements as the central criterion for dyslexia is that if the eye movements ceased to be erratic one would have to say that person was no longer dyslexic'. 'Eye movements are not the cause of dyslexia,' according to Rayner (1983), but 'rather, eye movements reflect an underlying cognitive or neurological problem'. Evans and Drasdo (1990) agreed and said 'indeed most researchers have found that in simple sequential tasks, dyslexic children's eye movements are not significantly different to those of controls'.

Research workers have continued to investigate this subject and Fischer and Biscaldi (1994) devised a test, dubbed the 'Freiburg Test' by Linnman (1995), which tests different eye movements. They claim that the test can determine whether or not the subject is dyslexic.

Binocular vision: The reference eye

Binocular vision describes the ability of the two eyes to work together in a co-ordinated way.

Ocular dominance has played an important role in the research into the possible visual causes of dyslexia. This has included work on a 'stable reference eye' (the dominant eye), for example the eye that would be used to look through a telescope. But Evans (1996a) pointed out that there are 'at least three different types of ocular dominance [for] sighting, motor and sensory'.

335

Much of the UK research into the significance of the reference eye was undertaken by Stein and Fowler at the Royal Berkshire Hospital in Reading. They hypothesized that children failed to learn to read normally because they lacked adequate control of the movements of the two eyes working together. Their work included the use of the Dunlop Test which had been developed in 1973 in Australia by researchers whose work suggested that it was possible to change the child's dominant eye and thus improve laterality. Stein and Fowler (1985) found that 68 per cent of dyslexic children had 'an unstable reference eye'. Riddell, Fowler and Stein (1988) suggested that 'poor vergence control interferes with the process of learning to read by disturbing the ability to determine the position of letters in words. This makes it difficult for the child to remember what the word looks like, and so impairs visual memory skill'. Their research findings were published in *The Lancet* and were taken up by the media. They caused great interest and as a result many children were referred by their GPs to the Royal Berkshire Hospital for treatment over a long period of time. The children with an unstable reference eye were prescribed a pair of glasses which had one eye occluded. In the early days this often consisted of sticking elastoplast over one lens. Later, glasses with a frosted lens were issued. Some children were also prescribed eye exercises which were to be carried out on a daily basis at home. Hopes were raised and the expectation was that once the eye problem was sorted out, the child's literacy problems would be solved. The media was largely responsible for the euphoria.

In the intervening years the Dunlop Test has been criticized on many grounds. The format of the test requires the child to respond orally to questions that have a heavy reliance on directionality and 'a language-disabled child may make inappropriate responses because of his inability to name the direction of movement correctly' (Wilsher and Taylor, 1986). If this is so, it must undermine the usefulness and reliability of the test results. Evans (1996b) reported that 'there is fairly wide agreement that the Dunlop Test is unreliable'.

Among those who have reviewed Stein and Fowler's work is Bishop (1989). She criticized it because she found that 'there was no evidence that monocular occlusion in children with an unfixed reference eye results in improved reading scores' and by 1989 Stein himself had reached the conclusion 'that visual confusion is not usually the sole cause of their problem' so 'alleviating their ocularmotor instability does not "cure" dyslexia' (Stein, 1990).

Coloured lenses or filters

Coloured lenses, filters or overlays have repeatedly been hailed in the press as the answer to the dyslexic's problems. *The Sunday Times* (1985) proclaimed 'Glasses Hope for Dyslexia' and by June 1993 the momentum of the lobby supporting these claims resulted in an article entitled 'Experts Hail Cure for Child Dyslexia' (Brace, 1993). In January 1995 the *Daily Mail* proclaimed 'Tinted Lenses Unravel Riddle of Dyslexia' (Hawking, 1995).

Interest in this field can be traced back to the realization that the use of coloured paper versus white paper had implications for some people with reading problems. One of the earliest mentioned cases in the literature was when Jansky (1958) reported on a girl who could read words on coloured cards, but was unable to read from white cards. In 1980 Meares broke new ground when she described children who found that the white gaps between the words on the page and the white spaces between the lines of the text caused problems, such as the words blurring and jumping around. She reported that these problems were alleviated if smaller print or coloured paper was used.

Scotopic Sensitivity Syndrome

Many of these features were echoed in 1983 by a psychologist called Helen Irlen when she presented a paper to the 91st Annual Convention of the American Psychological Association in California. Irlen claimed to have discovered a new syndrome that affected people with learning disorders and which she dubbed the 'Scotopic Sensitivity Syndrome'. It is now often referred to as the Irlen Syndrome although Evans (1996a) argued that 'this term is probably etymologically inappropriate and "Meares-Irlen Syndrome" may be a suitable alternative'. Meares was the first to report the features of the condition in scientific journals and therefore, in Evans' opinion, her name should be acknowledged.

Chief features of the Scotopic Sensitivity Syndrome

- **Light sensitivity (photophopia)**
  Sensitivity to bright light, especially fluorescent lighting, and glare, such as that from glossy white paper. This may make reading uncomfortable and as a result the letters and shapes may become distorted.

- **Visual resolution**
  Difficulty seeing print clearly, especially black print on a white background, because 'the white gaps between the words and lines mask the print' (Evans, 1996). This causes the words to blur, and the letters may move or jump about on the page.

- **Sustained focus**
  An inability to see groups of letters or words clearly at the same time because the eyes water, itch or burn as a result of reading. Blinking and straining may cause eye strain.

- **Sustained attention**
  A difficulty in maintaining concentration when reading. Blinking and straining may cause eye strain.

Irlen's Syndrome is regarded as being present when subjects report a 'sustained benefit from using coloured filters when reading' (Evans et al, 1995).

Claims were made by Irlen (1983) that 'between 50 per cent to 75 per cent of learning-disabled people suffer from this syndrome'. Irlen prescribes coloured lenses to treat the problem. The Irlen Institute reported on a survey of 155 people who had worn the lenses in Australia for twelve months and '43 per cent had less eye strain, 37 per cent less tendency to skip lines and 35 per cent improved concentration'. It claimed that 'the symptoms of eye strain and fatigue have been totally eliminated [by wearers of their lenses]' and that children can read better. Centres have been established and assessments offered worldwide. Part of the attraction is that the person needing the treatment can be tested and prescribed lenses designed to make reading easier and more comfortable. This is appealing to dyslexic people and their parents.

Irlen (1994) offered the following hints for the parents of children who appear to have problems with their eyes:

- Change the lighting – some lighting may be better than others.
- Use coloured paper – pink, blue or green for photocopies, not yellow or red.

Criticisms of the Irlen Syndrome
There is little published research to substantiate the claims of the Irlen Institute, and Miles (1993) said 'that some of the investigations into the effectiveness of tinted lenses have been poorly controlled'. Irlen's methods and claims have been criticized for the following reasons:

- There are many possible explanations for the symptoms Irlen describes. For example, there are over 40 different potential causes for discomfort around the eyes.
- There have been few double-blind placebo-controlled trials (when two groups of subjects are tested, one group being given the treatment and the other a placebo. Neither tester nor subject know who is actually receiving the treatment).

- Many of the reports of success have come from wearers of the lenses themselves. Many authorities attribute this to the Hawthorne Effect, that is, improvement is made because the subject expects improvement rather than because there actually is improvement. Evans (1993) opined that 'if children are given a pair of grey lenses to compare with a pair of tinted lenses, it would not be surprising if they preferred the coloured lenses'.

- Rosner and Rosner (1987) reviewed the majority of the published studies on tinted lenses and criticized the extremely unsatisfactory experimental designs in use.

- Much of the evidence of success does not come from an unbiased scientific investigation. Doubts have also been cast on the objectivity of a Medical Research Council study in 1989 by Neary and Wilkins (1991). They ran various trials on twenty wearers of the Irlen lenses. The twenty subjects had been selected by the Irlen Institute for inclusion in the trials because they found their lenses beneficial. The results lack objectivity not least because the subjects had paid over £200 for their glasses. 'Using subjects selected according to the Irlen profile does not provide compelling scientific support for the Irlen therapy', according to Stanley (1994). Cotton and Evans (1990) conducted scientific tests that did meet the rigorous standards of design to enable clear conclusions to be drawn and concluded that 'the effect of the lenses may be both motivational and attributional', that is, interest in and expectation of improvement and a physical solution which can be bought by wearing the coloured glasses.

- Hedderly (1981) conducted research on 200 pupils at a Dyslexia Institute in Yorkshire. He questioned the pupils about 'whether they found that words jumped about on the page' which Irlen claimed happens and professed to be able to cure. Only 3 per cent of the pupils reported that they had experienced this.

Intuitive Colorimeter

The optometry profession has become increasingly aware of the public's interest in coloured overlays and glasses and in the Irlen Syndrome. Wilkins, with funding from the Medical Research Council, invented the Intuitive Colorimeter. This can measure children's responses to colour filters and enabled further research by Wilkins et al (1994) on the efficiency of the coloured filter therapy. The Intuitive colorimeter is a piece of apparatus that allows children to view texts that are illuminated by coloured light. The child or examiner can adjust the hue or saturation (depth of colour) of the light that falls on the texts to be read. Coloured lenses can then be prescribed based on the results. The research was conducted initially on 68 children (42 boys and 26 girls), of whom

15 did not finish and 16 failed to complete the tests. The results of the study showed that some children experienced a reduction in the symptoms of visual discomfort, such as headaches and eyestrain, on the days when they wore their glasses with the prescribed lenses.

Response to the issue of coloured overlays and tinted lenses

The College of Optometrists was concerned about the risk of over prescription of lenses because 'the whole procedure is very subjective and, in the final analysis, amounts to asking the patient whether they can see better with the tinted lenses than without' (Evans, 1994b). It offered a simple, inexpensive alternative and suggested that children should be given coloured overlays (sheets of see-through coloured plastic to place over the text being read) for about a month. To check which overlay to use takes about five minutes and overlays are inexpensive to buy. If these prove effective the coloured lenses may then be prescribed.

Some opticians who use the Intuitive Colorimeter state in their literature that 'approximately one in two people who are "dyslexic" have found that specially coloured spectacle lenses independent of any optical correction or eye exercises can help them considerably to read more fluently and easily'. This claim is completely unfounded and unsubstantiated, either by clinical experience or by scientific research. Evans (1994a), a lecturer at the Institute of Optometry, considered that 'tinted lenses are unlikely to change a dyslexic child into a good reader but they may reduce asthenopia [sore, tired eyes, headaches] and hence encourage the child to try to read'. Coloured lenses may ameliorate the visual discomfort of a dyslexic child but they cannot teach him to read or spell.

Summary and conclusions

1   There continues to be debate and argument over the significance of the eyes when attempts are made to find the cause and a cure for dyslexia. As long ago as 1958 Tinker concluded that 'erratic eye movements are the result, not the cause, of reading difficulties' and his conclusions have been supported by many subsequent experiments.

2   Investigations continue into possible visual problems that may be associated with dyslexia. But much of the research has been discredited and 'does not provide compelling scientific support' (Stanley, 1994). Many dyslexic people have visual problems, but many people who are not dyslexic also have visual problems. The most prevalent disorder experienced by dyslexics is a lack of co-ordination between the two eyes. This may lead to eye strain

and discourage children from reading, but should not be said to account for an inability to read.

3   Miles (1993), when speaking of coloured lenses, said that in his opinion 'it is unethical for optometrists not to point out to parents the controversial nature of the treatment being offered'. This advice is in stark contrast to the claims that 'thousands of dyslexic children could be cured by simply wearing tinted lenses' (Brace, 1993). Pennington (1989) argued that 'clearly some treatments for dyslexia are targeted at symptoms that are only artificially related to the disorder. Effective treatments must address the underlying causes of dyslexia'. In his opinion, 'the primary symptom in dyslexia is a deficit in the phonological coding of written language'.

4   Evans and Drasdo (1991) surveyed most of the literature on tinted lenses and related therapies (108 papers were listed by them in their references) and concluded that 'at present there is no conclusive proof from vigorous scientific studies that tinted lenses can help poor reading performance'. A major criticism of the many studies has been the (small) size of the samples and, according to Pumfrey and Reason (1991), 'small group studies can produce positive (or negative) results by chance'.

5   On the other hand there have been reports from people who find coloured lenses helpful. Parents and teachers can conduct their own experiments by going to a stationer and buying coloured overlay sheets. They can experiment and find out if a blue or yellow or pink sheet helps the child to read with greater ease and fluency. This costs pence rather than pounds.

6   Wilkins (1996) conceded that 'the physiological basis for the beneficial effects of colour remains uncertain and contentious'. Researchers such as Vellutino (1979) concluded that 'disordered language processing, and not a visual deficit, is the main cause of reading disability'. Pennington and Stanovich agree that 'the predominant view to date is that dyslexia is associated with phonological difficulties originating within spoken language processes' (Snowling, 1987) and not with visual difficulties.

Chapter 15

Towards a better understanding . . .

Introduction

Much has been written about the gifted or the inspired teachers who recognized and nurtured the talents of a struggling pupil. Unfortunately there are also many reports from pupils for whom most of their education has been a source of embarrassment, bewilderment, confusion and pain. Evidence of resentment of their school days is found in eight teenage boys interviewed by Edwards (1994). The interviews chronicle the anger, frustration and embitterment of these boys, whose case histories show an educational system that has failed them. This 'fly on the wall' reporting documents institutions where pupils suffered violence, humiliation and neglect because of wholesale obliviousness of their needs and difficulties.

Bryant (1978) reiterated that 'it is a matter of common experience that repeated failure, especially in the face of great effort to learn and to do well, is one of the most destructive and devastating experiences a child can have'. The words of an individual pupil summed this up when he wrote:

> *In my primary school none of my teachers 'believed' in dyslexia. These were the people I was looking up to for encouragement and support, yet they openly implied that I was stupid. Do you wonder that I am angry?*

Source: Brown P. (1994) 'Halfway up the mountain'. *Times Educational Supplement*, 14 October.

This seventeen-year-old pupil's words reflect the emotional turmoil and traumas that many dyslexic pupils have endured during their school days. The educational system has clearly failed pupils such as these by not identifying their special educational needs.

There is more and more evidence to show that millions of people have problems with basic literacy and numeracy and that this seriously affects their lives, their personal relationships and their employment prospects.

Children today stand a better chance of being assessed and having their learning difficulties identified. The plight of young adults, including students, is gaining more attention and colleges and universities are making vigorous attempts to identify these people, despite a lack of adequate or appropriate diagnostic tools (either manual or technological) and a paucity of specialist knowledge among their teaching staff. Employers are becoming more alert and anxious to do something about the enigmatic employee who is good at many aspects of his job but who is often let down by inexplicable lapses, such as an inability to write coherent reports or follow instructions in a manual. Organizations such as the CBI have focused the attention of employers on their responsibilities under the new legislation in the Disability Discrimination Act 1995 which, among other things, gives disabled people new rights in the area of employment.

Dyslexia and the needs of dyslexic people are no longer the concerns of the minority. It has become a national issue. November 7th, 1996 marked the centenary of the first reported case of congenital word-blindness by Dr Pringle Morgan. Parliament enacted legislation as long ago as 1970 to deal with the problem. Further legislation culminated in the Special Educational Needs *Code of Practice* (1994) which opens the door and shows the way forward for all who strive to meet the needs of children with special educational needs.

The teacher's key role in management

Morgan (1983) reminded us that 'the person most directly involved with implementing any curriculum enabling students to learn – the key person – is the classroom teacher'. The *Code of Practice* (1994) imposes huge demands and responsibilities on classroom teachers and school governors, stating that all children with special educational needs should be identified and assessed. It also states that 'the child's class teacher or form/year tutor has overall responsibility'. Strauss (1978) made an emotional plea that 'dyslexia is real and it can be dealt with, and the most important thing a person with dyslexia can have is the understanding of the people around him'. Moreover, 'as teachers we have a legal responsibility to teach all children, but more important, we have a moral responsibility to teach all children' (Steingard and 'Gail', 1975). Dyslexic pupils 'learn when they have teachers who know how to teach them' (Bryant, 1978). The teaching profession is becoming increasingly aware of this and has responded positively to the statutory demands made upon it. In the Director of the BDA's view it is 'axiomatic that teachers with designated responsibilities for SEN should possess, or be working towards, the acquisition of recognized competencies and qualifications in special needs education' (Cann, 1996).

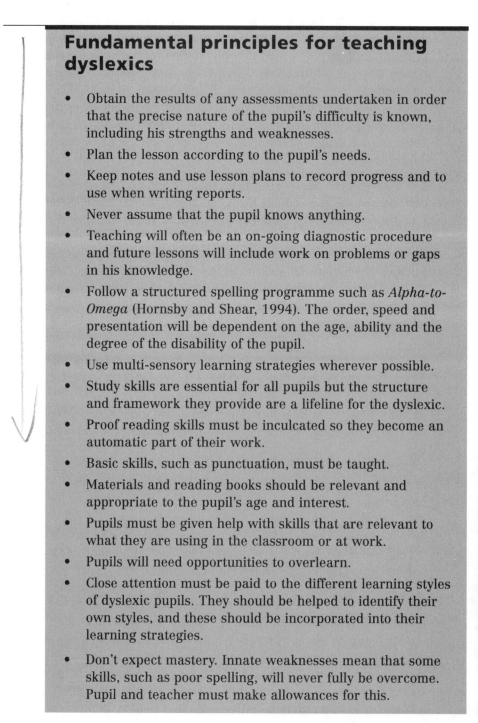

Fundamental principles for teaching dyslexics

- Obtain the results of any assessments undertaken in order that the precise nature of the pupil's difficulty is known, including his strengths and weaknesses.
- Plan the lesson according to the pupil's needs.
- Keep notes and use lesson plans to record progress and to use when writing reports.
- Never assume that the pupil knows anything.
- Teaching will often be an on-going diagnostic procedure and future lessons will include work on problems or gaps in his knowledge.
- Follow a structured spelling programme such as *Alpha-to-Omega* (Hornsby and Shear, 1994). The order, speed and presentation will be dependent on the age, ability and the degree of the disability of the pupil.
- Use multi-sensory learning strategies wherever possible.
- Study skills are essential for all pupils but the structure and framework they provide are a lifeline for the dyslexic.
- Proof reading skills must be inculcated so they become an automatic part of their work.
- Basic skills, such as punctuation, must be taught.
- Materials and reading books should be relevant and appropriate to the pupil's age and interest.
- Pupils must be given help with skills that are relevant to what they are using in the classroom or at work.
- Pupils will need opportunities to overlearn.
- Close attention must be paid to the different learning styles of dyslexic pupils. They should be helped to identify their own styles, and these should be incorporated into their learning strategies.
- Don't expect mastery. Innate weaknesses mean that some skills, such as poor spelling, will never fully be overcome. Pupil and teacher must make allowances for this.

- Encourage the pupil to make use of information technology where appropriate, particularly word processing.

- Practise skills wherever possible. Ignore failures and encourage the pupil to set standards for himself.

Evidence of success

Perceptive teachers and parents have known for some time that there are dyslexic people who have outstanding skills, sometimes artistic, creative, spatial or musical, but who have struggled with literacy. Geschwind (1982) pointed this out when he observed that 'it has become increasingly clear in recent years that dyslexics themselves are frequently endowed with high talents in many areas' and he went on to say that 'there have been in recent years an increasing number of studies that have pointed out that many dyslexics have superior talents in certain areas of non-verbal skills, such as art, architecture, engineering and athletics'.

The successes of well-taught dyslexic pupils set an example for the present generation of pupils. Many pupils have overcome their dyslexia sufficiently to succeed academically and/or to pursue successful careers in a wide variety of disciplines. There are successful engineers, plumbers, dental technicians ... Others have overcome their dyslexia sufficiently to take up places to study at Oxford or Cambridge universities.

Dyslexia and the gifted pupil

Dyslexia is no respector of age, intellectual ability or class. It is therefore not surprising that some dyslexics are very bright. A National Association for Gifted Children (NAGC) survey (1981) noted 'that very few of the parents interviewed considered their child to be gifted. They preferred to use such terms as "very able", "able" or "above average" to describe their child, the latter term being the most common'.

Definition of 'giftedness'

The US Federal Government in 1978 defined giftedness as follows:

Children, and where applicable, youth, who are identified at the pre-school, elementary, or secondary level as possessing demonstrative or potential abilities that give evidence of high performance capability in areas such as intellectual, creative, or in the performing and visual arts, and who by reason thereof require services or activities not ordinarily provided by school.

Source: Marland S. (1971) *Education of the Gifted and Talented (Marland Report).* US Office of Education, Department of Health, Education and Welfare, Washington DC.

Researchers in the USA have produced evidence that there are 'two different kinds of giftedness – schoolhouse giftedness and creative-productiveness giftedness. This distinction is essential in understanding students who can be learning-disabled and gifted at the same time' (Baum, Owen and Dixon, 1991).

According to Bryant (1978), 'some are gifted in intelligence, many are gifted in other ways – in abstract mathematical thinking, in music, in art and architecture, some are even gifted in the use of the spoken word – in verbal expression'. These talents are often not recognized while the pupil is at school, even though recognition of superior skill or talent is essential to bolster the low morale of the pupil who is struggling academically. Fortunately nowadays there is more understanding and value attached by society to those who have creative skills, some of whom are gifted but learning disabled.

Dyslexia successfully managed

The successes and achievements of many dyslexics prove that difficulties with literacy need not prevent anyone finding fame and fortune in many walks of life. According to West (1992), 'dyslexics often showed heightened abilities in performing, acting, or in lively speech, full of voice modulation, hand gestures, and animated facial expression, all abilities thought to be largely controlled by the right hemisphere [of the brain]'.

Susan Hampshire made her struggles public in the early 1970s, and she continues to campaign and crusade for fellow dyslexics. Many adults empathize with her when she recounts personal experiences such as when 'I ruined a dinner party because I left food in the oven for three to four hours instead of three-quarters of an hour' (*Hello!*, 1994).

Cher, singer, dancer and film star, who was not diagnosed until she was 30 years old, recalled 'I couldn't keep up with everybody else at school'. Film star Tom Cruise says that he had a dreadful time at school. Whoopi Goldberg too is dyslexic.

The world of sport has a long list of talented and outstanding sportsmen who are dyslexic. Duncan Goodhew, Moscow Olympic Gold Medallist, is a tireless campaigner for the cause of dyslexia.

Greg Louganis, the American diver, won a handful of gold medals at the Los Angeles Olympics in the diving events. He is on record as saying that he turned to sport to prove to his school mates who taunted him with being 'dumb and retarded' that they were wrong (cited in Smith, 1987). Bruce Jenner, Olympic Decathlon Champion, made a stunning admission when he said that 'reading aloud in the classroom was much more frightening and harder for him than any decathlon' (cited in Smith, 1987). The British Olympic oarsman, Steve Redgrave, who has represented his country so successfully, is dyslexic.

The architect of the acclaimed Pompidou Centre in Paris and the Lloyds of London Building, Sir Richard Rogers, is proof that dyslexia need not be a bar to a successful career. The 'enfant terrible' and Three Starred Michelin Chef, Marco Pierre White, has shown that dyslexia and success can go together in the competitive world of catering and cooking.

History books provide further proof that difficulties with literacy and later success is not a recent phenomenon. Leonardo da Vinci clearly had difficulties, as can be seen from his writings and drawings. Several scholars observed that his spellings were 'bizarre' or 'inconsistent' and Leonardo da Vinci himself stated that 'you should prefer a good scientist without literary abilities than a literate [one] without scientific skills' (Sartori, 1987). Another scientist to add to the list is Albert Einstein, who was described by West (1991) 'as probably the best-known scientist of any country and in any field'. There have been many great scientists whose difficulties give rise to a retrospective diagnosis of dyslexia. The physicist Michael Faraday had 'early problems with speech and some notable deficiencies in spelling, punctuation and capitalization' (West, 1991). One may speculate on Faraday's motives for initiating the Royal Institution's Annual Christmas Lectures which continue a century and a half later to attract and inspire future scientists each year. Was it because he realized that there were aspiring scientists who needed the stimulation of seeing and hearing the leading figures in the field and not just reading about their work in textbooks?

The Rodin Remediation Academy, which sponsors international conferences on learning disabilities, was named after the father of the sculptor, Auguste Rodin, because of his encouragement of his dyslexic son. Hans Christian Andersen, who failed to learn to read and write despite the help of ten royal tutors at the Danish Royal Court, dictated his stories to a scribe. He said that even at the age of 66 he still woke up with nightmares about a school master trying to teach him to read (cited in Smith, 1987). Eileen Simpson drew our attention to the plight of others, such as the Nobel Literature Laureate and twentieth century poet, William Butler Yeats who recalled that a string of relatives were called in to help him, and 'my father was an angry and impatient teacher and flung the reading book at my head' when he failed to read and 'he had come to think that I had not all my faculties' (Simpson, 1979). She also reported that Agatha Christie, author of 68 novels and 17 plays, had revealed in her autobiography that 'writing and spelling were always terribly difficult for me' and 'I was still an extraordinarily bad speller and have remained so until the present day'. Virginia Woolf's editors complained of her poor spelling and the lack of punctuation in her work.

Brilliant mathematicians, including the Rev C. L. Dodgson (whose pen name was Lewis Carroll and who is better known as the author of *Alice in Wonderland*) was a lecturer in mathematics at Oxford, yet according to West (1991) 'he had great difficulty in remembering numbers'. The French Mathematician Henri Poincaré is another whose 'drawing was notoriously poor ... his handwriting was poor as well'.

The lives and careers of these successful people show that poor literacy, whether identified or acknowledged, is not to be confused with lack of ability and there are indications that 'many dyslexics carry remarkable talents that benefit their society enormously' (Geschwind, 1982).

Summary and conclusions

1   Many people experience psychological pain which endures for life because their learning difficulties were not recognized while they were at school.

2   Dyslexia is not a myth. Scientific research and anecdotal evidence from dyslexic children and adults, and from their parents and teachers confirm that it is a reality. Its symptoms are manifold and the difficulties labyrinthine for those who experience it.

3   There is a general consensus that the best management for dyslexics is in mainstream education where they can be withdrawn for one-to-one specialist tuition. A very small percentage of severely dyslexic pupils may need to attend special schools for dyslexics.

4   The informed classroom teacher can create a supportive and

constructive learning environment when she accepts and understands that dyslexic children have different learning styles and that they are more prone to errors and defects, such as poor spelling and short term memory problems. Teaching a dyslexic pupil requires skill, knowledge, patience, flexibility and the ability to listen. Sympathy and good intentions do not teach a dyslexic. Structured, systematic, cumulative multi-sensory teaching does. Theoretical knowledge needs to be supported by practical experience.

5   There is evidence that some pupils may be dyslexic yet gifted. West (1991) argued that 'when the gift is there, the disability should not be allowed to prevent its recognition or development, especially when those with the greatest gifts may also have some of the greatest difficulties'.

6   The success stories of dyslexic people with special talents or skills can been a source of inspiration and pride and often make excellent role models for the struggling pupil.

7   Scientists with the help of functional magnetic resonance imaging (f MRI) can now study brain function in a non-invasive way and without using radioisotopes. They can see on a scanner which part of the brain performs a particular task, for example, 'The identification of brain sites dedicated to phonological processing in reading ... The isolation of such a signature brings with it the future promise of more precise diagnosis of dyslexia' (Shaywitz, 1996).

8   Medical science, particularly genetics, is moving towards a better understanding of the biological bases of dyslexia and is entering a new era with the new millennium. It will surely soon provide the educationalists with new evidence about the causes of this enigmatic condition which has been the subject of much debate. This can then lead to better detection and management of dyslexia worldwide.

Chapter 1

BDA (1979) 'Dyslexia: The child and the teacher'. *Cambridge Conference Proceedings 1974*. BDA, Reading

Booth T. and Goodey C. (1996) 'Playing for the sympathy vote'. *The Guardian*, 21 May

British Medical Association (1980) 'Dyslexia is not a medical problem'. *British Medical Association News Review*, January: 70

Code of Practice (1994) *Code of Practice on the Identification and Assessment of Special Educational Needs*. Department for Education and Employment, Central Office of Information, London

Crabtree T. (1975) Letter to *The Guardian*, 30 December

Crisfield J. (ed) (1996) *The Dyslexia Handbook*. BDA, Reading

Critchley M. (1966) *Developmental Dyslexia*. Heinemann, London

Critchley M. (1970) *The Dyslexic Child*. Heinemann, London

Critchley M. (1981) 'Dyslexia - an overview'. In Pavlidis G. Th. and Miles T. R. (eds) *Dyslexia Research and its Applications to Education*. John Wiley and Sons Ltd, Chichester

Critchley M. (1996) Personal communication

European Dyslexia Association (1994) Pamphlet. EDA, Brussels

Geschwind N. (1982) 'Why Orton was right'. *Annals of Dyslexia*, 32: 13–30, Orton Dyslexia Society, Baltimore MD

Gillingham A. and Stillman B. (1956) *Remedial Training for Children with Specific Language Disability in Reading, Spelling, and Penmanship* (1st edition). Educators Publishing Service Inc., Cambridge MA

Hammill D. D. (1990) 'On Defining Learning Disabilities: An Emerging Consensus'. *Journal of Learning Disabilities*, 23: 74–84

Hickey K. (1997) *Dyslexia: A Language Training Course for Teachers and Learners*. Private publication

Hinshelwood J. (1895) 'Word-blindness and visual memory'. *The Lancet*, 21 December: 1564–70

Hinshelwood J. (1912) 'The treatment of word-blindness acquired and congenital'. *British Medical Journal* 2: 1033–5

Hinshelwood J. (1917) *Congenital Word-blindness*. H. K. Lewis, London

Hornsby B. and Shear F. (1975) *Alpha-to-Omega*. Heinemann, Oxford

Kerr J. (1897) 'School hygiene, in its mental, moral and physical aspects'. Howard Medical Prize, *Journal of the Royal Statistical Society*, 60: 613–680

Kussmaul A. (1877) 'Disturbances of Speech'. In von Ziemssen H. (ed) and McCreery J. A. (trans) *Cyclopedia of the Practice of Medicine*. 14. Wood Wm. and Co, New York

M^{C}Nair-Scott A. (1991) *An Account of the Events and Achievements during the 25 Years since the Foundation of the First Dyslexia Association*. BDA, Reading

Masland R. (1989) 'Neurological aspects of dyslexia'. In Hales G., Hales M., Miles T. R. and Summerfield A. (eds) *Meeting Points in Dyslexia*: *Proceedings of the First International Conference of the British Dyslexia Association*. BDA, Reading: 20–8

Miles T. R. (1974) *The Dyslexic Child*. Priory Press Ltd, Hove

Miles T. R. (1991) 'On determining the prevalence of dyslexia'. In Snowling M. J. and Thomson M. (eds) *Dyslexia: Integrating Theory and Practice*. Whurr Publishers Ltd, London: 144–53

Miles T. R. (1993) *The Pattern of Difficulties* (2nd edition). Whurr Publishers Ltd, London.

Miles T. R. and Miles E. (1990) *Dyslexia: A Hundred Years On.* Open University Press, Milton Keynes

Naidoo S. (1972) *Specific Dyslexia.* Pitman Publishing, London

Naidoo S. (1979) 'Dyslexia: The child and the teacher'. *Cambridge Conference Proceedings 1974.* BDA, Reading: 4–6

Newton M. (1996) Personal communication

Newton M. and Thomson M. (1976) *The Aston Index: A Screening Procedure for written Language Dificulties.* Learning Development Aids, Wisbech

Orton J. L. (1963) 'The Orton story'. *Bulletin of Orton Society,* 13: 1–8

Orton J. L. (1966) 'The Orton–Gillingham approach'. In Money J. (ed) *The Disabled Reader: Education of the Dyslexic Child.* The Johns Hopkins Press, Baltimore: 119–45

Orton S. T. (1928) 'Specific reading disability – Strephosymbolia'. *Journal of the American Medical Association,* 90: 1095–9

Orton S. T. (1937) *Reading, Writing and Speech Problems in Children.* Norton, New York

Pennington B. F. (1989) 'Using genetics to understand dyslexia'. *Annals of Dyslexia,* 39: 81–93

Pringle Morgan W. (1896) 'A case of congenital word-blindness'. *British Medical Journal,* 7 November: 13–18

Pumfrey P. (1994) 'The management of specific learning difficulties (dyslexia): Challenges and Responses'. Unpublished paper. *Towards a Wider Understanding. Third International Conference of the British Dyslexia Association, Manchester*

Pumfrey P. and Reason R. (1991) *Specific Learning Difficulties (Dyslexia). Challenges and Responses.* Routledge, London

Rawson M. B. (1986) 'The many faces of dyslexia'. *Annals of Dyslexia,* 36: 179–91

Reid Lyon G. (1995) 'Toward a definition of dyslexia'. *Annals of Dyslexia,* 45: 3–27

Snowling M. J. (1987) *Dyslexia: A Cognitive Developmental Perspective.* Blackwell, Oxford

Thomson M. (1990) *Developmental Dyslexia: Studies in Disorders of Communication* (3rd edition). Whurr Publishers Ltd, London

Tomkins C. (1963) 'The last skill acquired'. *New York Times,* 13 September

US Office of Education (1977) *The Education for All Handicapped Children Act (Public Law 94–142)*

Vail P. (1990) 'Gifts, talents and the dyslexic: Wellsprings, springboards, and finding Foley's Rocks'. *Annals of Dyslexia,* 40: 13–17

Waites L. (1968) 'Dyslexia International World Federation of Neurology. Report of Research Group on Developmental Dyslexia and World Illiteracy'. *Bulletin of the Orton Society,* 18: 21–2

White Franklin A. (1979) Dyslexia: The child and the teacher. *Cambridge Conference Proceedings 1974.* BDA, Reading: 9–12

Willis T (1672) *De Anima Brutorum.* Apud Joannem Blaeu, Amsterdam

Chapter 2

Augur J. (1985) 'Guidelines for teachers, parents and learners'. In Snowling M. J. (ed) *Children's Written Language Difficulties: Assessment and Management,* NFER – Nelson, Windsor: 147–69

Badian N. A. (1988) 'The prediction of good and poor reading before kindergarten entry: A nine year follow-up'. *Journal of Learning Disabilities*, 21: 98–123

Badian N. A. (1995) 'Predicting reading ability over the long term: The changing roles of letter naming, phonological awareness and orthographic processing'. *Annals of Dyslexia*, 45: 79–96

Bradley L. (1989) 'Specific Learning Disability prediction – intervention – progress'. Paper presented to the *Rodin Remediation Academy International Conference on Dyslexia, University College of North Wales, Bangor. September*

Bradley L. and Bryant P. E. (1983) 'Categorising sounds and learning to read – A causal connection'. *Nature*, 301: 419–21

Brady S., Fowler A., Stone B. and Winburg N. (1994) 'Training phonological awareness: A study with inner-city Kindergarten children'. *Annals of Dyslexia,* 44: 26–59

Bryant P. E. (1985) 'The question of prevention'. In Snowling M. J. (ed) *Children's Written Language Difficulties: Assessment and Management*. NFER – Nelson, Windsor: 43–56

Cann P. (1996) 'Walking the corridors of power'. *Dyslexia Contact*, 15 (1)

Carlisle J. (1994) Personal communication

Carlisle J. (1995) Personal communication

Catts H. W. (1989) 'Defining dyslexia as a developmental language disorder'. *Annals of Dyslexia,* 39: 50–64

Chasty H. (1996) Review of 'Dyslexia: An avoidable national tragedy'. *Channel 4 documentary*. Hopeline Videos, London

Code of Practice (1994) *Code of Practice on the Identification and Assessment of Special Educational Needs*. Department for Education and Employment, Central Office of Information, London

De Fries J. C. (1991) 'Genetics and dyslexia: An overview'. In Snowling M. J. and Thomson M. (eds) *Dyslexia: Integrating Theory and Practice*. Whurr Publishers Ltd, London: 3–20

Duane D. D. (1991) 'Neurobiological issues in dyslexia'. In Snowling M. J. and Thomson M. (eds) *Dyslexia: Integrating Theory and Practice*. Whurr Publishers Ltd, London: 21–30

Ellis A. W. (1993) *Reading, Writing and Dyslexia: A Cognitive Analysis* (2nd edition). Lawrence Erlbaum Associates Ltd, Hove

Fawcett A. (1994) 'A wobble now means less work later'. *The Independent*, 26 April

Finucci J. M. and Childs B. (1976) 'Dyslexia: Family studies'. In Ludlow C. L. and Cooper J. A. (eds) *Genetic Aspects of Speech and Language Disorders*. Academic Press, London

Finucci J. M., Guthrie J. T., Childs A. L., Abbey H. and Childs B. (1976) 'The genetics of specific reading disability'. *Annals of Human Genetics,* 40: 1–23

Galaburda A. M., Sherman G. F. and Rosen G. D. (1989) 'The neural origin of developmental dyslexia: Implications for medicine, neurology and cognition'. In Galaburda A. M. (ed) *From Reading to Neurons*. Educators Publishing Service Inc., Cambridge MA: 337–88

Gardner P. (1994) 'Diagnosing dyslexia in the classroom: A three stage model. In Hales G. (ed) *Dyslexia Matters*. Whurr Publishers Ltd, London

Geschwind N. (1982) 'Why Orton was right'. *Annals of Dyslexia*, 32: 13–30

Hallgren B. (1950) 'Specific dyslexia ('congenital word-blindness'): A clinical genetic study'. *Acta Psychiatrica et Neurologica Scandinavica*, Supplement 65: 1–287

Hamilton-Fairley D. (1976) *Speech Therapy and the Dyslexic*. The Helen Arkell Dyslexia Centre, London

Hinshelwood J. (1917) *Congenital Word-blindness*. H. K. Lewis, London

Hiscock M. and Kinsbourne M. (1995) 'Progress in the measurement of laterality and implications for dyslexia researchers'. *Annals of Dyslexia*, 45: 249–68

Hornsby B. (1993) 'Early identification and remediation'. *Dyslexia Contact*, 12 (2): 12–15

Hutchins J. (1996) 'Computer Corner'. *The Bulletin, BDA Newsletter*, May

Lenneberg N. A. (1967) *Biological Foundations of Language*. John Wiley and Sons Inc., New York

Lubs H. A., Rabin M., Feldman E., Jallad B. J., Kusch A. and Gross-Glenn K. (1993) 'Familial dyslexia: Genetic and medical findings in eleven three generation families'. *Annals of Dyslexia*, 43: 44–60

Miles T. R. (1974) *The Dyslexic Child*. Priory Press Ltd, Hove

Miles T. R. (1993) *Dyslexia: The Pattern of Difficulties* (2nd edition). Whurr Publishers Ltd, London

Miles T. R. and Miles E. (1984) *Teaching Needs of Seven Year Old Dyslexic Pupils*. Department for Education and Science, London

Miles T. R. and Miles E. (1990) *Dyslexia: A Hundred Years On*. Open University Press, Milton Keynes

Nicolson R. I. and Fawcett A. J. (1994) 'Dyslexia and skill: Theoretical studies'. In Hales G. (ed) *Dyslexia Matters*. Whurr Publishers Ltd, London

Nicolson R. I. and Fawcett A. J. (1995) 'Balance, phonological skill and

dyslexia: Towards the Dyslexia Early Screening Test'. *Dyslexia Review,* 7 (1): 8–11

Pennington B. F. (1989) 'Using genetics to understand dyslexia'. *Annals of Dyslexia*, 39: 81–93

Reid G. (1990) 'Specific Learning Difficulties: Attitudes towards assessment and teaching'. Fife Region Psychological Service. In Hales G., Hales M., Miles T. R. and Summerfield A. (eds) *Meeting Points in Dyslexia: Proceedings of the First International Conference of the British Dyslexia Association*. BDA, Reading

Richardson S. O. (1989) 'Specific developmental dyslexia: Retrospective and prospective views'. *Annals of Dyslexia*, 39: 3–24

Rudel R. G. (1985) 'The definition of dyslexia: Language and motor deficits'. In Duffy F. H. and Geschwind N. (eds) *Dyslexia: A Neuroscientific Approach to Clinical Evaluation*. Little Brown, Boston

Singleton C., Thomas K. and Leedale R. (undated*) Final report on the Humberside Early Screening Research Project*. Dyslexia Computer Resource Centre, University of Hull

Smith S. (1992) 'Origins, patterns and prognoses – Familial patterns of learning disabilities'. *Annals of Dyslexia,* 42: 143–58

Smith S. D. Kimberling W. J., Pennington B. F. and Lubs H. A. (1983) 'Specific reading disability: Identification of an inherited form through linkage analysis'. *Science*, 219: 1345–7

Snowling M. J. (1987) *Dyslexia: A Cognitive Developmental Perspective*. Blackwell, Oxford

Squire R. (1996) 'Vouchers – Exploding the Myth'. *Nursery World*, 11 April: 26

Vogler G. P., De Fries J. C. and Decker S. N. (1985) 'Family history as an indicator of risk for reading disability'. *Journal of Learning Disabilities*, 18: 419–21

Warnock M. (1993) Foreword to *Opening the Door*. BDA, Reading

White Franklin A. (1979) 'Dyslexia: The child and the teacher'. *Cambridge Conference Proceedings 1974*. BDA, Reading: 9–12

Wolff P. H., Michel G. F. and Ovrut M. (1990) 'Rate and timing precision of motor co-ordination in developmental dyslexia'. *Developmental Psychology*, 26: 349–59

Chapter 3

Bishop D. and Adams C. (1990) 'A prospective study of the relationship between specific language impairment, phonological disorders and reading retardation'. *Journal of Child Psychology and Psychiatry*, 30: 1027–50

Blacock, J. (1982) 'Persistent auditory language deficits in adults with learning disabilities'. *Journal of Learning Disabilities*, 15: 604–9

Bloom L. (1980) 'Language development, language disorders and learning disabilities : L D'. *Bulletin of the Orton Society*, 30: 115–33

Borwick C. and Townend J. (1993) *Developing Spoken Language Skills*. The Dyslexia Institute, Staines

Bradley L. and Bryant P. E. (1983) 'Categorising sounds and learning to read – A causal connection'. *Nature*, 301: 419–21

Bullock A. (1975) *A Language for Life*. HMSO, London

Bush C. S. (1979) *Language Remediation and Expansion. 100 Skill-building Reference Lists*. Communication Skill Builders Inc., Tucson AR

Calfee R. (1983) 'The mind of the dyslexic'. *Annals of Dyslexia*, 33: 9–28

Catts H. W. (1989) 'Defining dyslexia as a developmental language disorder'. *Annals of Dyslexia*, 39: 50–64

Chasty H. (1985) 'What is dyslexia?'. In Snowling M. J. (ed) *Children's Written Language Difficulties: Assessment and Management*. NFER – Nelson, Windsor: 11–27

Chinn S. and Ashcroft R. (1993) *Mathematics for Dyslexics: A Teaching Handbook*. Whurr Publishers Ltd, London

Cox A. (1982) Personal communication

Croall J. (1995) 'A code without a key'. *The Guardian*, 28 March

Danwitz M. W. (1975) 'Early speech and language problems'. *Bulletin of the Orton Society*, 25: 86–90

Denckla M. B. and Rudel R. G. (1976) 'Rapid automatized naming (RAN): Dyslexia differentiated from other learning disabilities'. *Neuropyschologia*, 4: 471–9

Duane D. D. (1991) 'Neurological issues in dyslexia'. In Snowling M. J. and Thomson M. (eds) *Dyslexia: Integrating Theory and Practice*. Whurr Publishers Ltd, London: 21–30

Freud S. (1891) *On Aphasia*. International Universities Press, New York (1953). Original work published in Germany

Gauntlett D. (1978) 'In another's shoes: A case study of a mature dyslexic'. *Dyslexia Review*, 2: 23–7

Geschwind N. (1982) 'Why Orton was right'. *Annals of Dyslexia*, 32: 13–30

Goswami U. (1991) 'Recent work on reading and spelling development'. In Snowling M. J. and Thomson M. (eds) *Dyslexia: Integrating Theory and Practice*. Whurr Publishers Ltd, London: 108–21

Haarhoff T. (1920) *Schools of Gaul*. Oxford University Press, London

Hamilton-Fairley D. (1976) *Speech*

Therapy and the Dyslexic. The Helen Arkell Dyslexia Centre, London

Heisler A. B. (1983) 'Psychological issues in learning disabilities'. *Annals of Dyslexia*, 33: 303–10

Hornsby B. (1988) *Overcoming Dyslexia: A Straightforward Guide for Families and Teacher.* Macdonald Optima, London

Hornsby B. (1989) *Before Alpha: Learning Games for the Under Fives.* Souvenir Press Ltd, London

Liberman I. and Shankweiler D. (1985) 'Phonology and the problems of learning to read and write'. *Remedial and Special Education,* 6: 8–17

Lundberg I., Frost J. and Petersen O–P. (1988) 'Effects of an extensive program for stimulating phonological awareness in pre-school children'. *Reading Research Quarterly*, 33: 263–84

Masland R. (1990) 'Neurological aspects of dyslexia'. In Hales G., Hales M., Miles T. R. and Summerfield B. (eds) *Meeting Points in Dyslexia: Proceedings of the First International Conference of the British Dyslexia Association.* BDA, Reading: 20–8

Miles T. R. (1974) *Understanding Dyslexia.* Hodder and Stoughton, Sevenoaks

Miles T. R. (1983) *The Bangor Dyslexia Test.* Learning Development Aids, Wisbech

Miles T. R. and Miles E. (eds) (1992) *Dyslexia and Mathematics.* Routledge, London

National Curriculum (1995) Department for Education and Employment. HMSO, London

Pennington B. F. (1990) 'Annotation: The genetics of dyslexia'. *Journal of Child Psychiatry,* 31: 193–201

Rome P. D. and Osman J. S. (1985) *Language Toolkit.* Educators Publishing Service, Cambridge MA

Phelps G. T. and Phelps T. D. (1982) In Snowling M. J. (ed) *Children's Written Language Difficulties.* NFER – Nelson, Windsor: 59–79

Royal College of Speech and Language Therapists (1996) 'Special Educational Needs: The working of the Code of Practice and the Tribunal'. *Education Committee Second Report.* HMSO, London

Sawyer J. and Butler K. (1991) 'Early language intervention: A deterrent to reading disability'. *Annals of Dyslexia,* 41: 55–79

Sheffield B. S. (1991) 'The structured flexibility of Orton–Gillingham'. *Annals of Dyslexia,* 41: 41–54

Snowling M. J. (1987) *Dyslexia: A Cognitive Developmental Perspective.* Blackwell, Oxford

Snowling M., Stackhouse J. and Rack J. (1986) Phonological dyslexia and dysgraphia: Developmental analysis'. *Cognitive Neuropsychology,* 3: 309–39

Sparks R. L. and Ganschow L. (1993) 'The effect of multi-sensory structured language instruction on native language and foreign language aptitude skills of at-risk high school foreign language learners: A replication and follow-up study'. *Annals of Dyslexia*, 43: 194–237

Stackhouse J. (1985) 'Segmentation, speech and spelling difficulties'. In Snowling M. J. (ed) *Children's Written Language Difficulties: Assessment and Management.* NFER – Nelson, Windsor: 96–115

Thomas C. J. (1905) 'Congenital "Word-blindness" and its treatment'. *Ophthalmoscope*, 3: 380–5

Treiman R. (1985) 'Onsets and rimes as units of spoken syllables: Evidence from children'. *Journal of Experimental Child Psychology*, 39: 255–82

US Office of Education (1977) 'Definition and criterion for defining students as learning disabled'. **Federal**

Register 42: 250 p. 65083. US Government Printing Office, Washington DC

Vellutino F. R. (1979) *Dyslexia Theory and Research*. The MIT Press, Cambridge MA

Chapter 4 _____

Aaron P. G., Kuchta S. and Grapenthin C. T. (1988) 'Is there a thing called dyslexia?'. *Annals of Dyslexia*, 38: 33–49

Anderson R. C., Hiebert E. H., Scott J. A. and Wilkinson I. A. (1985) *'Becoming a NATION of Readers'. The Report of the Commission on Reading*. US Department of Education

Augur J. (1985) 'Guidelines for teachers, parents and learners'. In Snowling M. J. (ed) *Children's Written Language Difficulties: Assessment and Management*. NFER – Nelson, Windsor: 147–69

Augur J. and Briggs S. (eds) (1992) *The Hickey Multi-sensory Language Course*. Whurr Publishers Ltd, London

Bannatyne A. D. (1971) *Language, Reading and Learning Disabilities*. Thomas, Springfield IL

BDA (1996) *Education Committee Second Report. 'Special Educational Needs: The Working of the Code of Practice and the Tribunal'*. HMSO, London

Bloomfield L., Barnhart C. L. and Barnhart R. K. (1964) *Let's Read*. Educators Publishing Service Inc., Cambridge MA

Bramley W. (1996) *Units of Sound*. The Dyslexia Institute, Staines

Brand V. (1993) *Spelling Made Easy* (2nd edition). Egon Press Publishers Ltd, Royston

Bullock A. (1975) *A Language for Life*. HMSO, London

Carless S. and Hearn B. (1990) 'Parental involvement with reading'. In Pinsens P. (ed) *Children with Literacy Difficulties*. David Fulton Publishers, London: 15–28

Chall J. S. (1987) 'Reading development in adults'. *Annals of Dyslexia*, 37: 240–63

Chasty H. (1981) 'Explanation of terms and processes'. *Dyslexia Review Supplement. Parent's Handbook*. Dyslexia Institute, Staines: 7–8

Clay M. (1991) *Becoming Literate. The Construction of Inner Control*. Heinemann Education, Oxford

Code of Practice (1994) *Code of Practice on the Identification and Assessment of Special Educational Needs*. Department for Education and Employment, Central Office of Information, London

Cooke A. (1993a) *Tackling Dyslexia: The Bangor Way*. Whurr Publishers Ltd, London

Cooke A. (1993b) 'Partnership in Learning'. *Dyslexia Sentence*. Conference of the British Dyslexia Association, London

Crombie M. (1994) 'Assessing dyslexia'. *Special Children*, September: 13–17

Douglas J. W., Ross J. M. and Simpson M. R. (1968*) All Our Future. National Survey in Health and Development*. Davies, London

Doyle J. (1996) *Dyslexia: An Introductory Guide*. Whurr Publishers Ltd, London

Elliot C. D. (1996) *The British Ability Scales: Second Edition (BAS II)*. NFER – Nelson, Windsor

Ellis A. W. (1993) *Reading, Writing and Dyslexia: A Cognitive Analysis* (2nd edition). Lawrence Erlbaum Associates Ltd, Hove

Fielding L., Wilson P. and Anderson M. (1986) 'A new focus on free reading: The role of trade books in reading instruction'. In Raphael T. and Reynolds R. (eds) *Contents of Literacy*

Frith U. (1985) 'Beneath the surface of developmental dyslexia'. In Patterson K. E., Marshall J. C. and Coltheart M. (eds) *Surface Dyslexia in Adults*. Routledge and Kegan Paul, London

Gillingham A. (1956) *Phonetic Word Cards (Jewel Case). Remedial Training for Children with Specific Disability in Reading, Spelling and Penmanship*. Educators Publishing Service Inc., Cambridge MA

Glynn T. and McNaughton S. (1985) 'The Mangere home and school remedial reading procedure: Continuing research on their effectiveness'. *New Zealand Journal of Psychology*, 14: 66–77

Gough P. and Tunmer W. (1986) 'Decoding, reading and reading disability'. *Remedial and Special Education,* 7: 6–10

Greenwood J. A. (1983) 'Adapting a college preparatory curriculum for dyslexic adolescents: The Rationale'. *Annals of Dyslexia*, 33: 235–42

Hagley F. (1987) *Suffolk Reading Scale*. NFER – Nelson, Windsor

Hewison J. and Tizard J. (1980) 'Parental involvement and reading attainment'. *British Journal of Educational Psychology*, 50: 209–15

Hickey K. (1977) *Dyslexia: A Language Training Course for Teachers and Learners*. Private publication

Hinshelwood J. (1912) 'The treatment of word-blindness acquired and congenital'. *British Medical Journal* 2: 1033–5

Hinson M. and Gains C. (1993) *The NASEN A–Z. A Graded List of Reading Books*. NASEN Enterprises Ltd, Staffordshire

Hornsby B. (1994) Personal communication

Hornsby B. and Pool J. (1990/1991/1992) *Alpha-to-Omega Activity Packs.*

Stages 1, 2 and 3. Heinemann Education, Oxford

Hornsby B. and Shear F. (1994) *Alpha-to-Omega* (4th edition). Heinemann Education, Oxford

Kline C. L. and Kline C. L. (1975) 'Follow-up study of 216 dyslexic children'. *Bulletin of the Orton Society* 25: 127–44

Makar B. W. (1976) *Primary Phonics*. Educators Publishing Service Inc., Cambridge MA

Miles E. (1993) *The Bangor Dyslexia Teaching System* (2nd edition). Whurr Publishers Ltd, London

Morgan R. (1983) *Helping Children Read*. Methuen Children's Books, London

Muter V. (1994) 'Influence of phonological awareness and letter knowledge on beginning reading and spelling development'. In Hulme C. and Snowling M. (eds) *Reading Development and Dyslexia*. Whurr Publishers Ltd, London: 45–62

Neale M. D. (1988) (British adaptation Christophers U. and Whetton C.) *Neale Analysis of Reading Ability. Revised British Edition*. NFER – Nelson, Windsor

NFER – Nelson (1990) *NFER – Nelson Group Reading Test. The Macmillan Test Unit*. NFER – Nelson, Windsor

Norrie E. *Edith Norrie Magnetic Letter Case* (1994). Helen Arkell Dyslexia Centre, Farnham

Peer L. (1996) 'Reading difficulty'. (Fogg Index). *The Bulletin, BDA Newsletter,* May

Plowden Report (1967) *Children and Their Primary Schools*. HMSO, London

Pring L. and Snowling M. (1986) 'Developmental changes in word recognition: An information processing account'. *Journal of Experimental Psychology*, 38A: 395–418

Pumfrey P. D. and Reason R. (1991) *Specific Learning Difficulties (Dyslexia). Challenges and Responses.* Routledge, London

Raven J. C. (1988) *Raven's Progressive Matrices and Vocabulary Scales: 1979 British Standardization and Revision (1988).* NFER – Nelson, Windsor

Rawson M. B. (1968) *Developmental Language Disability.* Johns Hopkins University Press, Baltimore

Reid G. (ed) (1993) *Specific Learning Difficulties (Dyslexia). Perspectives on Practice.* Moray House Publications, Edinburgh

Richardson S. O. (1990) 'Specific developmental dyslexia: A language learning disability'. In Hales G., Hales M., Miles T. R. and Summerfield A. (eds) *Meeting Points in Dyslexia: Proceedings of the First International Conference of the British Dyslexia Association.* BDA, Reading: 2–10

Rutter M., Tizard J. and Whitmore K. (eds) (1970) *Health, Education and Behaviour.* Longmans, London

Schonell F. J. (1961) 'Schonell Graded Word Reading Test'. In *The Psychology and Teaching of Reading.* Oliver and Boyd, Edinburgh

Sheffield B. (1991) 'The structured flexibility of Orton–Gillingham'. *Annals of Dyslexia*, 41: 41–54

Simpson G. B., Lorsback T. C. and Whitehouse D. C. (1983) 'Encoding and contextual components of word recognition in good and poor readers'. *Journal of Experimental Child Psychology*, 35: 161–71

Singleton C. (1995) 'Dyslexia in higher education'. *Dyslexia Contact,* 14 (2): 7–9

Smith F. (1973) *Psycholinguistics and Reading.* Holt, Rinehart and Winston, New York

Snowling M. (1987) *Dyslexia: A Cognitive Developmental Perspective.* Blackwell, Oxford

Stanovich K. E. (1985) 'Explaining the variance in reading ability in terms of psychological processes: What have we learned?' Paper presented to the New York Branch of the Orton Dyslexia Society

Stanovich K. E. (1988) 'The right and wrong places to look for the cognitive locus of reading disability'. *Annals of Dyslexia*, 38: 154–77

Stanovich K. E. (1991) 'The theoretical and practical consequences of discrepancy definitions of dyslexia'. In Snowling M. and Thomson M. (eds) *Dyslexia: Integrating Theory and Practice.* Whurr Publishers Ltd, London: 125–43

Terman L. M. and Merrill M. A. (1960) *Stanford-Binet Intelligence Scale.* Harrap, London

The Independent (1993) Kerper T. 'Stand your ground Mr Patten: Tony Kerpel argues that teachers views matter less than those of "education consumers"' *The Independent* 7 May

Thomson M. (1984) *Developmental Dyslexia.* Edward Arnold, Leeds

Thomson M. (1990) *Developmental Dyslexia: Studies in Disorders of Communication* (3rd edition). Whurr Publishers Ltd, London

Thomson M. E. and Watkins E. J. (1990) *Dyslexia: A Teaching Handbook.* Whurr Publishers Ltd, London

Tizard J., Schofield W. N. and Hewison J. (1982) 'Collaboration between teachers and parents in assisting children's reading'. *British Journal of Educational Psychology*, 52: 1–15

Townend J. (1994) *Understanding Dyslexia: A Teacher's Perspective.* The Dyslexia Institute, Staines

Turner M. (1993) 'Testing times'. *Special Children.* April: 12–16

Vincent D. and de la Mare M. (1990) *New Macmillan Reading Analysis.* NFER – Nelson, Windsor

Wechsler D. (1990) *Wechsler Pre-school and Primary Scale of Intelligence – Revised UK Edition (WPPSI-R^{UK})*.

Wechsler D. (1992) *Wechsler Intelligence Scale for Children – Third UK Edition (WISC-III^{UK})*. The Psychological Corporation Ltd, London

Wilkinson G. S. (1993) *Wide Range Achievement Test (WRAT 3)*. Wide Range Inc. Delaware

Young D. (1992) *Cloze Reading Tests*. Hodder and Stoughton, London

Chapter 5

Alston J. (1989) *Writing Left-handed*, Dextral Books, Manchester

Alston J. and Taylor J. (1987) *Handwriting: Theory, Research and Practice*. Routledge, London

Augur J. and Briggs S. (eds) (1992) *The Hickey Multi-sensory Language Course*. Whurr Pulishers Ltd, London

Bannatyne A. (1968) 'Diagnosis and remedial techniques for use with dyslexic children'. *Academic Therapy*, 3 (4): 213–24

Beery K. E. (1982) *Revised Administration, Scoring, and Teaching Manual for the Developmental Test of Visual-Motor Integration*. Modern Curriculum Press, Cleveland, Toronto

Bentley D. and Stainthorpe R. (1993) 'The needs of the left-handed child in the infant classroom. Writing is not always right'. *Reading*, 27 (2): 4–8

Bramley W. (1996) *Units of Sound: Teachers' Notes*. The Dyslexia Institute, Staines. Note: all quotes herewith are from the 1984 edition.

Brown R. (1992) *Ginn Handwriting: Motor Skills and Letter Formation*. Ginn and Co., Aylesbury

Bullock A. (1975) *A Language for Life*, HMSO, London

Burt C. (1937) *The Backward Child*. University of London Press, London

Chasty H. (1995) 'Obtaining a professional assessment of dyslexic students'. In *Lost for Words*. BBC Educational Developments, London: 18–20

Cox A. R. (1992) *Foundations for Literacy: Structures and Techniques for Multi-sensory Teaching of Basic Language Skills* (Revised edition. Note: all quotes herewith are from the 1980 edition.). Educators Publishing Service Inc., Cambridge MA

Critchley M. (1970) *The Dyslexic Child*. Heinemann, London

Cruickshank W. M., Bentzen F., Ratzeburt F. and Tamhouser M. (1961) *A Teaching Method for Brain-injured and Hyperactive Children*. Syracuse University Press, Syracuse NY

Enstrom E. E. (1962) *The Relative Efficiency of Various Approaches with the Left Handed*. The Peterson System Inc., Dallas

Faludy T. and Faludy A. (1996) *A Little Edge of Darkness*. Jessica Kingsley Publishers, London

Fellgett P. (1986) 'Living with dyslexia'. *Dyslexia Contact,* 5 (1)

Galaburda A. M. (1990) 'The Testosterone Hypothesis: Assessment since Geschwind and Behan 1982'. *Annals of Dyslexia*, 40: 18–38

Geschwind N. (1983) 'Biological associations of left-handedness'. *Annals of Dyslexia*, 33: 29–40

Geschwind N. and Behan P. O. (1982) 'Left-handedness: Association with immune disease, migraine, and developmental disorder'. *Proceedings of the National Academy of Sciences* (USA), 79: 5097–100

Haskell S., Barrett E. and Taylor H. (1977) *The Education of Motor and Neurologically Handicapped Children*. Croom Helm, Australia

Hickey K. (1977) *Dyslexia: A Language Training Course for Teachers and Learners*. Private Publication

Johnson S. (1984) 'The writing problem: Whatever became of Palmer'. *New York Times*, 8 January

Johnson W. T. (1976) *How to Teach Handwriting: The Johnson Handwriting Program*. Educators Publishing Service Inc., Cambridge MA

Kephart N. (1960) *The Slow Learner in the Classroom*. Merrill, Columbus OH

Luria A. R. (1973) *The Working Brain*. Penguin Books, London

Murray J. A. H., Bradley H., Cragie W. A. and Onions C. T. (eds) (1970) The Oxford English Dictionary. Oxford University Press, Oxford

National Curriculum (1995). Department for Education and Employment. HMSO, London

Paul D. (1990) *Living Left Handed*. Bloomsbury Publishing Co., London

Paul D. (1996) 'Left handers do not get equal help'. *Times Educational Supplement*. 17 May

Phelps J. and Stempel L. (1987) 'Handwriting: Evolution and evaluation'. *Annals of Dyslexia*, 37: 228–39

Richardson M. (1935) *Writing and Writing Patterns*. University of London Press, London

Sassoon R. (1983) *The Practical Guide to Children's Hand-writing*. Thames and Hudson, London

Smith S. L. (1979) *No Easy Answers: Teaching the Learning Disabled Child*. Winthrop Publishers, Cambridge MA

Strauss A. E. and Lehtinen L. (1947*) The Psychopathology and Education of the Brain-injured Child*. Grune and Stratton, New York

Taylor H. (1994) Personal communication

Thomson M. J. and Watkins B. (1990) *Dyslexia: A Teaching Handbook*. Whurr Publishers Ltd, London

Tyrer N. (1992) 'How to help the left-handed child. You and your family'. *Daily Mail*, 16 October

Waites L. (1982) Personal communication

Wise M. (1924) *On the Techniques of Manuscript Writing*. Scribner's Sons, New York.

Chapter 6

Aaron P. G. (1993) 'Is there a visual dyslexia?' *Annals of Dyslexia*, 43: 110–24

Augur J. and Briggs S. (eds) (1992) *The Hickey Multi-sensory Language Course*. Whurr Publishers Ltd, London

Bramley W. (1996) *Units of Sound*. The Dyslexia Institute, Staines

Brand V. (1992) *Spelling Made Easy. Books 0–3* (2nd edition) Egon Press Publishers Ltd, Royston

Bryant P. and Bradley L. (1985) *Children's Reading Problems*. Blackwell, Oxford

Calfee R. (1984) 'Applying cognitive psychology to education practice: The mind of the reading teacher'. *Annals of Dyslexia*, 34: 219–40

Cook L. (1981) 'Misspelling analyses in dyslexia: Observation of developmental strategy shifts'. *Bulletin of the Orton Society*, 31: 123–34

Cook M. and Cook Moats L. (1983) 'A comparison of the spelling errors of older dyslexic and second grade normal children'. *Annals of Dyslexia*, 33: 121–40

Cotterell G. C. (1970) 'The Fernald Auditory-Kinaesthetic technique of teaching reading and spelling'. In White Franklin A. and Naidoo S. (eds) *Assessment and Teaching of Dyslexic Children*. Invalid Children's Aid Association, London: 97–100

Cox A. R. and Hutcheson L. (1988) 'Syllable division: Prerequisite to dyslexics' literacy'. *Annals of Dyslexia*, 38: 226–42

Crystal D. (1987) *The Cambridge Encyclopaedia of Language*. Cambridge Reference, Cambridge

Denckla M. and Rudel R. (1976) 'Naming of pictured objects by dyslexic and other learning disabled children'. *Brain and Language*, 3: 1–15

Dyslexia Institute (1993) *The Dyslexia Institute Literacy Programme*. The Dyslexia Institute, Staines

Farrer M. (1993) 'Introduction to spelling rules'. In *Hornsby Correspondence Course Module 2* (3rd edition). Hornsby International Dyslexia Centre, London

Fernald G. M. (1943) *Remedial Techniques in the Basic Subjects*. McGraw Hill, New York

Frith U. (1985) 'Beneath the surface of developmental dyslexia'. In Marshall J. C., Patterson K. E. and Coltheart M. (eds) *Surface Dyslexia in Adults and Children*. Routledge and Kegan Paul, London

Gillingham A. and Stillman B.W. (1956) *Remedial Training for Children with Specific Disability in Reading, Spelling and Penmanship*. Educators Publishing Service Inc., Cambridge MA

Goodman K. S. (1969) 'Analysis of reading miscues: Applied psycholinguistics'. *Reading Research Quarterly*, 5: 9–30

Goswami U. (1991) 'Recent work on reading and spelling development'. In Snowling M. J. and Thomson M. (eds) *Dyslexia: Integrating Theory and Practice*. Whurr Publishers Ltd, London: 108–21

Hornsby B. and Miles T. R. (1980) 'The effects of a dyslexia-centred teaching programme'. *British Journal of Educational Psychology*, 50: 236–42

Hornsby B. and Pool J. (1990/1991/1992) *Alpha-to-Omega Activity Packs. Stages 1, 2 and 3*. Heinemann Educational, Oxford

Hornsby B. and Shear F. (1994) *Alpha-to-Omega* (4th edition). Heinemann Educational, Oxford

Kibel M. and Miles T. R. (1994) 'Phonological errors in the spelling of taught dyslexic children'. In Hulme C. and Snowling M. J. (eds) *Reading Development and Dyslexia*. Whurr Publishers Ltd, London: 105–27

Kline C. L. and Kline C. L. (1975) 'Follow-up study of 216 dyslexic children'. *Annals of Dyslexia*, 25: 127–45

Koontz A. (1994) 'Multi-sensory teaching.' Unpublished paper. *Towards a Wider Understanding. Third International Conference of the British Dyslexia Association, Manchester*

Miles E. (1993) *The Bangor Dyslexia Teaching System* (2nd edition). Whurr Publishers Ltd, London

Miles E. (1994) Personal communication

Miles T. R. (1993) *Dyslexia: The Pattern of Difficulties* (2nd edition). Whurr Publishers Ltd, London

Miles T. R. and Miles E. (1983) *Help for Dyslexic Children*. Methuen, London

National Curriculum (1995). Department for Education and Employment. HMSO, London

Peters M. (1967) *Spelling: Caught or Taught*. Routledge and Kegan Paul, London

Pollock J. (1980) *Signposts to Spelling*. Heinemann Educational, London

Pollock J. and Waller E. (1994) *Day-to-Day Dyslexia in the Classroom*. Routledge, London

Rak E. T. (1972) *Spellbound: Phonic Reading and Spelling*. Educators Publishing Service Inc., Cambridge MA

Russel U. (1993) 'Test reveals poor spelling standards'. *The Sunday Times*, 1 May

Schonell F. J. (1932) *Essentials in Teaching and Testing Spelling* (New edition 1969). Macmillan and Company Ltd, London

Schonell F. J. (1971) *Schonell Graded Word Spelling Test*. Oliver and Boyd, Edinburgh

Scragg D. G. (1974) *A History of English Spelling*. Manchester University Press, Manchester

Sheffield B. B. (1991) 'The structured flexibility of Orton–Gillingham'. *Annals of Dyslexia,* 41: 41–54

Sloboda J. A. (1980) 'Visual imagery and individual differences in spelling'. In Frith U. (ed) *Cognitive Processes in Spelling.* Academic Press, London

Snowling M. (1987) *Dyslexia: A Cognitive Developmental Perspective*. Blackwell, Oxford

Stanback M. L. (1992) 'Syllable and rime patterns for teaching reading: Analysis of a frequency-based vocabulary of 17,602 words'. *Annals of Dyslexia*, 42: 196–221

Steere A., Peck C. Z., Kahn L. (1971) *Solving Language Difficulties: Remedial Routines* (Revised edition). Educators Publishing Service Inc., Cambridge MA

Stirling E. (1990) 'The adolescent dyslexic: Strategies for spelling'. In Hales G., Hales M., Miles T. R. and Summerfield A. (eds) *Meeting Points in Dyslexia: Proceedings of the First International Conference of the British Dyslexia Association*. BDA, Reading: 153–60

Sykes J. B. (1982) *Concise Oxford Dictionary* (7th edition). Clarendon Press, Oxford

Thomson M. E. (1981) 'An analysis of spelling errors in dyslexic children'. *First Language*, 2: 141–50

Thomson M. (1990) *Developmental Dyslexia: Studies in Disorders of Communication* (3rd edition). Whurr Publishers Ltd, London

Thomson M. (1991) 'The teaching of spelling using techniques of Simultaneous Oral Spelling and Visual Inspection'. In Snowling M. and Thomson M. E. (eds) *Dyslexia: Integrating Theory and Practice.* Whurr Publishers Ltd, London

Thomson M. E. and Watkins E. J. (1990) *Dyslexia: A Teaching Handbook*. Whurr Publishers Ltd, London

Vellutino F. R. (1979) *Dyslexia: Theory and Research*. The MIT Press, Cambridge MA

Vernon P. E. (1983) *The Graded Word Spelling Test*. Hodder and Stoughton, Sevenoaks

Wilkinson G. S. (1993) *Wide Range Achievement Test 3 (WRAT–3)*. Wide Range Inc., Delaware

Wood E. (1982) *Exercise Your Spelling Workbooks I, II, III*. Hodder and Stoughton, London

Chapter 7

Barcham C., Bushell R., Lawson K. and McDonnell C. (1986) *The Staffordshire Mathematics Test*. NFER – Nelson Windsor

Bath J. B. and Knox D. E. (1984) 'Two styles of performing mathematics.' In Bath J. B., Chinn S. J. and Knox D. E. (Eds) *Dyslexia: Research and its Application to the Adolescent*. Better Books Ltd, Bath

BDA (1981) *Your Questions Answered*. BDA, Reading

Chinn S. J. (1992) 'Individual diagnosis and cognitive style'. In Miles T. R. and Miles E. *Dyslexia and Mathematics*. Routledge, London: 23–41

Chinn S. J. (1994) 'A dual study: Basic number facts, recall and compensatory strategies and comparative speed in simple numeracy work'. Paper presented to *Towards a Wider Understanding. Third International*

Conference of the British Dyslexia Association, Manchester

Chinn S. J. and Ashcroft J. R. (1993) *Mathematics for Dyslexics: A Teaching Handbook*. Whurr Publishers Ltd, London

Code of Practice (1994) *Code of Practice on the Identification and Assessment of Special Educational Needs*. Department for Education and Employment, Central Office of Information, London

Critchley M. (1970) *The Dyslexic Child*. Heinemann, London

Eade T. (1995) Personal communication

Fellgett P. (1986) 'Living with dyslexia'. *Dyslexia Contact*, 5 (1)

Gillham B. (1980) *Basic Number Diagnostic Test*. Hodder and Stoughton, Sevenoaks

Gillham B. and Hesse K. A. (1976) *Basic Number Screening Test*. Hodder and Stoughton, Sevenoaks

Henderson A. (1989) *Maths and Dyslexics*. St David's College, Llandudno

Joffe L. (1980) 'Dyslexia and attainment in school mathematics'. *Dyslexia Review*, 3 (1): 10–14 *and* 3 (2): 12–18

Joffe L. (1983) 'School mathematics and dyslexia: a matter of verbal labelling, generalizations, horses and carts'. *Cambridge Journal of Education,* 13 (3): 22–7

Kavanagh J. K. and Truss T. J. Eds (1988) *'Learning Disabilities'. Proceedings of the National Conference*. York Press, Parkton MD

Lever I. M. (1994) 'The assessment and diagnosis of children's mathematical understanding.' Unpublished paper *Towards a Wider Understanding. Third International Conference of the British Dyslexia Association, Manchester*

Miles E. (1992) 'Reading and writing in mathematics'. In Miles T. R. and Miles E. *Dyslexia and Mathematics*. Routledge, London

Miles T. R. (1974) *Understanding Dyslexia*. Hodder and Stoughton, Sevenoaks

Miles T. R. (1992) 'Some theoretical considerations'. In Miles T. R. and Miles E. (eds) *Dyslexia and Mathematics*. Routledge, London: 1–22

Miles T. R. and Miles E. (1983) *Help for Dyslexic Children*. Methuen, London

Miles T. R. and Miles E. (eds) (1992) *Dyslexia and Mathematics*. Routledge, London

Nash L.-J. (1996) Personal communication

O'Leary J. (1995) 'Crunching numbers'. *The Times*, 30 November

Pollock J. and Waller E. (1994) *Day-to-Day Dyslexia in the Classroom*, Routledge, London

Sharma M. (1989) *Mathematics Learning Personality. Math Notebook 7 (1, 2). 1–10*. Centre for Learning and Teaching Mathematics, Framingham MA

Steeves K. J. (1983) 'Memory as a factor in the computational efficiency of dyslexic children with high abstract reasoning ability'. *Annals of Dyslexia*, 33: 141–52

Street J (1976) 'Sequencing and directional confusion in arithmetic'. *Dyslexia Review,* 15 (Summer): 16–19

Vernon P. E. and Miller K. M. (1986) *Graded Arithmetic – Mathematics Test: Junior Form*. Hodder and Stoughton, London

Vernon P. E., Miller K. M. and Izard J. F. (1986) *Mathematics Competency Test,* Hodder and Stoughton, London

Waddon A. (1975) 'Problems of numeracy in dyslexia'. *Dyslexia Review*, 14: 11–14

West T. (1995) 'Skills for the future'. In Phillips M. (ed) *QED: Lost for Words*. BBC Educational Developments, London

Chapter 8 _____

BDA (1996) *National Dyslexia Survey in conjunction with the Professional Association of Teachers*. BDA, Reading

Buzan T. (1982) *Using your Head*. Ariel Books, BBC Publications, London

Charlton M. (undated) *Model Compositions for Certificate Forms*. James Brodie, Bath

Chinn S. (1994) 'Whole school provision for the whole child'. In Hales G. (ed) *Dyslexia Matters.* Whurr Publishers Ltd, London

Denckla M. (1982) 'Dealing with dyslexia'. *Newsweek*, 22 March

Devlin A. (1995) *Criminal Classes*. Waterside Press, Winchester

Dinklage K. (1971) 'Inability to learn a foreign language'. In Blaine G. and McArthur C. (eds) *Emotional Problems of the Student*. Appleton-Century-Crofts, New York

Edwards J. (1994) *The Scars of Dyslexia: Eight Case Studies in Emotional Reactions*. Cassell, London

Farrer M. (1990) 'Study skills: Background theory'. In *Hornsby Correspondence Course*. Hornsby International Dyslexia Centre, London

Gillingham E. (1994) Personal communication

Gilroy D. E. and Miles T. R. (1996) *Dyslexia at College* (2nd edition). Routledge, London

Glasser W. (1969) *Schools without Failure*. Harper Row, New York

Greenwood J. A. (1983) 'Adapting a college preparatory curriculum for dyslexic adolescents: The Rationale'. *Annals of Dyslexia*, 33: 235–42

Hamblin D. (1981) *Teaching Study Skills*. Blackwell, Oxford

Hamblin D. (1986) *Starting to Teach Study Skills*. Blackwell, Oxford

Joint Forum for the GCSE and GCE (1996) *Candidates with Special Assessment Needs: Special Arrangements and Special Consideration*. Manchester

Miles E. (1996) 'Languages and the dyslexic'. In Crisfield J. (ed) *The Dyslexia Handbook*. BDA, Reading: 46–54

Morris G. (1983) 'Adapting a college preparatory curriculum for dyslexic adolescents II: The focus. Confronting the problems of what to teach'. *Annals of Dyslexia*, 33: 243–50

Myklebust H. (1965) *Development and Disorders of Written Language*. Grune and Stratton, New York

Newton M. P. and Thomson M. (1976) 'Dyslexia: A guide to examinations'. *Dyslexia Review*, 16: 16–19

Nicolson R. and Fawcett A. (1995) 'Balance, phonological skill and dyslexia: Towards the dyslexia early screening test'. *Dyslexia Review*, 7 (1): 8–13

Northedge A. (1990) *The Good Study Guide*. Open University Press, Milton Keynes

Pauk W. (1974) *How to Study in College*, Houghton Mifflin Co., Boston

Scott P. (1986) *Countdown to GCSE English*. NFER – Nelson, Windsor

Scottish Examination Board (1996) *Scottish Certificate of Education and Certificate of Sixth Year Studies Examinations Arrangements for Candidates with Special Educational Needs*. Guidance for Centres for Examinations in and after 1996

Snowling M. J. (1985) *Children's Written Language Difficulties: Assessment and Management*. NFER – Nelson, Windsor

Sparks R. L. and Ganschow L. (1993) 'The effects of multi-sensory structured language instruction on native language and foreign language aptitude skills of at-risk High School foreign language learners: A replication and follow-up study'. *Annals of Dyslexia*, 43: 194–216

Sparks R. L., Ganschow L., Kenneweg S., Kenneweg S. and Miller K. (1991) 'Use of an Orton-Gillingham approach to teach a foreign language to dyslexic/learning-disabled students: Explicit teaching of phonology in a second language'. *Annals of Dyslexia*, 41: 96–118

Stirling E. G. (1985) *Help for the Dyslexic Adolescent*. Private publication, Sheffield

The Times (1996) 'How to pass classroom tests'. 11 May

Thomson M. (1990) *Developmental Dyslexia* (3rd edition). Whurr Publishers Ltd, London

Thomson M. E. and Watkins E. J. (1990) *Dyslexia: A Teaching Handbook*. Whurr Publishers Ltd, London

Vail P. (1992) *Learning Styles*. Modern Learning Press, New York

Chapter 9 _____

Aaron P. G. and Phillips S. (1986) 'A decade of research with dyslexic college students: A summary of findings'. *Annals of Dyslexia*, 36: 44–63

Brand V. (1990) 'The RSA link between the UK and the antipodes'. In Hales G., Hales M., Miles T. R. and Summerfield A. (eds) *Meeting Points in Dyslexia: Proceedings of the First International Conference of the British Dyslexia Association*. BDA, Reading: 279–81

BTEC (1993) *BTEC GNVQ External Tests: Provision for Candidates with Special Requirements*. BTEC Publications, London

Burton G., Diana J. and Gennosa E. W. (1991) 'Self-esteem: Nothing succeeds like success'. In Stracher D. A. (ed) *A Manual of Successful Strategies for Learning-disabled College Students*. Dowling College, New York: 26–34

Carman R. A. and Adams W. R. Jr (1972) *Study Skills: A Student's Guide for Survival*. John Wiley and Sons Inc., New York

Clayton P. (1996) *Access Students and Dyslexia: A Guide to Good Practice*. University of Kent, Canterbury

Dearing R. (1993) 'Sowing the seeds of change'. *The Times*, 4 October

Dearing R. (1996) *Review of Qualifications for 16–19 year olds*. Whittaker, London

Department for Education and Employment (1996) *Guidance Notes for Disabled Students in Higher Education*. HMSO, London

Dreyer P. P., Gennosa E. W., Schneld M. K. and Ventimiglia K. G. (1991) 'Writing: If you can't write it, you can't think it'. In Stracher D. A. (ed*) A Manual of Successful Strategies for Learning-disabled College Students*. Dowling College, New York: 105–26

Fennell E. (1993) 'How to release hidden talent'. *The Times*, 4 October

Gilroy D. (1994) Personal communication

Gilroy D. E. and Miles T. R. (1996) *Dylsexia at College* (2nd edition). Routledge, London

Joint Forum for the GCSE and GCE (1996) *Candidates with Special Assessment Needs: Special Arrangements and Special Considerations*, Manchester

Miller G. A. (1974) 'The Magical Number Seven Plus or Minus Two: Some limits in our capacity for processing information'. *Psychological Review*, 63: 81–97

Pauk W. (1974) *How to Study in College*. Houghton Mifflin Co., Boston

Schneld M. K., Haber C. J. and Vincent G. (1991) 'Organization: Framework for learning'. In Stracher D. A. (ed) *A Manual of Successful Strategies for Learning-disabled College Students*. Dowling College, New York: 35–45

Scottish Examination Board (1996) *Scottish Certificate of Education and Certificate of Sixth Year Studies Examinations. Arrangements for Candidates with Special Educational Needs*. Guidance for Centres for Examinations in and after 1996

Singleton C. (1993) 'Computer support for adult dyslexics'. In Crisfield J. (ed) *BDA Handbook 1993/4*. BDA, Reading: 108–12

Singleton C. (1995) 'Dyslexia in higher education'. *Dyslexia Contact*, 14 (2): 7–9

SKILL (1990) *Financial Assistance for Students with Disabilities in Higher Education*. The National Bureau for Students with Disabilities, London

Smyth J. and Wallace K. (1996) *The Educational Grants Directory. 1996/97 Edition*. Directory of Social Change, London

The Sunday Times (1995) quoting Nicholls J. cited in Scott-Clark C. (1995) 'Universities face inquiry on low I-Q entrants' *The Sunday Times* 10 September

UCAS (1995) Personal communication

Welch M. and Bowman M. (1996) *How can the Classroom Teacher use the Dyslexia Archive Effectively?* University of Kent, Canterbury

Zdzienski D. (1996) *Diagnostic Assessments for Students in Higher Education*. Script submitted for publication to Dyslexia Computer Resource Centre, University of Hull

Chapter 10

Birkle J. (1994) Personal communication

Brown P. (1996) 'Why don't we teach them to type? A parent's guide'. *The Times*, 24 May

Clayton P. and Lillywhite C. (1993) *Maths Programs: Using Computers with Dyslexics*. Dyslexia Computer Resource Centre, University of Hull

Code of Practice (1994) *Code of Practice on the Identification and Assessment of Special Educational Needs*. Department for Education and Employment, Central Office of Information, London

Evans K. and Welch M. (1996) *A Software Tool for Aiding Study in Dyslexic Students in Higher Education*. University of Kent, Canterbury

Gauntlett D. (1991) *A Review of Spelling Aids for the Dyslexic*. BDA, Reading

Hanbury King D. (1985) *Writing Skills for the Adolescent*. Educators Publishing Service Inc., Cambridge MA

Heppell S. (1995) 'Weaned on the screen'. *The Sunday Times*, 7 May

Higgins E. L. and Zvi J. C. (1995) 'Assistive technology for post secondary students with learning disabilities: From research to practice'. *Annals of Dyslexia*, 45: 123–42

Hutchins J. (1992) 'Using computers with dyslexics'. *Computer Users. Bulletin & Supplement*. Dyslexia Computer Resource Centre, University of Hull

Hutchins J. (1994a) 'Report on three presentations made at the symposium'. *Dyslexia Contact. Special Edition*, 13 (4): 21–2

Hutchins J. (1994b) 'Talking computers'. *Dyslexia Contact*, 13 (2): 23

Ingram E. (1984) *Computer Assisted Learning*. BDA, Reading

Innes P. (1990) *Defeating Dyslexia: A Boy's Story*. Kyle Cathie Ltd, London

Joint Council for the GCSE and GCE (1996) *Candidates with Special Assessment Needs: Special Arrangements and Special Consideration*, Manchester

Moseley D. (1991) 'Designing software for word study and for mastery of spelling'. In Singleton C. (ed) *Computers and Literacy Skills.* Dyslexia Computer Resource Centre, University of Hull: 60–86

National Curriculum (1995). Department for Education and Employment. HMSO, London

Pottage T. (1996) *Word Processing and Spell Checking* (2nd edition). Dyslexia Computer Resource Centre, University of Hull

Scheib B. and Lillywhite C. (1994) 'Keyboard skills and laptop word processing.' In Singleton C. (ed) *Computers and Dyslexia: Educational Applications for New Technology.* Dyslexia Computer Resource Centre, University of Hull: 88–98

Singleton C. (1993) 'Computer support for adult dyslexics'. In Crisfield J. and Smythe I. (eds) *The Dyslexia Handbook 1993/4.* BDA, Reading: 108–12

Singleton C. (ed) (1994) *'Computers and Dyslexia: Educational Applications of New Technology'.* Dyslexia Computer Resource Centre, University of Hull: 88–98

Stoecker J. (1985) *Touch Typing Instruction in the Elementary School: Current Practice. A Proposed Research-based Inservice Program* (unpublished PhD Thesis). University of Oregon

Terrell C. (1994) Personal communication

Welch M. and Bowman M. (1996) *A Computer-based Archive to Aid Adult Dyslexics.* University of Kent, Canterbury

Wentke R. (1996) 'The A to Z of the world of multimedia: A parent's guide'. *The Times*, 24 May

Chapter 11 ——————————

Associated Board of the Royal Schools of Music (1995) *Guidelines for the Examining of Dyslexic Candidates.* London

Atkinson J. (1991) 'The musical ability of children with dyslexia and its relationship to visual function'. Paper to Rodin Conference, Berne

Atkinson J., Watkins K., and Fowler-Watts S. (1992) *A preliminary investigation into musical ability in children with dyslexia*, unpublished paper

Backhouse G. (1994) 'Dyslexia in a professional musician'. In Miles T. R. and Augur J. (eds) *Music and Dyslexia. Cambridge Conference Proceedings 1992*. BDA, Reading: 24–37

BDA (1992) 'Music and Dyslexia'. *Papers produced by the BDA Music and Dyslexia Working Party*. BDA, Reading

Beaumont C. (1994) 'Teaching music to dyslexic children'. In Miles T. R. and Augur J. (eds), *'Music and Dyslexia'. Cambridge Conference Proceedings 1992*. BDA, Reading: 11–19

Bradley L. and Bryant P. E. (1983) 'Categorising sounds and learning to read: A causal connection'. *Nature*, 301: 419–21

Brand V. (1993) 'Music and dyslexia'. In Crisfield J. and Smythe I. (eds) *The Dyslexia Handbook 1993/4*. BDA, Reading: 77–80

Brand V. (1995) Personal communication

Cantwell A. (1992) 'Object naming ability of adults with written language difficulties'. *Annals of Dyslexia,* 42: 179–95

Crisfield J. and Smythe I. (1993) *The Dyslexia Handbook 1993/4*. BDA, Reading

Done D. J. and Miles T. R. (1978) 'Learning, memory, and dyslexia'. In Gruneberg M. M., Morris P. E. and Sykes R. N. (eds) *Practical Aspects of Memory*. Academic Press, London

Ganschow L., Miles T. R. and Lloyd-Jones J. (1994) 'Dyslexia and musical notation'. *Annals of Dyslexia*, 44: 185–202

Geschwind M. D. (1984) 'The brain of a learning-disabled individual'. *Annals of Dyslexia,* 34: 319–27

Hazeley J. (1994) Personal communication

Hubicki M. (1994) 'Musical problems? Reflections and suggestions'. In Hales G. (ed) *Dyslexia Matters*. Whurr Publishers Ltd, London

Hubicki M. (1996) Personal communication

Miles T. R. and Augur J. (eds) (1994) 'Editors' Foreword'. In *Music and Dyslexia. Cambridge Conference Proceedings 1992*. BDA, Reading: ii

Oglethorpe S. S. (1996) *Instrumental Music for Dyslexics. A Teaching Handbook*. Whurr Publishers Ltd, London

Oldfield C. (1987) 'Some problems incurred by a dyslexic flute player ... as she finds it'. *The Journal of the British Flute Society*, 5 (2): 18

Pollack C. and Branden A. (1982) 'Odyssey of a 'mirrored' personality'. *Annals of Dyslexia*, 32: 275–88

Chapter 12 ⎯⎯⎯⎯⎯⎯⎯⎯

ALBSU (1994) *Basic Skills in Prisons: Assessing the Need*. Adult Literacy and Basic Skills Unit, London

Anderson R. C., Hiebert E. H., Scott J. A. and Wilkinson I. A. (1985) *'Becoming a NATION of Readers'. Report of the commission on Reading*. US Department of Education

Beare D. (1975) 'Self-concept and the adolescent L/LD student'. *Journal of Texas Personnel and Guidance Association*, 4 (1): 29–32

Bradford P. (1993) *Dyslexia: An Avoidable National Tragedy*. Channel 4

Bryant T. R. (1978) 'The effect of student failure on the quality of family life and community mental health'. *Bulletin of the Orton Society* 28: 8–14

CBI (1995) *Dyslexia: The Hidden Resource. Conference Proceedings*. Felicity Patterson, Confederation of British Industry, London

Chall J. S. (1986) 'The Development of Reading in Children and Adults'. Paper presented to the *37th Annual Conference of the Orton Dyslexia Society, Philadelphia*

Cox A. (1983) 'Programming for teachers of dyslexics'. *Annals of Dyslexia*, 33: 221–3

Critchley M. (1966) *Developmental Dyslexia*. Heinemann, London

Daily Mail (1996) 'Dyslexic's despair at the golf club tee-hees'. 15 May

Department of Social Security (1995) *Disability on the Agenda* (cassette). Department of Social Security, Bristol

Gauntlett D. (1978) 'In another's shoes. A case study of a mature dyslexic'. *Dyslexia Review*, 1 (2): 23–7

Guyer B. P. and Sabatino D. (1989) 'The effectiveness of multi-sensory alphabetic phonetic approach with college students who are learning disabled'. *Journal of Learning Disabilities*, 23: 43–4

HMSO (1996) *Complete Theory Test for Cars and Motorcycles*. HMSO, London

Johnson D. J. (1980) 'Persistent auditory disorders in young dyslexic adults'. *Bulletin of the Orton Society*, 30: 268–76

Kershaw J. (1974) 'People with dyslexia'. *Report of a Working Party commissioned by the British Council for the Rehabilitation of the Disabled under the chairmanship of Dr John Kershaw, British Council for Rehabilitation of the Disabled,* London

Klein C. (1993) *Diagnosing Dyslexia*. Adult Literacy and Basic Skills Unit, London

Klein C. (1994) 'Setting up a learning programme for adult dyslexics'. In

Snowling M. and Thompson M. (eds) *Dyslexia: Integrating Theory and Practice*. Whurr Publishers Ltd, London: 293–301

Lilleyman S. A. (1996) 'Report on the DriveSafe open day, Coventry, 29 May 1996'. *The Bulletin, BDA Newsletter*, June

Margolis J. (1995) 'Spellbound'. *Tatler*, February

McLoughlin D., Fitzgibbon G. and Young V. (1994) *Adult Dyslexia Assessment, Counselling and Training*. Whurr Publishers Ltd, London

Moseley D. (1995) *The ACE Spelling Dictionary: Find Words Quickly and Improve Your Spelling*. Learning Development Aids, Wisbech

Oppenheim P. (1995) 'Draft speaking note: Dyslexia – Conference'. Institute of Directors, 28 February

Peer L. (1994) 'Telling tales'. *Dyslexia Contact*, 13 (1)

Renwick, The Lord (1990) 'Unstarred question on illiteracy in House of Lords'. Hansard, 4 April

Saunders R. (1990) 'Dyslexia as a factor in the young adult offender'. In Hales G., Hales M., Miles T. R. and Summerfield A. (eds) *Meeting Points in Dyslexia: Proceedings of the First International Conference of the British Dyslexia Association*. BDA, Reading: 232–9

Scarborough H. S. (1984) 'Continuity between childhood dyslexia and adult reading'. *British Journal of Psychology*, 75: 329–48

Simpson E. (1979) *Reversals: A Personal Account of Victory Over Dyslexia*. Houghton Mifflin Co., Boston

Singleton C. (1992) 'Computer support for adult dyslexics'. In Crisfield J. (ed) *The Dyslexia Handbook 1992/3*. BDA, Reading: 108–112

Thomson M. (1990) *Developmental Dyslexia* (3rd edition). Whurr Publishers Ltd, London

Tizard J. (1972) *Children with Specific Reading Difficulties*. HMSO, London

Vellutino F. R. (1987) 'Dyslexia'. *Scientific American,* 256 (3): 20–7

West T. G. (1991) *In the Mind's Eye*. Prometheus Books, New York

Chapter 13

[Unless otherwise specified, quotes in this chapter are taken from the Code of Practice 1994]

Advisory Centre for Education (1996) *Special Educational Handbook: The Law on Children with Special Needs* (7th edition). Advisory Centre for Education, London

Augur J. and Briggs S. (eds) (1992) *The Hickey Multi-sensory Language Course*. Whurr Publishers Ltd, London

BDA (1996a) 'Special Educational Needs: The working of the Code of Practice and the Tribunal'. Memorandum submitted to *House of Commons Education Committee Second Report*. Appendix 10. HMSO, London: 28–33

BDA (1996b) 'Time taken in processing statements'. *The Bulletin, BDA Newsletter*, May

Brereton A. (1994) Personal communication

Brereton A. (1995) Personal communication

Circular No 4/96 (1996) *Children and Young Persons with Special Educational Needs Assessment and Recording Circular No 4/96 (1996)* Scottish Office Education and Industry Department, Edinburgh

Code of Practice (1994) *Code of Practice on the Identification and Assessment of Special Educational Needs*. Department for Education and Employment, Central Office of Information, London

Department for Education and Employment (1992) *Special Educational Needs: Access to the System*. HMSO, London

Department for Education and Employment (1994) *Special Educational Needs: A Guide for Parents*. HMSO, London

Devon County Council (1996) 'Special Educational Needs: The Working of the Code of Practice and the Tribunal'. Memorandum submitted to *House of Commons Education Committee Second Report*. Appendix 15. HMSO, London: 42–3

Education Act 1981. HMSO, London

Education Act 1993. HMSO, London

Educational Law Association (1995) 'Factsheet'

Friel J. (1995) *Children with Special Needs. Assessment, Law and Practice – Caught in the Acts*. (3rd edition). Jessica Kingsley Publishers, London

Healey T. (1996) Letter to the Clerk of the House of Commons Education Committee Second Report, 'Special Educational Needs: The working of the Code of Practice and the Tribunal' following the Evidence Session of 7 February. HMSO, London

Hornsby B. and Shear F. (1994) *Alpha-to-Omega* (4th edition). Heinemann Educational, Oxford

Miles E. (1993) The Bangor Dyslexia Teaching System (2nd edition). Whurr Publishers Ltd, London

Minister of State (1993)

Office for Standards in Education (1996) *The Implementation of the Code of Practice for Pupils with Special Educational Needs*. HMSO, London

Orton C. (1996) Personal communication

Pumfrey P. (1994) 'The management of specific learning difficulties (dyslexia): Challenges and responses'. Unpublished paper. *Towards a Wider Understanding. Third International Conference of the British Dyslexia Association, Manchester*

The Sunday Observer (1994) 11 September

Scottish Office Education and Industry Department (1996) *A Parent's Guide to Special Educational Needs*. Scottish Office Industry and Education Department, Edinburgh

Warnock M. (1978) 'Special Educational Needs'. *Report of the Committee of Enquiry into the Education of Handicapped Children and Young People*. HMSO, London

Warnock M. (1994) Opening address (unpublished). *Towards a Wider Understanding. Third International Conference of the British Dyslexic Association, Manchester*

Chapter 14

Aaron P. G. (1993) 'Is there a visual dyslexia?'. *Annals of Dyslexia*, 43: 110–24

Bishop D. V. M. (1989) 'Unfixed reference, monocular occlusion and developmental dyslexia – A critique'. *British Journal of Opthalmology*, 73: 209–15

Boder E. (1971) 'Developmental dyslexia: Prevailing diagnostic concepts and a new diagnostic approach'. In Myklebust H. (ed) *Progress in Learning Disabilities*. Grune and Stratton, New York: 293–321

Brace A. (1993) 'Experts hail cure for child dyslexia'. *Mail on Sunday*, 27 June

Cotton M. M. and Evans K. M. (1990) 'An evaluation of the Irlen Lenses as a treatment for specific reading disorders'. *Australian Journal of Psychology*, 42: 1–12

Critchley M. (1966) *Developmental Dyslexia*. Heinemann, London

Evans B. J. W. (1993) 'Dyslexia, eye movements, controversial optometric therapies, and the transient visual system'. *Optometry Today*, 33: 17–19

Evans B. J. W. (1994a) 'The Intuitive Colorimeter: Friend or foe? Part 1'. *Optician*, 207 (5436): 18–22

Evans B. J. W. (1994b) 'The Intuitive Colorimeter: Friend or foe? Part 2'. *Optician*, 207 (5439): 24–6

Evans B. J. W. (1996a) 'Assessment of visual problems in reading'. In Beech J. and Singleton C. (eds) *Problems in Reading*. Routledge, London

Evans B. J. W. (1996b) 'Visual problems and dyslexia'. *Dyslexia Review*, 8 (1): 4–7

Evans B. J. W. and Drasdo N. (1990) 'Review of ophthalmic factors in dyslexia'. *Ophthalmic and Physiological Optics*, 10: 123–32

Evans B. J. W. and Drasdo N. (1991) 'Tinted lenses and related therapies for learning disabilities: An overview'. *Ophthalmic and Physiological Optics,* 2: 206–17

Evans B. J. W., Wilkins A. J., Brown J., Busby A., Wingfield A., Jeanes R. and Bald J. (1995) 'A preliminary investigation into the aetiology of Meares-Irlen Syndrome'. *Ophthalmic and Physiological Optics,* 16 (2): 1–11

Fischer B. and Biscaldi M. (1994) *'Eye Movements in Reading*. Pergamon Press, Oxford

Geschwind N. (1982) 'Comments made on the occasion of the dedication of Samuel Torrey Orton Library College of Physicians and Surgeons, Columbia University'. *Annals of Dyslexia*, 32: 13–30

Hawking L. (1995) 'Tinted lenses unravel riddle of dyslexia'. *Daily Mail*, 17 January

Hedderly R. (1981) 'Characteristics of a clinical example of dyslexic children'. Unpublished study, Dyslexia Institute, Huddersfield

Hinshelwood J. (1912) 'The treatment of word-blindness acquired and congenital'. *British Medical Journal 2*: 1033–5

Irlen H. (1983) 'Successful treatment of learning disabilities'. Paper presented to the *91st Annual Convention of the American Psychological Association at Anaheim, California*

Irlen H. (1994) 'Irlen seminar'. Special Needs Exhibition 1994, London

Jansky J. J. (1958) 'A case of severe dyslexia with aphasia-like symptoms'. *Bulletin of the Orton Society*, 8: 8–10

Johnson D. J. and Myklebust H. (eds) (1967) *Learning Disabilities: Educational Principles and Practices*. Grune and Stratton, New York

Linnman J. (1995) 'Recording, stimulation and analysis of human eye movements'. Unpublished Phd Thesis

Miles T. R. (1993) 'On current research: Tinted lenses'. *Dyslexia Contact*, 12 (2): 8

Miles T. R. and Miles E. (1990) *Dyslexia: A Hundred Years On*. Open University Press, Milton Keynes

Neary C. and Wilkins A. (1991) 'Effects of phosphor persistence and the control of eye movements'. *Perception*, 18: 257–64

Newman S. (1989) Ocular dominance, saccadic eye movements and reading'. *Dyslexia Contact*, 8 (1): 12–13

Orton S. T. (1925) 'Word-blindness in schoolchildren'. *Archives Neurology and Psychiatry*, 14: 581

Orton S. T. (1937) *Reading, Writing and Speech Problems in Children*. Norton, New York

Orton S. T. (1946) *Word-blindness in School Children and Other Papers on Strephosymbolia*. Orton Society, Baltimore

Pavlidis G. Th. (1981) 'Do eye movements hold the key to dyslexia?'. *Neuropsychologia*, 19: 57–64

Pennington B. F. (1989) 'Using genetics to understand dyslexia'. *Annals of Dyslexia*, 39: 81–93

Pumfrey P. D. and Reason R. (1991) *Specific Learning Difficulties (Dyslexia). Challenges and Responses.* Routledge, London

Rayner K. (1983) 'Eye movements, perceptual span, and reading disability'. *Annals of Dyslexia,* 33: 163–73

Riddell P., Fowler S. and Stein J. (1988) 'Vergence eye movements and dyslexia'. *Dyslexia Contact,* 7, (2): 5

Rosner J. and Rosner J. (1987) 'The Irlen Treatment: A review of the literature'. *Optician,* 25: 26–33

Snowling M. J. (1987) *Dyslexia: A Cognitive Developmental Perspective.* Blackwell, Oxford

Stanley G. (1994) 'Visual deficit models of dyslexia'. In Hales G. (ed) *Dyslexia Matters.* Whurr Publishers Ltd, London: 19–29

Stanovich K. E. (1985) 'Explaining the variance in reading ability in terms of psychological processes: What have we learned?'. *Annals of Dyslexia,* 35: 67–9

Stein J. (1990) 'Unstable binocular control in dyslexic children'. In Hales G., Hales M., Miles T. R. and Summerfield A. (eds) *Meeting Points in Dyslexia: Proceedings of the First International Conference of the British Dyslexia Association.* BDA, Reading

Stein J. and Fowler S. (1985) 'Effect of monocular occlusion on visuomotor perception and reading in dyslexic children'. *The Lancet,* 13 July: 69–73

Sunday Times (1985) 'Glasses hope for dyslexia'. 22 December

Tinker M. (1958) 'Recent studies of eye movements in reading'. *Psychological Bulletin,* 55: 215–31

Vellutino F. R. (1979) *Dyslexia: Theory and Research.* The MIT Press, Cambridge MA

Wilkins A. (1996) 'Helping reading with colour'. *Dyslexia Review,* 7: 3

Wilkins A. J., Evans B. J. W., Brown J. A., Busby A. E., Wingfield A. E., Jeanes R. J. and Bald J. (1994) 'Double-masked placebo controlled trial of precision spectral filters in children who use coloured overlays'. *Ophthalmic and Physiological Optics,* 14: 365–70

Wilsher C. and Taylor J. A. (1986) 'Remedies for dyslexia: Proven or unproven'. *Early Child Development and Care,* 27: 287–99

Zangwill O. L. and Blakemore C. (1972) 'Dyslexics' reversal of eye movements during reading'. *Neuropsychologia,* 51: 526–34

Chapter 15

Baum S. M., Owen S. V. and Dixon J. (1991) *To be Gifted and Learning Disabled.* Creative Learning Press Inc., Mansfield Center CO

Brown P. (1994) 'Halfway up the mountain'. *Times Educational Supplement,* 14 October

Bryant T. E. (1978) 'The effect of student failure on the quality of family life and community mental health'. *Bulletin of the Orton Society,* 28: 8–14

Cann P. (1996) 'Useful words about teacher training'. *The Bulletin. BDA Newsletter.* June

Code of Practice (1994) *Code of Practice on the Identification and Assessment of Special Educational Needs.* Department for Education and Employment, Central Office of Information, London

Edwards J. (1994) *The Scars of Dyslexia: Eight Case Studies in Emotional Reactions.* Cassell, London

Geschwind N. (1982) 'Why Orton was right'. *Annals of Dyslexia,* 32: 13–30

Hello! (1994) *Susan Hampshire.* October

Hornsby B. and Shear F. (1994) *Alpha-to-Omega* (4th edition). Heinemann Educational, Oxford

Marland S. (1971) *Education of the Gifted and Talented* (Marland Report). US Office of Education, Department of Health, Education and Welfare, Washington DC

Morgan C. G. (1983) 'Adapting a college preparatory curriculum for dyslexic adolescents: Applications for the classroom'. *Annals of Dyslexia*, 33: 251–68

National Association for Gifted Children (1981) *According to their Needs: A Survey of Good Practice in Schools with a Description and Commentary*

Sartori G. (1987) 'Leonardo DaVinci Omo Sanzo Lettere: A case of surface dysgraphia?'. *Cognitive Neuropsychology*, 4: 1–10

Shaywitz S. E. (1996) 'Dyslexia: A new model of this reading disorder emphasizes defects in the language-processing rather than the visual system. It explains why some very smart people have trouble learning to read.' *Scientific American*, 275: 5, 78: 84, New York

Simpson E. (1979) *Reversals: A Personal Account of Victory Over Dyslexia*. Victor Gollancz Ltd, London

Smith S. L. (1987) 'Masking the feeling of being stupid'. *American University Newsletter*

Steingard P. and 'Gail' (1975) 'The unheard cry – Help me! A plea to teachers of dyslexic children'. *Bulletin of the Orton Society*, 25: 178–84

Strauss R. (1978) 'Richard's story'. *Bulletin of the Orton Society*, 28: 181–5

West T. G. (1991) *In the Mind's Eye*. Prometheus Books, New York

West T. G. (1992) 'A future of reversals: Dylsexic talents in a world of computer visualization'. *Annals of Dyslexia*, 42: 124–39

Appendices ————————

Baddeley A. D., Wilson B. A. and Watts F. N. (Eds), (1995) *Handbook of Memory Disorders*, John Wiley & Sons Ltd, Chichester

Cox A. R. (1992) *Foundations for Literacy: Structures and Techniques for Multi-sensory Teaching of Basic Language Skills* (Revised edition). Educators Publishing Service Inc., Cambridge MA

Chomsky C. (1970) 'Reading, writing and phonology'. *Harvard Education Review*, 40: 287–309

Critchley M. and Critchley E. (1978) *Dyslexia Defined*. Heinemann, London

Crystal D. (1987) *The Cambridge Encyclopaedia of Language*. Cambridge Reference, Cambridge

Ellis A. W. (1993) *Reading, Writing and Dyslexia: A Cognitive Analysis* (2nd edition). Lawrence Erlbaum Associates Ltd, Hove

Evans B. J. W. (1996) 'Visual problems and dyslexia'. *Dyslexia Review*, 8 (1): 4–7

Joffe L. (1980) 'Dyslexia and attainment in school mathematics'. *Dyslexia Review*, 3 (1): 10–14 *and* 3 (2): 12–18

Liberman I. and Shankweiler D. (1985) 'Phonology and the problems of learning to read and write'. *Remedial and Special Education*, 6: 8–17

Miles T. R. and Miles E. (eds) (1992) *Dyslexia and Mathematics*. Routledge, London

Orton J. L. (1966) 'The Orton–Gillingham approach' in *The Disabled Reader; Education of the Dyslexic Child*, Money J. (Ed.) John Hopkins Press, Baltimore, Maryland

Treiman R. (1985) 'Onsets and rimes as units of spoken syllables: Evidence from children'. *Journal of Experimental Child Psychology*, 39: 255–82

Waites L. (1968) 'Dyslexia International World Federation of Neurology. Report of Research Group on Developmental Dyslexia and World Illiteracy'. *Bulletin of the Orton Society*, 18: 21–2

Acquired dyslexia occurs due to damage to the brain which can be caused by cerebrovascular accident such as a head injury or a brain tumour. There are four types with varying symptoms and specific features.

1 Deep dyslexia: includes semantic errors which relate to meaning when reading.
2 Phonological dyslexia: includes an inability to read nonsense words.
3 Surface dyslexia: includes a disturbance between the person's visual word recognition and the semantic knowledge.
4 Word-form dyslexia, also known as Deterine's syndrome: includes the patients who can only understand what they read aloud by reading one letter at a time.

Agnomia A difficulty with naming objects – the word seems to be on the 'tip of the tongue', but can't be recalled rapidly.

Agnosia A loss in the ability to recognize persons or things seen. They can see and describe what they see, but they have difficulties in describing what they have seen.

Alexia An acquired reading difficulty that occurs as a result of illness or injury to the brain. It can arise along with difficulties in speech comprehension or vocabulary selection or with writing difficulties and only mild disturbances of speech.

Alliteration This is when two or more words close together begin with the same letter or the same sound, e.g. 'sing a song of sixpence' or a group of words that begin with the same sounds, e.g. ship – shop – shed.

Analogy This is used to look at words and to give a parallel form such as 'day is to week as month is to year'.

Antonym A word of opposite meaning such as hot – cold.

Aphasia The partial or total loss of the ability to speak or understand written or spoken language as a result of, for example, a stroke, head injury or a brain tumour. Expressive aphasics cannot express the words they want to use. Receptive aphasics cannot understand the speech which they can hear.

Apraxia An inability to perform a task when requested although the activity can be performed perfectly well spontaneously.

Articulation The process of producing speech sounds by the movement of the lips, jaw, tongue or throat.

Assimilations The conformation of a sound, usually a consonant, to a neighbouring sound. It means that a sound is changed because of the influence of another sound next to it, e.g. /ng/ as 'bang'.

Attainment tests Reveal how much the pupil knows and how he performs when he is tested in a particular subject such as spelling.

Auditory analysis An ability to identify sounds in the initial position (beginning of a word), in the medial position (middle of a word), or the final position (at the end of a word).

Auditory discrimination An ability to detect the differences or similarities between individual sounds in words when presented orally at the beginning, middle or end of pairs of words, e.g. bat, cat; ship, shop; pat, pad.

Auditory memory An ability to recall material presented orally, such as sounds in a word. This is necessary to spell a word because the sequence of the sounds has to be remembered, and this has then to be converted into the correct letter that represents the sound. It also applies to a sequence of words in a sentence such as in a sentence given for dictation.

Auditory perception The ability to understand and make sense of sounds which are heard such as an ability to tell the difference between 'fan', 'van' or 'than'. For someone with an auditory perception difficulty, this may cause a problem. It does not mean that there is a problem with the person's hearing or ability to hear loud or soft sounds which is a different type of hearing skill.

Auditory sequential memory An ability to recall in a particular order, sounds, groups of words, numbers, facts, etc., such as the days of the week or times tables.

Blends These are letters found next to each other. They sound quickly but separately, therefore they blend. Blending is also the bringing together of the constituent sounds of a word to make a whole word. There are consonant blends, such as bl, cl, tw, dr. There are also vowel blends such as ee, ai which are more correctly described as diphthongs.

Breve A code mark ˘ placed over a vowel denoting that it is a short vowel, e.g. băt.

Centiles Used to describe percentile rankings in psychometric tests. They relate to and help compare the child's achievement test scores to the proportion of the comparative population who can be expected to achieve less than that score.

Cerebral damage Brain damage which can be either acquired or congenital.

Cerebral dominance The dominant side of the body for certain tasks. Dominance refers to the superiority of one side of the body for carrying out or performing certain functions involving the eyes, ears, hands or feet.

Cerebral hemispheres The brain has two hemispheres (sides): left and right. The left hemisphere is the dominant hemisphere for the majority of people. It controls the right side of the body, and it contains the language centres of the brain. The right hemisphere contains the centres controlling rhythm, artistic skills and creativity.

Circumlocution Speaking in a roundabout or long-winded fashion or to use several words instead of one to describe an object or act, for example 'thingummyjig'; 'What's it called, thing with legs, ears and a tail' (a dog); or, when asked to say what a tree is, to reply 'A bit like the end of a broom with green leaves on.'

Closed syllable Ends in a consonant. The vowel is short so therefore it says its sound.

Closed tests Tests carried out by people who usually have to be specifically trained to use the particular test such as the Wechsler Intelligence Scale for Children (WISC) test which may only be administered by a chartered psychologist.

Cloze procedure Exercise that involves filling in missing letters, missing words or missing parts of sentences.

Code of Practice on the Identification and Assessment of Special Educational Needs Issued by the UK Government as a result of the Education Act 1993 and sets out fundamental principles about the education of children with special educational needs.

Comprehension When applied to reading is an ability to understand and recall the contents of what has been read. It requires fluent decoding skills (reading with automaticity), knowledge of word meanings and an ability to use previous experience or contextual cues to understand the meaning which is being conveyed by the words.

Congenital Comes from the Latin and means 'appearing at birth', as distinct from hereditary which means something that is transmitted by parents to their offspring.

Consonants All the letters of the alphabet except the vowels.

Contextual cues Additional information such as syntax or grammar that may help the reader to make sense of what he reads.

Contraction When letters or groups of letters are omitted from words to make a shortened form. An apostrophe is used to show where the letters have been omitted such as they are/they're.

Cross-laterality Refers to someone using different sides of the body for different tasks such as using the right hand for *all* handed tasks, but using the left eye for *all* eyed tasks.

Cursive Handwriting which is joined up and is a continuous flowing movement. The lower case letters begin on the line and the pen is not raised until the whole word is written.

Developmental dyscalculia Literally, a difficulty with calculation. A broader concept, according to Miles and Miles (1992), implies an impairment of mathematical skills.

Diacritical marks These are the code marks or signs used on the vowels to show whether vowels are short or long. Short vowels are coded with a breve (˘): hăt, pĕt, rĭg. Long vowels are coded with a macron (¯): trāin, wēēd.

Diagnostic tests Tests used to identify strengths and weaknesses, for example, in spelling.

Digit span test A series of digits (numbers) are given. The person is asked to repeat these after the tester: first in the forward position such as 2, 9, 6, 4; then the person is asked to repeat a series of numbers in the reverse order to which they were given. The span refers to the maximum number of digits the person can say either in the forward or backward position. This is regarded as a test of short term auditory memory.

Digraph Consonant digraphs are two consonants which, when side by side, make one sound, e.g. /sh/, /ch/, /ph/, /th/, /wh/, as in ship, chum, phone, thumb, when. Vowel digraphs are two vowels which, when side by side, make one sound – /ee/ or /ai/ as in 'speed' or 'train'.

Diphthongs Two vowels together producing a glide from one position to another to make one vowel sound such as /oi/ or /ou/ as in 'boil' or 'couch'.

Dominant hand Usually implies the preferred hand particularly the hand used to write with.

Double-masked placebo-controlled trial Scientific trials carried out to test drugs or medical procedures. A placebo (a dummy pill or treatment) is given to one patient while the real treatment is given to the other. To be 'double-masked', neither the practitioner nor the patients should know which patient has received the genuine treatment.

Dysarthria An articulatory disorder that occurs because of a dysfunction in the central nervous system in the motor musculature of speech.

Dyscalculia According to Joffe (1980), 'difficulty in dealing with numbers and calculation as an aspect of dyslexia'. But Critchley and Critchley (1978) maintained that the usage of the word 'dyscalculia' in relation to dyslexics who have arithmetical difficulties is inappropriate, since to the neurologist, it describes a concomitant of acquired brain disease. Miles and Miles (1992) criticized Joffe's definition as too narrow because 'suffers from dyscalculia' would mean no more than 'is weak at Mathematics'.

Dyseidectic dyslexia A poor visual memory for words. Each word is read as if it has not been seen before. The same words are not recognized from one line to the next. Often every word needs to be sounded out letter by letter before it can be read.

Dyslalia A functional speech defect due to defects in the organs of speech or motor nerves.

Dyslexia Difficulty with words. It is derived from the Greek prefix '*dys*' meaning difficulty or malfunction and the root '*lexis*' meaning language. See pages 1–4 for full definitions.

Dysphonetic dyslexia Describes dyslexics who have major phonological problems but who can learn a small sight vocabulary of words which helps them when they are reading. Elena Boder is credited with first describing this as well as two other types.

Dysphonetic-dyseidectic dyslexia Those who have difficulties with phonological awareness and visual memory.

Dysphonia Difficulty in pronouncing vocal sounds.

Dyspraxia Comes from the Greek word *praxis* for 'doing, acting', 'deed and practice', and is used to describe people who have difficulty planning and carrying out non-habitual motor skills. They have 'an impairment in the ability to perform unfamiliar or familiar motor skills' with automaticity.

Fine motor skills Skills that are performed by the fingers and the hands such as using a pencil.

Fogg Index A test of readability. It is a quick method which can be used to check how difficult it is to read material of 100 words or more, and from this it is possible to then calculate the reading age of the passage or book.

Formes frustes A medical term which describes variants of a condition or a disease which are atypical or incomplete such as the dyslexia syndrome.

Grapheme The name of the letters of the alphabet such as 'Bee' for B, 'Dee' for D.

Gross motor skills Skills that are associated with the arms and the legs such as catching a ball or kicking a ball.

Hawthorne effect This is used by the scientific community when results of an experiment are not based on scientific investigation, but rather on the subjective responses of the individual on whom the tests are conducted. Elton Mayo and his associates carried out experiments on a group of workers at the Hawthorne Western Electric Plant to examine the effects of different working practices on their performance and output, and discovered that work productivity was increased as a result of the psychological stimulus of being singled out and made to feel important.

Homograph A word which is spelt the same as another, but is pronounced differently: Reading and reading; minute, minute.

Homonym A word that is spelt the same but has different meanings: Pole and pole.

Homophone A word that sounds the same, but has a different spelling and a different meaning: right, rite, write; pair, pear, pare.

Individual Education Plan Written record as prescribed by the *Code of Practice 1994* which describe strategies for supporting the child's progress and monitoring and review arrangements.

IQ Relates to the intelligence quotient as obtained on an intelligence test. It is calculated as follows:

$$IQ = \frac{MA \text{ (Mental Age)}}{CA \text{ (Chronological Age)}} \times 100$$

Italic Letters in printing that slope to the right. Often used to emphasize a word or series of words.

Key Stages Refers to pupils' ages and year groups as applied by the National Curriculum to pupils in maintained schools.

	Ages	Year group
Key Stage 1	5–7	1–2
Key Stage 2	7–11	3–6
Key Stage 3	11–14	7–9
Key Stage 4	14–16	10–11

Keyword A word that is used consistently to help recall, for example, when teaching the letter–name–sound association. The key word 'apple' would be used to practise saying '/a/ apple', while at the same time looking at a picture of an apple and saying its sound.

Kinesthetic The use of the sense of touch such as tracing the letters in a word using a finger and feeling it when doing so. The sense of movement can form a pattern and the motor memory may help some people to then reproduce the word when asked to write it.

Language Implies the acquired use of conventional symbols, usually audible (speech) or visible (writing), for the purpose of communication.

Laterality The side of the body used for a set task or function. It can apply to the eyes, ears, hands or feet. Most people are completely right-lateralized. Those people who, for example, use their right hand to write and their left hand for one or more other tasks such as to unscrew a jar or to bat are described as of 'mixed laterality'.

Learning difficulties The Education Act 1993 says that a child with learning difficulties has 'significantly greater difficulty in learning than the majority of children his age'.

Linguistics Chomsky (1970) defines linguistics as 'the study of language as represented in the brain of the speaker'. It also applies to the knowledge of the language.

Long vowel A long vowel says its name such as 'Amy' in the name, or 'navy' in the colour.

Macron A horizontal code mark placed over a long vowel to denote that it is a long vowel, e.g. sōlō.

Magic 'e' A mnemonic devised to describe the lengthening processes of the letter 'e' after a vowel at the end of a word. The word 'hat' has a short vowel. If 'e' is added to the end of the word, it then becomes the word 'hate'. The vowel 'a' has been changed to a long vowel (saying its name). 'e' is silent but has had the 'magic' effect of changing the vowel sound (see page 116).

Mental age This is calculated using an intelligence test and the child's chronological age. It tells how much above or below a child's intelligence is, in comparison to children of the same age.

Miscue analysis This is made by keeping a 'running record' of the errors made by someone when reading or spelling. The written record of these may be analysed later for diagnostic purposes.

Mnemonic A memory device to help remember letters in a word to aid spelling such as '**are rats evil**?' to help remember that a-r-e spells 'are'.

Morpheme The smallest meaningful part of a word. It can include an affix, preposition or conjunction.

Morphology The study of the structure of words.

Motor skills Skills that are performed by the muscles. They are controlled by the brain.

Multi-sensory learning The simultaneous use of the eyes, ears, hands and lips to utilize all the pathways to the brain when learning.

National Curriculum A programme of study for each Key Stage and which should be taught to the great majority of pupils in ways appropriate to their abilities. It is compulsory and applies to pupils in maintained schools, including grant-maintained schools and grant-maintained special schools. It sets out a programme of study and attainment targets for each of the stages.

Onset According to Treiman (1985) this is the initial consonant or consonant cluster of letters in words, e.g. tr(ip), dr(um).

Open syllable Ends in a vowel, so the vowel is long and, therefore, usually says its name, e.g. mē.

Ophthalmologist A medically qualified doctor with postgraduate specialist training in the examination, and medical and surgical treatment of defects and diseases in the eye.

Optician Makes and supplies glasses and contact lenses.

Optometrist Trained to detect and manage defects in vision and to dispense glasses and contact lenses.

Orthography The art of writing words with the proper letters according to the standard usage in spelling. It includes the way the words are conventionally written.

Palindrome Words that are spelt the same way backwards or forwards, e.g. 'madam', 'Eve'. It can apply to words, sentences or phrases.

Parallel forms of tests Alternative or equivalent forms of a test that may be used to re-test and evaluate progress without the risk of introducing the 'practice effect' which can affect the reliability of a test.

Perception The interpretation of a sensation such as noise. This would be auditory perception; visual perception would be interpreting something by using the eyes.

Phoneme The smallest unit of sound that distinguishes one word from another, thus changing the meaning of a word, e.g. c, b or f before 'at' makes 'cat', 'bat', 'fat'.

Phonetics Crystal (1987) says that 'the general study of human sound-making and reception is known as phonetics', in other words, human speech.

Phonics The teaching of reading and spelling by sounding out the individual letter sounds, then blending and synthesizing the sounds to produce a word when learning to read.

Phonological awareness An ability to recognize different sounds – 'bun', 'pun', 'fun'. Liberman and Shankweiler (1985) said 'phonological awareness is the explicit awareness of the sound segments in words'. Ellis (1993) gave a fuller definition and said that much research has focused in this field and that it 'is the capacity to reflect upon and manipulate the sound structure of words and is assessed in tasks which range from deciding whether or not two words rhyme through deciding whether or not two words have the same initial sounds (phonemes) to removing phonemes from words and saying what is left'. In other words, a realization that words are made up of a number of sounds, e.g. /c/ /a/ /t/.

Phonology The study of the sound system and the speech sounds in relation to meaning, including syllables and phonemes produced, and the rules governing the combining of sounds in a given language.

Prefix A letter or a group of letters that go at the beginning of a word and usually change the meaning of a word, e.g. **il**legal, **mis**pronounce.

Psychiatrist A medically qualified doctor with post-graduate specialist training in psychiatry who studies behavioural and personality disorders as well as mental disease and emotional difficulties.

Psycholinguistics The examination of the mental processes used in the acquisition and use of language.

Psychologist A person who studies the human mind and mental characteristics. Educational psychologists are graduates, usually with a degree in psychology and with experience of teaching, who specialize in the assessment of children by means of psychometric tests. The tests usually predict ability including skills and weaknesses.

Pun A play on words, e.g. 'Our business is developing' (could mean making progress or could mean processing photographs); 'Mr Tennant is a good tenant'.

Reading age/Spelling age A pupil's reading/spelling attainment which has been measured on a standardized reading/spelling test and compared to that of children of a similar age. The scores are usually given in years and months.

Record of Needs A confidential folder opened by a Scottish education authority after a child has been assessed and identified as having 'specific or complex special educational needs'. It details the difficulties and explains the educational measures proposed to meet the needs.

Rhyme Usually refers to words which sound the same at the end of a line such as in a poem. It can also refer to individual words such as in speak, shriek, streak.

Rhythm Describes a beat such as in a marching song.

Riddle Does not describe something as it seems. It has a puzzle which has to be worked out to get the answer.

Rime According to Treiman (1985) corresponds to the vowel and final consonant(s) –, e.g. dr(ip), tr(ap), sp(ot). Rimes may also be single phonemes, e.g. tr(ee).

Root The main part of a word. It is the base or primary word from which other words can be derived, e.g. 'form' → deform, forming.

Scotopic Sensitivity Syndrome Described by Helen Irlen in 1983 and based on the discoveries of Olive Meares. 'The condition is characterized by symptoms of eyestrain and visual perceptual distortions when reading, which can be alleviated with coloured filters' (Evans, 1996). Also known as Irlen Syndrome.

Semantics Relates to the meaning of language. It makes sense of words.

SENCO The teacher who is responsible for organizing the school's arrangements and provision for pupils with special educational needs is called the Special Educational Needs Co-ordinator (SENCO).

Short term memory (STM) Where a small amount of material is held in mind over a period of several seconds. STM is described as involving 'primary memory' if the material is held passively and then given back as a response in the same form as it was presented, and as 'working memory' if the information must be reorganized while being held, or integrated with further incoming information or with previously learned material. (Baddeley et al, 1995)

Short vowels Say their sound.

Sight vocabulary A bank of words that are instantly recognizable from visual inspection when reading.

Simultaneous Oral Spelling (SOS) Devised by Orton to teach spelling in a multi-sensory way. According to Cox (1992), there are five precise steps:

1 The teacher says the word while the pupil listens using his ears and watches the teacher's mouth using his eyes.

2 The pupil repeats the word using his lips.

3 The pupil then spells the word aloud.

4 The pupil writes the word using his kinesthetic (motor) memory and auditory memory.

5 The pupil reads aloud the word he has written (proof reading).

Special Educational Needs (SEN) According to the Education Act 1993 'a child has special educational needs if he has a learning difficulty which calls for special educational provision to be made for him'.

Specific developmental dyslexia According to the World Federation of Neurology, it is 'A disorder manifested by difficulty in learning to read, despite conventional instruction, adequate intelligence, and socio-cultural opportunity. It is dependent upon fundamental cognitive disabilities which are frequently constitutional in origin' (Waites, 1968).

Specific learning difficulty The word 'specific' denotes that there are particular learning difficulties which affect certain cognitive skills such as memory, sequencing or perception, rather than a general learning difficulty which affects most aspects of learning.

Spoonerism Takes its name from the scholar, the Reverend W. A. Spooner (1844–1930), who had a tendency to accidental or deliberate transposition of the initial sounds, or other parts of two or more words, and who in 1879 in the chapel of New College, Oxford announced the hymn 'Kinquering Congs Their Titles Take'.

Standardized reading or spelling test A test that has been tested on a large sample of pupils. A scale of averages can then be worked out from these results. A standardized reading or spelling test can reveal a pupil's attainment level in comparison with others of a similar age.

Statement A document which is issued by a LEA after a child has been assessed and who is found to have significant special educational needs. It describes these needs and lists the appropriate provision to be made to meet them.

Strephosymbolia Literally, twisted symbols. Coined by Orton from the Greek to describe 'a specific characteristic of reading impairment in the children he studied – the instability in recognition and recall of the orientation of letters and the order of letters in words' (J. L. Orton, 1966).

Suffix A letter or a group of letters that go at the end of a word and usually change the use of the word, e.g. wal<u>ked</u>, walk<u>er</u>, walk<u>ing</u>.

Syllable A word or part of a word with one vowel sound. It is sometimes described as a beat, thus 'dot', 'peg' have one syllable, 'den|tist' has two syllables, and 're|mem|ber' has three syllables.

Synonym A word of exactly the same meaning, e.g. father/daddy, circular/round.

Syntax Rules concerning the grammatical ordering of words in speech or written language to make sentences.

Synthesize The ability to put parts of sounds together to produce a whole word, e.g. b – a – t = 'bat'.

Visual discrimination The ability to detect the differences in shape, size and conformation of letters and objects.

Visual memory The ability to recall or retain a mental picture of a letter, word or object including its shape, length and the order of letters.

Visual sequential memory The ability to recall a series of letters or objects in the order in which they were presented. It involves orientation as well as sequences. For example, if a pupil is shown a card with three faces on it and then is asked to reproduce the sequence of cards from a choice of six cards, he must be able to put them in the correct order with the profiles either left or right as in the original card.

Vowels There are five vowels: a, e, i, o, u. The letter y is sometimes described as a vowel in words such as 'my' or 'try'. There are two kinds of vowels: short vowels and long vowels. Short vowels say their sounds. Long vowels say their names.

Word-blind This term was coined in 1877 by Adolf Kussmaul to describe people who 'lost' their ability to read as a result of an accident or illness. It is now regarded as outmoded, but still survives in popular mythology. In 1972 Meredith said 'the expression "word-blind" is unfortunate. It is a misleading metaphor. The child sees the printed word and can sometimes say what it is. If he were "blind to words", as he might be blind to colours, he would never see any words'.

Acronyms

ACE	Advisory Centre for Education
ADAR	The Art and Design Admissions Registry
ALBSU	Adult Literacy and Basic Skills Unit
AMBDA	Associate Member of the British Dyslexia Association
BAS	British Ability Scales
BDA	British Dyslexia Association
BMA	British Medical Association
BTEC	Business and Technology Education Council
CA	Chronological Age
CAL	Computer Assisted Learning
CBI	Confederation of British Industry
CCETSW	Central Council for Education and Training in Social Work
COP	Code of Practice on Special Educational Needs
CoPS 1	Cognitive Profiling System
CReSTeD	Council for the Registration of Schools Teaching Dyslexic Pupils
CV	Curriculum Vitae
DDA	Disability Discrimination Act
DES	Department of Education and Science
DEST	Dyslexia Early Screening Test
DfE	Department for Education
DfEE	Department for Education and Employment
DI	Dyslexia Institute
EP	Educational Psychologist
FE College	Further Education College
FEFC	Further Education Funding Council
GCE	General Certificate of Education (refers to 'A' level)
GCSE	General Certificate of Secondary Education
GNVQ	General National Vocational Qualifications
HEFC	Higher Education Funding Council for England and Wales
HND	Higher National Diploma
ICAA	Invalid Children's Aid Association
IEP	Individual Education Plan
INSET	In-Service Education of Teachers
IQ	Intelligence Quotient
LEA	Local Education Authority
MA	Mental Age
Mb	Megabytes
NAGC	National Association for Gifted Children
NASEN	National Association of Special Educational Needs
NCVQ	National Council for Vocational Qualifications

NFER	National Foundation for Educational Research
NHS	National Health Service
NVQ	National Vocational Qualification
OFSTED	Office for Standards in Education
OU	Open University
PACT	Placing, Assessment and Counselling Team
PATOSS	Professional Association of Teachers and Students with Specific Learning Difficulties
PTA	Parent Teachers' Association
RAM	Random Access Memory
REHAB	British Council for the Rehabilitation of the Disabled
RSA	Royal Society of Arts
SATS	Standard Achievement Tests
SEN	Special Educational Needs
SENCO	Special Educational Needs Co-ordinator
SKILL	National Bureau for Students with Disabilities
SOED	Scottish Office Education Department
SOS	Simultaneous Oral Spelling
SpLD	Specific Learning Difficulties
SRG	State Research Grant
UCAS	Universities and Colleges Admissions Services
VR	Verbal Reasoning
WAIS	Wechsler Adult Intelligence Scale
WISC	Wechsler Intelligence Scale for Children
WPPSI	Wechsler Pre-school and Primary Scale of Intelligence

General

The British Dyslexia Association (BDA)
98 London Road, Reading, Berkshire RG1 5AU.
Tel: 0118 966 2677 (Administration)
Tel: 0118 966 8271 (National Helpline)

This is the national organization. It has a network of *Local Associations and Support Groups* throughout the country. Most are run by local volunteers who offer advice and counselling. Some associations also arrange specialist teaching, run courses (e.g. computer workshops) and provide specialist knowledge of the Local Education Authority provision for dyslexic children. Names and telephone numbers of local groups are available from the BDA at Reading on the National Helpline listed above.

The Council for the Registration of Schools Teaching Dyslexic Pupils (CReSTeD)
Tel: 00 35 31 679 0276

The organization provides parents with a list of schools which have been inspected and registered by them, offering help to dyslexic pupils.

Dyslexia Association of Northern Ireland
31 High Street, Hollywood, Co. Down.
Tel: 101 6790276

The European Dyslexia Association (EDA)
Avenue Charles Woeste Bt. 7, 1090 Brussels, Belgium
Tel: 00 32 242 717 36

The European Dyslexia Association is a forum for support for dyslexic children, adolescents and adults. It promotes discussion, dialogue and co-operation within the European Union and in the countries belonging to the Council of Europe. It has two categories of membership:

Effective members who represent the National Dyslexia Associations of independent sovereign states: Austria, Belgium, Croatia, Denmark, France, Germany, Great Britain, Greece, Hungary, Ireland, Netherlands, Norway, Poland and Spain.

Adherent members, comprising countries in and outside Europe who wish to co-operate with those countries that share their language: Brazil, Catalonia, Cyprus, Gilbraltar, India, Isle of Man, Israel, Luxembourg, Malta, Quebec, Scotland, Sweden, Switzerland, United Kingdom

Joint Forum for the GCSE and GCE
Devas St., Manchester M15 6EX.

Scottish Dyslexia Association
Head Office, Unit 3, Stirling Business Centre,
Wellgreen Place, Stirling FK8 2DZ.
Tel: 01786 446650

Teaching and Assessment Centres

Helen Arkell Dyslexia Centre
Helen Arkell Centre, Frensham, Farnham, Surrey GU10 3BW.
Tel: 01252 792400

The Helen Arkell Dyslexia Centre offers assessments, specialist
teaching and training courses, including the RSA Diploma in
Specific Learning Difficulties (three terms, one day a week). Also
two-term RSA certificates and courses for classroom assistants.

The Dyslexia Institute
133 Gresham Road, Staines, Middlesex TW18 2AJ.
Tel: 01784 463851 Fax: 01784 460747
Training Office: 01785 819497

The Dyslexia Institute provides assessments, specialist teaching and
training courses for teachers, including a post-graduate diploma in
the teaching of pupils with Specific Learning Difficulties and a wide
range of specialist short courses, awareness courses and INSET
tailored to individual needs. It has a Network of Centres offering
these services nationwide, details of which can be obtained
contacting The Dyslexia Institute on the telephone number above.

Hornsby International Dyslexia Centre
261 Trinity Road, London SW18 3SN.
Tel: 0181 874 1844

The Hornsby International Dyslexia Centre offers assessments,
specialist teaching and training courses, including a diploma (one
year part-time, one term full-time), RSA courses in specific learning
difficulties, study skills linked to the National Curriculum,
foundation courses and a post-graduate diploma in Certificate of
Further Professional studies (SpLD).

University of Wales
Aberystwyth
Old College, UCW, Aberystwyth SY23 2AX.
Tel: 01970 622144

Aberystwyth offers two dyslexia modules of a MEd course
(part-time).

Bangor
Faculty of Education, University of Wales, Bangor LL57 2DG.

Bangor offers a Certificate of Further Professional Studies (SpLD) as a one-year part-time course. This course is also available at Cumbria, Ambleside. (Contact: The Administrator, Bebbington Dyslexia Centre, Friends Meeting House, Rydal Road, Ambleside, Cumbria.) Bangor also offers a four-module, two-year part-time course with two modules leading to a Diploma or, on completion of a dissertation, to the degree of MEd.

Other centres which run the RSA Diploma and Certificate in Specific Learning Difficulties

Adult Dyslexia and Skills Development Centre, Tavistock Place, London WC1H 9SN

Amersham and Wycombe College, High Wycombe Campus, Spring Lane, Flackwell Heath, Buckinghamshire HP10 9HE

Barnsley College, Old Mill Site, Church St, Barnsley, South Yorkshire S70 2AX

Basingstoke College of Technology, Basingstoke, Worthing Rd, Hampshire RG21 8TH

Beechwood Dyslexia Centre, Meopham School Campus, Wrotham Rd, Meopham, Kent DA13 0AH

Bexley Local Education Support and Training, Bexley Education Directorate, Hillview, Hillview Drive, Welling, Kent OA16 3RY

Bournemouth and Poole College of Further Education, North Rd, Parkstone, Poole, Dorset BH11 9JJ

Bridgwater College, Bath Rd, Bridgwater, Somerset TA6 4PZ

Bromley Adult Education Training College, Church Lane, Prince's Plain, Bromley, Kent BR2 8LD

Broxbourne Dyslexia Unit, The Priest's House, 90 High Rd, Broxbourne, Hertfordshire EN10 70Z

Chippenham College, Cocklebury Rd, Chippenham, Wiltshire SN15 3QD

Cleveland Tertiary College, Corporation Rd, Redcar, Cleveland TS10 1EZ

Cornwall Learning Support Services, Dalvenie House, New County Hall, Truro, Cornwall TR1 3BA

Education Service, Silver Centre, Stocksfield, Newcastle-upon-Tyne, Tyne and Wear NE5 2DX

Education Training and Support Division, Education Development Centre, Church Lane, Prince's Plain, Bromley, Kent BR2 8LD

Evesham College, Cheltenham Rd, Evesham, Hereford and Worcestershire WR11 6LP

Fareham College, Bishopsfield Rd, Fareham, Hampshire PO14 1NH

Faversham Adult Education Centre, Church Rd, Faversham, Kent ME13 8AL

Greenwich Professional Development Centre, 1a Middle Park Avenue, Eltham, London SE9 5HH

George Watson's College, Colinton Rd, Edinburgh, Lothian EH10 5EG

Hertfordshire Education Centre, Butterfield Rd, Wheathampstead, Hertfordshire AL4 8PY

Hertfordshire Regional College, Ware Centre, Scotts Rd, Ware, Hertfordshire SG12 9JF

Integrated Support Service, Special Services, Blenheim Centre, Crowther Place, Leeds, West Yorkshire LS6 2ST

Learning Support Service, County Hall, North Allerton, North Yorkshire DL7 8AE

Leeds Metropolitan University Faculty Office, James Building, Beckett Park Campus, Leeds, West Yorkshire LS6 305

Long Rd VI Form College, Long Rd, Cambridge, Cambridgeshire CB2 2PX

Medway Dyslexia Centre, 1 The Close, Rochester, Kent ME1 1SD

The National Hospitals, Chandler House, College of Speech Sciences, 2 Wakefield St, London WC2N 1PG

Nene College, Broughton Green Rd, Northhamptonshire NN2 7AL

Norfolk County Council Education, The Greenwood Centre, Greenwood Rd, Tuckswood, Norwich, Norfolk NR4 6BN

North Hertfordshire College, Letchworth Centre, Cambridge Rd, Hitchin, Hertfordshire SG4 0JD

North West Institute of Further and Higher Education, Strand Rd, Londonderry, Co. Londonderry, Northern Ireland BT48 7BY

Oxford Dyslexia Foundation, Stroud Court, Oxford Rd, Farmoor, Oxfordshire OX2 9NN

Selly Oak School, Oak Tree Lane, Selly Oak, Birmingham, West Midlands B29 6HZ

Shrewsbury College of Arts and Technology, London Rd, Shrewsbury, Shropshire SY2 6PR

South Nottinghamshire College, College Rd, Nottingham, Nottinghamshire NG 7GA

Stafford College, Earl St, Stafford, Staffordshire ST16 2QR

Tile Hill College of Further Education, Tile Hill Lane, Coventry, West Midlands CV4 9SU

Weald College, Brookshill, Harrow Weald, Harrow, Middlesex HA3 6RR

West Hertfordshire College, Watford Campus, Hampstead Rd, Watford, Hertfordshire WB1 3EZ

West Sussex Centre, Horsham Professional Centre, Clarence Rd, Horsham, West Sussex, RH13 5SQ

Support for adults with dyslexia

Adult Dyslexia and Skills Development Centre
5 Tavistock Place, London WC1H 9SN.
Tel: 0171 388 8744

Adult Dyslexia Association
336 Brixton Road, London SW9 7AA.
Tel: 0171 737 7646

Adult Literacy and Basic Skills Unit (ALBSU)
7th Floor, Commonwealth House, 10–19 New Oxford St, London WC1A 1NU.
Tel: 0171 405 4017

British Dyslexia Association (see page 386)

Dyslexia Adult Support Group
94(a) Market St, Chorley, Lancashire PR7 2SF.
Tel: 01257 269301

Dyslexia Institute (see page 387)

The Dyslexia Teaching Centre
23 Kensington Square, London W8 5HN.
Tel: 0171 937 2408

The Prince's Youth Business Trust
(education grants)
The Green Park Centre, Stablebridge Rd, Aston Clinton, Aylesbury, Buckinghamshire HP22 5NE.
Tel: 01296 631779

The books and resources listed in this section should be available from the specialist suppliers listed on pages 399–400.

Teaching manuals

Alpha-to-Omega: The A-Z of Teaching Reading, Writing and Spelling
B. Hornsby and F. Shear (1994, fourth edition)
Heinemann Educational, Oxford.

The Bangor Dyslexia Teaching System
E. Miles (1993, second edition)
Whurr Publishers Ltd, London.

Dyslexia: A Teaching Handbook
M. E. Thomson and E. J. Watkins (1990)
Whurr Publishers Ltd, London.

Foundations for Literacy: Structures and Techniques for Multi-sensory Teaching of Basic Written English Language Skills (Revised edition)
A. R. Cox (1992).
Educators Publishing Service Inc., Cambridge MA

The Hickey Multi-Sensory Language Course
J. Augur and S. Briggs (eds) (1992, second edition)
Whurr Publishers Ltd, London.

Remedial Training for Children with Specific Disability in Reading, Spelling and Penmanship
A. Gillingham and B. W. Stillman (1956)
Educators Publishing Service Inc., Cambridge MA

Units of Sound
W. Bramley (1996)
The Dyslexia Institute, Staines.

Teaching aids including spelling and phonic resource material

Alpha-to-Omega Activity Packs, Stages 1, 2 and 3
B. Hornsby and J. Pool (1990, 1991, 1992)
Heinemann Educational, Oxford.

Edith Norrie Magnetic Letter Case
Helen Arkell Dyslexia Centre, Farnham.

Exercise Your Spelling Workbooks I, II, III
E. Wood (1982)
Hodder and Stoughton, London.

Remedial Spelling
V. Brand (1985)
Egon Press Publishers Ltd, Royston.

Signposts to Spelling
J. Pollock (1980)
Heinemann Educational, Oxford.

Spelling Made Easy. Books 0–3
V. Brand (1992, second edition)
Egon Press Publishers Ltd, Royston.

Spellbound: Phonic Reading and Spelling Workbook and Teacher's Manual
E. Rak (1972)
Educators Publishing Service Inc., Cambridge MA

Solving Language Difficulties
A. Steere, C. Z. Peck and L. Kahn (1971)
Educators Publishing Service Inc., Cambridge MA

Phonic reading books

Let's Read (nine readers)
L. Bloomfield, C. Barnhart and R. Barnhart (1964)
Educators Publishing Service Inc., Cambridge MA

One Way With Words
A. M. Gillam
Bath Educational Publishers Ltd, Bath.

Primary Phonics; More Primary Phonics (10 readers in each)
B. Makar (1976)
Educators Publishing Service Inc., Cambridge MA

Sounds Easy (17 readers plus Workbooks)
R. Birkett
Egon Publishers Ltd, Baldock.

Reading books for children

Hummingbirds Series (9 books)
S. McCullagh
Harper Collins, London

Happy Families (16 books)
A. Ahlberg and C. McNaughton
Highly amusing with excellent illustrations.
Penguin Books Ltd, London.

Animal Crackers (12 titles)
Bright, funny short stories with delightful illustrations based on real-life animal stories.
Orchard Books, London.

Banana Books
Bright lively stories written by popular authors.
Reed Children's Books, London

Jet Series Young Lions
Harper Collins, London

Puddle Lane Readers
S. McCullagh
Ladybird, Leics

High interest/low reading age books for teenagers and adults

Bulls Eye Books
Abridged versions of the classics.
Stanley Thornes Ltd, Cheltenham

Spirals
Short and pithy, appeal to the most reluctant of readers, not least for their brevity.
Stanley Thornes Ltd, Cheltenham

Longman Classics
Abridged versions of the classics, grouped into four stages of difficulty.
Addison Wesley Longman, Harlow.

Wellington Square
Stories based on a 'real' neighbourhood. Grouped into five levels of difficulty.
Thomas Nelson, Andover

Heinemann New Wave
  Readers/Heinemann Guided
  Readers
  Heinemann Educational, Oxford.

Impact
  Ginn and Co., Aylesbury.

Reference books

Developmental Dyslexia
  M. E. Thomson (1990, third
  edition)
  Whurr Publishers Ltd, London

**Specific Learning Difficulties
(Dyslexia). Challenges and
Responses**
  P. D. Pumfrey and R. Reason
  (1991)
  Routledge, London

The Pattern of Difficulties
  T. R. Miles (1993)
  Whurr Publishers Ltd, London.

In the Mind's Eye
  T. G. West (1991, second edition)
  Prometheus Books, New York.

**Dyslexia: A Cognitive
Developmental Perspective**
  M. J. Snowling (1987)
  Blackwell, Oxford.

The Dyslexia Handbook
  J. Crisfield (ed) (1996)
  BDA, Reading.

Overcoming Dyslexia
  B. Hornsby (1988)
  Optima Macdonald, London

This Book Doesn't Make ~~snes eens sceens sns~~ Sense
  J. Augur (1995, reissued)
  Whurr Publishers Ltd, London.

**Day-to-Day Dyslexia in the
Classroom**
  J. Pollock and E. Waller (1994)

**Developing Spoken Language
Skills**
  C. Borwick and J. Townend
  (1993)
  The Dyslexia Institute, Staines.

Dyslexia at College
  D. E. Gilroy and T. R. Miles
  (1996, second edition)
  Routledge, London.

**Adult Dyslexia Assessment,
Counselling and Training**
  D. McLoughlin, G. Fitzgibbon
  and V. Young (1994)
  Whurr Publishers Ltd, London.

**Dyslexia: Signposts to Success. A
Guide for Dyslexic Adults**
  J. Matty (1995)
  BDA, Reading.

**Children with Special Needs:
Assessment, Law and Practice
– Caught in the Acts**
  J. Friel (1995, third edition)
  Jessica Kingsley Publishers Ltd,
  London.

**Young Adults with Special Needs:
Assessment, Law and Practice
– Caught in the Acts**
  J. Friel (1995, third edition)
  Jessica Kingsley Publishers Ltd,
  London.

**Special Educational Needs
Handbook: The Law on
Children with Special Needs**
  Advisory Centre for Education
  (1996)
  London.

**Special Educational Needs: A
Guide for Parents**
  DfEE (1994)
  London.

Handwriting

Handwriting Helpline
J. Alston and J. Taylor
Routledge, London.

Handwriting: Theory, Research and Practice
J. Alston and J. Taylor (1987)
Routledge, London.

Left-handed Helpline
D. Paul (1993)
Dextral Books, Manchester.

Handwriting materials

Grippy Pencil Grips
Better Books, Dudley.

Pencil Grips
Learning Development Aids
(LDA), Cambridge.

Multigrips
Taskmaster Ltd, Leicester.

Right Line Paper with Raised Lines
Stop-Go Paper
Taskmaster Ltd, Leicester.

Maths

Basic Numeracy
V. Burge
Helen Arkell Dyslexia Centre,
Farnham.

Dyslexia and Mathematics
T. R. Miles and E. Miles (eds)
(1992)
Routledge, London.

Maths and Dyslexics
A. Henderson (1989)
St David's College,
Llandudno.

Mathematics for Dyslexics: A Teaching Handbook
S. Chinn and R. Ashcroft (1993)
Whurr Publishers Ltd,
London.

What To Do When You Can't Learn the Times Tables
S. Chinn (1996)
Marko Publishing, Mark College,
Somerset.

Assessment and attainment tests

Screening tests

The Bangor Dyslexia Test
T. R. Miles (1983)
Preliminary indicator of the
classic signs.
Learning Development Aids,
Wisbech.

Cognitive Profiling System (CoPS 1)
C. Singleton, K. Thomas and R.
Leedale (1996)
Identifies dyslexia and SEN
Chameleon Educational Ltd,
Nottinghamshire.

Dyslexia Early Screening Test (DEST)
R. Nicolson and A. Fawcett
(1995)
Age 4.6–6.5 years.
The Psychological Corporation,
London.
Tel: 0171 267 4466

Dyslexia Screening Test (DST)
R. Nicolson and A. Fawcett
(1996)
Age 6.6–16 years.
The Psychological Corporation,
London.
Tel: 0171 267 4466

Assessment tests

The Aston Index (Revised)
M. E. Thomson and M. Newton
(1982)
16 tests for diagnosing strengths
and weaknesses associated with
SEN and dyslexia.
Age 5–14 years.
Learning Development Aids,
Wisbech.

Cognitive Profiling System (CoPS1)
C. Singleton, K. Thomas and R.
Leedale (1996)
Identifies dyslexia and SEN
Chameleon Educational Ltd,
Nottinghamshire.

General intellectual cognitive ability tests
The following may only be used by psychologists:

Wechsler Adult Intelligence Scale (WAIS–R^{UK})
Age 16–74 years.
The Psychological Corporation,
London.

Wechsler Intelligence Scale for Children (WISC–III^{UK})
Age 6–16 years.
The Psychological Corporation,
London.

Wechsler Pre-School and Primary Scale of Intelligence (WPPSI–R^{UK})
Age 3–7 years.
The Psychological Corporation,
London.

British Ability Scales: Second edition (BAS II)
C. D. Elliot (1996)
Age 2.6–17.11 years.
NFER – Nelson, Windsor.

Teachers may use the following:

Raven's Progressive Matrices and Vocabulary Scales: 1979 British Standardization and Revision (1988)
J. C. Raven (1988)
Age 5–adult.
NFER – Nelson, Windsor.

Reading tests

Graded Word Reading Test. The Macmillan Test Unit
(1990)
Age 6–14 years.
NFER – Nelson, Windsor.

Wide Range Achievement Test 3 (WRAT 3)
G. S. Wilkinson (1993)
Age 5–75 years.
Wide Range Inc., Delaware.
Also available from The
Dyslexia Institute, Staines.

Reading accuracy

Neale Analysis of Reading Ability: Revised British Edition
M. D. Neale with U. Christophers
and C. Whetton (1988)
Also includes a comprehension
test.
Age 5–13 years.
NFER – Nelson, Windsor.

New Macmillan Reading Analysis
D. Vincent and M. de la Mare
(1990)
Age 7–9 years.
NFER – Nelson, Windsor.

Reading comprehension tests

The NFER – Nelson Group Reading Test
The Macmillan Test Unit (1990)
Age 8.3–15.3 years.
NFER – Nelson, Windsor.

Sentence completion tests

Cloze Reading Tests
D. Young (1992)
Age 7.6–12.6 years.
Hodder and Stoughton, London.

Suffolk Reading Scale
F. Hagley (1987)
Age 6.4–13.11 years.
NFER – Nelson, Windsor.

Spelling tests

Graded Word Spelling Test
P. E. Vernon (1983)
Age 6.0–16 years.
Hodder and Stoughton, London.

Wide Range Achievement Test (WRAT 3)
G. S. Wilkinson (1993)
Age 5.0–75 years.
Wide Range Inc., Delaware.

British Spelling Test Series
D. Vincent and M. Crumpler (1996)
Age 5–24 years.
NFER – Nelson, Windsor.

Maths tests

Basic Number Diagnostic Test
B. Gillham (1980)
Age 5.0–7.0 years.
Hodder and Stoughton, London.

Basic Number Screening Test
B. Gillham and K. A. Hesse (1976)
Age 7–12 years.
Hodder and Stoughton, London.

The Staffordshire Mathematics Test
C. Barcham, R. Bushell, K. Lawson and C. McDonnell (1986)
Age 7–8.7 years.
NFER – Nelson, Windsor.

Graded Arithmetic-Mathematics Test: Junior Form
P. E. Vernon and K. M. Miller (1986)
Age 6–11 years.
Hodder and Stoughton, London.

Mathematics Competency test
P. E. Vernon, K. M. Miller and J. F Izard (1986)
Age 11–adult.
Hodder and Stoughton, London.

Wide Range Achievement Test 3 (WRAT 3)
G. S. Wilkinson (1993)
Age 5–75 years.
Wide Range Inc., Delaware
Also available from the Dyslexia Institute, Staines.

Dictionaries

The ACE Spelling Dictionary: Find Words Quickly and Improve Your Spelling
D. Moseley (1995)
Readership: children, teenage, adult.
Learning Development Aids, Wisbech.

Cassell Spelling Dictionary
D. Firnberg (1995)
Readership: children, adult.
Cassell, London.

Spelling Checklist
E. Stirling
114 Westbourne Rd,
Sheffield S10 2QT
726 words frequently misspelt by the dyslexic child.

The Word Hunter's Companion
A First Thesaurus
J. Green (1976)
Blackwell, Oxford.

Computer software and literature

This is a huge market that is constantly changing. The list of materials available is often out of date before the ink is dry. However, help is at hand from the British Dyslexia Association Computer Committee. The Committee, which works in conjunction with the Dyslexia Computer Resource Centre at the University of Hull, consists of practitioners and academics who evaluate new materials as they come onto the market.

Sources of information

The Dyslexia Computer Resource Centre
Department of Psychology,
University of Hull, Hull HU6 7RX.
Tel: 01482 465589

This contains a wide range of software that has been evaluated by the Computer Committee members of the BDA. It also publishes a series of booklets:

How Computers Can Help
Word Processing & Spell Checking
Maths Programs
IBM PCs and Compatibles
Acorn Computers (BBC and Archimedes)
Early Literacy and Numeracy Skills

Singleton C. (ed) (1994) *Computers and Dyslexia: Educational Applications of New Technnology*

The National Council for Educational Techonology
Milburn Hill Rd, Science Park,
Coventry CV4 7JJ.
Tel: 01203 416994

The National Federation of Access Centres
Hereward College of FE,
Bramstone Crescent,
Tile Hill Lane, Coventry CV4 9SW.
Tel: 01203 461231

Access centres assess the needs of disabled students, advise on equipment and run courses.

ACE Centre
Ormerod School,
Waynflete Rd, Headington,
Oxford OX3 8DD.
Tel: 01865 63508

Provides training and evaluates software.

Computability Centre
IBM Warwick, PO Box 94,
Warwick CV34 5WS.
Tel: 01800 269545

Provides information, education and training for people with disabilities.

National Association for Special Educational Needs (NASEN)
4–5 Amber Business Village,
Amber Close, Amington
Tamworth, Staffordshire
B77 4RR.
Tel: 01827 311500

Web sites and email

On the British Dyslexia Association Web site you will find a full list of dyslexia web sites on the Internet.

BDA home page address is:
http://www.dur.ac.uk/~dot7da/Web_e-dres/links.html

Dyslexia Archive email address is: m16@unix.hensa.ac.uk

ADA Dyslexia 2000 Network email address is: dyslexia.hq@dial.pipex.com

Computer software compatible with multi-sensory teaching programmes

Alpha-to-Omega
Workshark 2
Whitespace.

The Bangor Dyslexia Teaching
System
Xavier Software.

Spelling Made Easy
Starspell Plus
Fisher-Marriott.

Handheld spell checkers

Franklin Elementary Spellmaster
Linked to *Oxford Children's Dictionary.*

The Franklin Spellmaster QE–95
Franklin Electronic Publishers (Europe) Ltd, Sunbury-on-Thames.

Electronic dictionaries and encyclopaedias

Collins Electronic English
Dictionary and Thesaurus (1995)
HarperCollins, London.

Microsoft Encarta 96
Encyclopaedia (1996)
Microsoft

Maths programs

Mathsblast and Kidworks
Age 6–10 years.
ABL AC, Newton Abbot.

The BDA Computer Committee publishes an updated list of useful maths programs. The specialist suppliers carry them in their catalogue.

Computer touch typing programs

MicroType: Fairley House:
Wombourne, Staffs
(see page 400)

Touch Typing Program: Fingers
for Windows: Type to Learn
Apt Projects (see page 400)

Talking packages

Talking Pendown
Longman Logotron.

Texthelp
iAnsyst Ltd

Videos

Understanding Dyslexia (1996)
Understanding Dyslexia: A Guide
for Parents (1996)
Understanding Dyslexia: A Guide
for Teachers (1996)
The Dyslexia Institute, Staines
(see page 387).

Channel 4 Dyslexia: An Avoidable
National Tragedy (1993)
Hopeline Videos,
PO Box 515,
London SW15 6LQ.
Tel: 0181 788 2718

I'm Not Stupid (1993)
Jackie Stewart's Story
MP Associates,
ABS House,
35 Chiltern Avenue,
Amersham, Buckinghamshire
HP6 5AE.
Tel: 01494 766082

Talking books on cassette

BBC Books
Woodlands, 80 Wood Lane,
London W12 OTT.
Tel: 0171 6366 1500

Listening Library
12 Lant St., London SE1.
Tel: 0171 4007 9417

Tapeworm Cassettes
Apsley House,
Apsely Rd,
New Malden,
Surrey KT3 3NJ.
Tel: 0181 942 7788

The Talking Book Shop
11 Wigmore St.,
London W1H 9LB.
Tel: 0171 491 4117

Specialist suppliers

Ann Arbor Publishers
PO Box 1, Bedford,
Northumberland NE70 7JX.
Tel: 01668 214460

Anything Left Handed Ltd
57 Brewer St,
London WIR 3FB.
Tel: 0171 437 3910

British Dyslexia Association
(See page 386).

Better Books
3 Paganel Drive, Dudley,
West Midlands DY1 4AZ.
Tel: 01384 253276

The Dyslexia Institute
(See page 387).

Educators Publishing Services Inc.
31 Smith Place, Cambridge MA,
02138–1000 USA
Tel: 001 800 225 5750

The Helen Arkell Centre
(See page 387).

The Hornsby International Dyslexia Centre
(See page 387).

Learning Development Aids (LDA)
Aware House, Duke St.,
Wisbech, Cambridgeshire
PE13 2AE.
Tel: 01945 63441

Left-handed Company
PO Box 52, South DO,
Manchester M20 8PJ.
Tel: 0161 445 0159

Special Educational Needs
9 The Close, Church Aston,
Newport, Salop TF10 9JL.
Te: 01948 770673

Taskmaster Ltd
Morris Rd, Leicester LE2 6BR.
Tel: 0116 270 4286

Suppliers of electronic packages (software/hardware)

ABLAC
South Devon House,
Station Rd, Newton Abbot,
Devon TQ12 2BP.
Tel: 01626 331 992

Apt Projects
PO Box 1066, Belton,
South Yorkshire DN8 1QX.
Tel: 01427 875103

MicroType Fairley House
77 Orton Lane,
Wombourne, Staffordshire
WV5 9AP.
Tel: 01902 892599

Fisher-Marriott
3 Grove Rd, Ansty, Coventry
CV7 9JD.
Tel: 01203 616325

**Franklin Electronic Publishers
(Europe) Ltd**
7 Windmill Business Village,
Brooklands Close,
Sunbury-on-Thames,
Middlesex TW16 7DY
Tel: 01932 770185

iAnsyst Ltd
United House, North Rd,
London N7 9PD.
Tel: 0171 607 5844

Longman Logotron
124 Cambridge Science Park,
Milton Rd, Cambridge CB4 4ZS.
Tel: 01223 435558

REM (Rickitt)
Great Western House, Langport,
Somerset TA10 9YL.
Tel: 01458 253636

Sherston Software
Swan Barton, Sherston,
Malmesbury, Wiltshire SN16 0LH.
Tel: 01460 57152

**Tandy Education Supplies and
Services**
Intertan UK Ltd, Tandy Centre,
Leamore Lane, Walsall, West
Midlands WS2 7PS.
Tel: 01922 434000

Whitespace
41 Mall Rd, London W6 9DG.
Tel: 0171 240 0208

Xavier Software
Department of Psychology,
UNCW, 37 College Rd, Bangor,
Gwynedd LL57 2DG.
Tel: 01248 382 616

List 1: One hundred most used words

in	was	is	I	he
it	a	the	that	to
and	of	are	for	you
had	so	have	said	as
not	they	with	one	we
on	his	at	him	all
but	old	be	up	do
can	me	came	my	new
get	she	here	has	her
will	an	no	or	now
did	by	if	go	down
just	out	your	into	our
went	them	well	there	were
big	call	back	been	come
from	only	first	off	over
must	make	more	made	much
look	little	some	like	right
then	their	when	this	two
see	about	could	before	other
which	what	where	who	want

Source: McNally J. and Murray W. (1984) *Keywords to Literacy and the Teaching of Reading.* The Teaching Publishing Co. Ltd, Kettering, Northants

List 2: One hundred next most used words

after	five	many	sit
again	fly	may	soon
always	found	men	stop
am	four	miss	take
another	gave	mother	tell
any	girl	Mr	ten
ask	give	Mrs	than
away	going	never	these
bad	good	next	thing
ball	got	once	think
because	green	open	three
best	hand	own	time
bird	have	play	too
black	head	put	three
blue	help	ran	under
boy	home	read	us
bring	house	red	very
day	how	room	walk
dog	jump	round	white
don't	keep	run	why
eat	know	sat	wish
every	last	saw	woman
far	left	say	work
fast	let	school	would
father	live	should	year
fell	long	sing	yes
find	man		

Words are arranged according to the number of times they were mis-spelled.

1 their	26 went	51 mother	76 interesting
2 too	27 where	52 another	77 once
3 there	28 stopped	53 threw	78 like
4 they	29 very	54 some	79 they're
5 then	30 morning	55 its	80 cousin
6 until	31 something	56 bought	81 all right
7 our	32 named	57 getting	82 happened
8 asked	33 came	58 going	83 didn't
9 off	34 name	59 course	84 always
10 through	35 tried	60 women	85 surprise
11 you're	36 here	61 animals	86 before
12 clothes	37 many	62 started	87 caught
13 looked	38 knew	63 that's	88 every
14 people	39 with	64 would	89 different
15 pretty	40 together	65 again	90 interesting
16 running	41 swimming	66 heard	91 sometimes
17 believe	42 first	67 received	92 friends
18 little	43 were	68 coming	93 children
19 things	44 than	69 to	94 an
20 him	45 two	70 said	95 school
21 because	46 know	71 wanted	96 jumped
22 thought	47 decided	72 hear	97 around
23 and	48 friends	73 from	98 dropped
24 beautiful	49 when	74 frightened	99 babies
25 it's	50 let's	75 for	100 money

Source: Johnson L. W. (1950) '100 words most often mis-spelled by children in the elementary grades' *Journal of Educational Research*, 44 (2): 154–5.

Index